Bishops and Bodies

CRITICAL ISSUES IN HEALTH AND MEDICINE

Edited by Rima D. Apple, University of
Wisconsin–Madison and Janet Golden, Rutgers University–Camden, and
Rana A. Hogarth, University of Illinois at Urbana–Champaign

Growing criticism of the U.S. healthcare system is coming from consumers, politicians, the media, activists, and healthcare professionals. Critical Issues in Health and Medicine is a collection of books that explores these contemporary dilemmas from a variety of perspectives, among them political, legal, historical, sociological, and comparative, and with attention to crucial dimensions such as race, gender, ethnicity, sexuality, and culture.

For a list of titles in the series, see the last page of the book.

Bishops and Bodies

Reproductive Care in American
Catholic Hospitals

Lori Freedman

RUTGERS UNIVERSITY PRESS
NEW BRUNSWICK, CAMDEN, AND NEWARK, NEW JERSEY
LONDON AND OXFORD

Rutgers University Press is a department of Rutgers, The State University of New Jersey, one of the leading public research universities in the nation. By publishing worldwide, it furthers the University's mission of dedication to excellence in teaching, scholarship, research, and clinical care.

Library of Congress Cataloging-in-Publication Data
Names: Freedman, Lori, 1973– author.
Title: Bishops and bodies : reproductive care in American Catholic hospitals /
    Lori Freedman.
Description: New Brunswick, New Jersey : Rutgers University Press, [2023] |
    Series: Critical issues in health and medicine | Includes bibliographical
    references and index.
Identifiers: LCCN 2022049494 | ISBN 9781978828865 (paperback) |
    ISBN 9781978828872 (hardback) | ISBN 9781978828889 (epub) |
    ISBN 9781978828896 (pdf)
Subjects: LCSH: Catholic hospitals—United States. | Maternal health services—
    United States. | Reproductive health services—United States. | Medical ethics—
    Religious aspects—Catholic Church.
Classification: LCC RA975.C37 F74 2023 | DDC 362.110973—dc23/eng/20230202
LC record available at https://lccn.loc.gov/2022049494

A British Cataloging-in-Publication record for this book is available from the British Library.

References to internet websites (URLs) were accurate at the time of writing. Neither the author nor Rutgers University Press is responsible for URLs that may have expired or changed since the manuscript was prepared.

♾ The paper used in this publication meets the requirements of the American National Standard for Information Sciences—Permanence of Paper for Printed Library Materials, ANSI Z39.48-1992.

rutgersuniversitypress.org

To my mother, Judy Freedman

Contents

Foreword by Debra Stulberg   ix
Prologue: Unsafe and Unequal   xiii

Introduction: Doctrinal Iatrogenesis   1

1   Growth: How Catholic Health Care Expanded   15

2   Inferior: How Catholic Directives Contradict Medical Standards   28

3   Consumer Medicine?: Patients and the Illusion of Choice   46

4   Emergencies: Patient Loss and Suffering   68

5   Mostly Above-Board Workarounds   87

6   Under-the-Radar Workarounds   111

7   Separation of Church and Hospital   126

Conclusion   144

Appendix: Positionality, Methods, and Scholarly Journey   159
Acknowledgments   163
Notes   165
Index   201

Foreword

"Did you hear we're going to be working for the pope?" I was a few months into my family medicine residency and working on the labor and delivery floor when one of the senior physicians asked me this question. We'd had a busy shift and were getting a quick bite to eat between deliveries. His question caught me off guard. I had selected this hospital for residency because of its strength in women's health and its commitment to serving the nearby low-income Chicago community with high-quality care. And while I knew the hospital was facing financial pressures and considering potential buyers, I had not heard that our leadership had agreed on a deal to be acquired by a large Catholic hospital system.

Driving home the next day, my thoughts turned to the implications of this deal. My first worry was about my ability to get abortion training. Like many people, I knew Catholic hospitals do not provide abortion care—this is a commonly understood reality. But our hospital actually had not been providing abortions when it was secular, so I had arranged with the hospital to allow me to use my elective time to go off-site for abortion training. Now I worried whether the new hospital owners would prohibit this. At this time, I had no idea of the other ways being Catholic would affect our hospital and the people who walked through its doors. (I later learned that my lack of awareness was very common. Most people do not have any sense of all the services Catholic hospitals prohibit.) I naively assumed that, with abortion already something we needed to refer our patients out for, the care our patients received would not change.

In wondering what this would mean for my abortion training, my first reaction was to call my mentor from medical school who worked on the national issue of abortion access. Her first reaction was to put me in touch with MergerWatch—the leading national organization dedicated to understanding and addressing Catholic-secular hospital mergers.

In talking with MergerWatch, I came to understand that my hospital was not alone, and that our patients were likely to suffer unanticipated consequences. Many of the services we provided on a regular basis would be lost: emergency contraception for rape victims in the emergency room, long-acting contraception in hospital-owned clinics, and sterilization procedures done in hospital offices or operating rooms—these would all go by the wayside. And patients facing pregnancy complications that require prompt treatment—such as ectopic pregnancies and miscarriages—would, at times, have their care compromised as well. These are among the effects I would learn about in coming months.

With the help of MergerWatch and local healthcare advocates, we organized inside the hospital and by hosting community forums on the impact this change in ownership would have. Nonetheless, the hospital acquisition still went forward. The first day of the new ownership, we had to start telling patients in labor that the postpartum tubal ligation they had planned for nine months could no longer be done. Within weeks, we had to decide if we would sneak and provide birth control devices for our patients.

I will never forget a patient I saw on the labor and delivery floor after the merger. She came to the hospital for cramping, where she learned she was six months pregnant. In taking her history, I found out she had only recently given birth, shortly after the hospital became Catholic. She had asked for a tubal ligation with her last birth, but because of the new hospital ownership she had been told no.

This crash education in Catholic hospitals was not something I sought out. But as I finished residency, I decided I wanted to study it more formally. I had so many questions, and I had learned that these questions did not yet have good answers. What do doctors nationally think about this issue? What about patients? How do they respond when their care is limited by the hospital's religion? And how does this square with modern medical ethics, which I always had learned emphasized patient autonomy and beneficence as its guiding principles? Finally, what could policymakers do to protect patients in these situations?

By the time I started my fellowship in medical ethics and healthcare research, I already had heard of Lori Freedman's work. During one of our hospital community forums, an obstetrician shared about how the new Catholic directives required doctors to transfer patients to other hospitals for treatment of miscarriages in which there was still a fetal heartbeat and how this change created unnecessary delays for patients in distress. One of the attorneys in our coalition said they had heard from patients at Catholic hospitals who also had treatment denied or delayed for the same reason. And the national experts from MergerWatch told us all: Yes, this is a common enough problem that there is a sociologist in California writing an article about it!

As it turned out, Lori's paper, called "When There's a Heartbeat: Miscarriage Management in Catholic Hospitals," was the first publication in the peer-reviewed literature to document this doctrinally mandated substandard care for miscarrying patients. And when these same physician interviews wove their way into Lori's first book, in which she elucidated doctors' myriad constraints in trying to provide abortion care, our field's understanding of the power of institutions within medicine (especially reproductive medicine) exploded.

Before long, I was introduced to Lori personally through a mutual friend, and the next time I made my way to the Bay Area we made plans to meet. What began as a coffee date has gone on to be the most fruitful and fulfilling collaboration of my career. The earliest interviews contained in this book emerged from the first project we worked on together, which was followed by several more.

As a physician, I can speak and write about the patient cases I know, and give a medical perspective on what it means when the bishops' directives tie doctors' hands. But it is Lori's sociological lens that has made our body of research possible. To interview hundreds of providers and patients, to elicit honest stories about some of the most distressing moments individuals have experienced, and to see the patterns that emerge from beneath the surface of these stories—I can only say that, to me, it feels like magic.

But Lori is not a magician. She is a skilled interviewer who thinks carefully about what questions to ask and then creates space for every interviewee to share experiences that uncover their vulnerability. She brings the utmost respect for people from every walk of life—doctors, ethicists, and patients from diverse personal and religious backgrounds. And she is an insightful qualitative analyst, diving deep into interviewees' narratives. Moving beyond simple descriptions of her subjects' common experiences, she observes how power structures and social norms undergird their storytelling. When doctors described crying in their on-call rooms before having to tell patients they could not provide medically necessary treatment, Lori saw the mismatch between how doctors were trained to see themselves (as benevolent experts acting on their patients' behalf) to their reality in practice (as agents of the institutions that employ them) and the distress this caused. When women patients repeatedly blamed themselves for failing to predict that their reproductive care would be restricted at a Catholic hospital ("I should have done my research," they would say), Lori recognized the gendered pattern of socialization: women are trained to have low expectations for reproductive care and to internalize the fault as their own.

Working with and learning from Lori has been a joy and privilege for me. But the greatest joy is that the rest of the world now gets to benefit as well. *Bishops and Bodies* is the place where all the interviews and analyses come together, and the widespread impact of Catholic hospital ownership on reproductive health becomes clear. In this post-*Roe* era, it is essential reading for anyone who cares about reproductive health. And, more broadly, we should all care about the lessons of this book: about who controls the care we all receive, what the growth of the bishops' control means, and who is most likely to be hurt.

Debra Stulberg, MD
Chair, Department of Family Medicine, University of Chicago

Prologue

UNSAFE AND UNEQUAL

For more than a decade, I have conducted research about how the policies of the United States Conference of Catholic Bishops (USCCB) that govern care inside Catholic health facilities affect patients' bodies and their reproductive wellbeing both with and without their knowledge. These policies are called the Ethical and Religious Directives for Catholic Health Care Services (ERDs), and they prohibit or restrict many treatments or services. The most well-known is abortion, but their reach is much broader.

While the Supreme Court decision *Dobbs v. Jackson Women's Health Organization* revoked the constitutional right to abortion in June 2022, Catholic hospitals have long operated under institutional policies that prohibited abortion as well as several other reproductive treatments, such as sterilization, other contraception, and in vitro fertilization. This book takes an intimate look at what happens when patients and physicians encounter the bishops' policies during medical care, and, through their stories, I demonstrate how the ERDs compel substandard practice. I show also how clinician strategies to work around the restrictions, while clever and patient-centered in a way, ultimately prove unreliable, insufficient, and unevenly distributed.

This book focuses on Catholic health care rather than religious health care generally because Catholic hospitals constitute about 70 percent of all religious hospitals in the United States,[1] and they have centralized religious authority with far more restrictive policies than the heterogenous remainder. Before I lay out my argument, there are five common myths I would like to dispel so we can dive deeper into this sociologically rich yet convoluted medical terrain.[2] I present these myths with some countering facts for which there will be more evidence in the rest of the book:

———

Myth 1: Catholic health care does not affect many people.
Fact: One of every six patients in the United States is treated in a Catholic hospital.

Catholic health care is not a niche medical realm for Catholic people. In fifteen states, Catholic hospitals operate over a quarter of the hospital beds. In fifty-two rural communities, a Catholic hospital is the only option for care. Many Catholic facilities are part of large networks, run by multiprovider, multistate corporations. As an example, the second largest health system in the United States, Common-Spirit, is Catholic. It operates 385 hospitals, and together with its urgent care, surgery centers, and physician practices, it operates 700 facilities in twenty-one states.[3] Catholic hospitals employ and treat millions of people from all religious backgrounds and walks of life.

Myth 2: Abortion is the only "issue."
Fact: Catholic hospitals restrict several aspects of reproductive and end-of-life care.
The ERDs mandate that Catholic hospital clinicians and employees restrict or prohibit common treatments and services, including care and referrals for contraception; sterilization; prenatal diagnosis; obstetric complications; infertility treatment; gender confirming procedures; and pregnancy loss. While this book focuses on reproductive care, it is worth noting that medical aid-in-dying is strictly prohibited, along with some other end-of-life medical services, as well.[4]

Myth 3: Catholic patients want care that adheres to Catholic doctrine.
Fact: Catholic patients use contraception, abortion, and other restricted services as much as other patients.[5]
Survey research shows that the majority of Catholic patients do not desire the Church's management of their medical options.[6] Relatedly, very few women consider a hospital's religious affiliation important when deciding where to go for reproductive care, and Catholic women, in particular, report more often trying to avoid a Catholic hospital (6 percent) than intentionally seeking one out (3 percent).[7]

Myth 4: Catholic hospitals care for lots of poor people with Church funding.
Fact: Catholic hospitals provide less health care to low-income people than average, and that care is financed by public insurance and public grants, not the Church.
While Catholic hospitals are religiously and spiritually sponsored by Church congregations and clergy, such as Little Sisters of the Poor, care is not financed by them. Nationally, Catholic hospitals provide less charity (2.7 percent) and Medicaid (7.2 percent) care than average (2.9 percent charity and 8.9 percent Medicaid).[8]

Myth 5: Patients can go elsewhere if they do not want Catholic care.
Fact: Patients do not necessarily know in advance, and many do not have other options.
Over a third of women whose primary hospital is Catholic do not know that it is. And, the vast majority of people do not know about *how* care is restricted in Catholic hospitals until they cannot get what they need. Those who do know and would like to avoid religiously restricted care often are unable to do so because of

the lack of other providers nearby or the fact that their insurance does not cover care in other hospitals.[9]

———

That patients do not know whether or how Catholic religious policies restrict their health care raises a host of bioethical issues. Four principles within medicine have dominated bioethics for decades—autonomy, beneficence, nonmaleficence, and justice—despite the occasional critiques and alternative framings offered.[10] Autonomy for a patient means having control over one's own treatment decisions without coercion by others. Ensuring that patients are informed and autonomous is ground zero in Western bioethics. Since the 1970s,[11] when the medical field reckoned with the concept that patients have rights that must be protected, ethicists and healthcare regulators have increasingly endeavored—almost to a fault—to ensure that patients understand and freely choose their medications and procedures, including more information than one usually wants related to potential side effects, as anyone who has seen a commercial for a brand name medication can attest. There is nothing so American as enjoying snacks and a football game while being warned that diarrhea, impotence, and death may all be potential "side effects" of a medication being advertised by aggressively happy actors.[12]

When it comes to ensuring that patients are both informed and autonomous decision makers about their reproductive health care, it can seem as if an entirely different ethical standard applies. Even though medical researchers have generated ample scientific expertise about how to best manage complex contraception, infertility, gender-affirming surgery, termination of pregnancies, and obstetric complications, patients are left uninformed. A physician is under no legal obligation to tell a patient in a Catholic hospital that they will not be offered some of the most common and safe treatments in these medical domains. And nearly every woman of reproductive age admitted to the hospital for any health concern has the potential to simultaneously need reproductive medical management—for example, she could be pregnant, or she may require contraception because her new medical treatment would endanger a pregnancy.

The American College of Obstetrics and Gynecology (ACOG), the leading professional organization for ob-gyns, considers patient autonomy an integral part of determining the standard of care; meaning that the standard is to offer patients a choice between safe options (for example, of contraception, of infertility treatment, of method of miscarriage management). "Standard of care" is a legalistic concept that generally means "that which a minimally competent physician in the same field would do under similar circumstances."[13] If resources are available, and there are preference-sensitive choices to be made between safe and standard treatments that have different bodily consequences, true patient autonomy means the patient chooses. Other major mainstream medical organizations, including the American Medical Association and American Public Health Association, emphasize the importance of autonomy as well.[14]

xvi   PROLOGUE

Research shows that reproductive autonomy—having the means to control when and whether one has children—leads to improved patient well-being and better outcomes in maternal and child health. In particular, when women are forced to carry unwanted pregnancies to term, the entire family's vulnerability to domestic violence and poverty increases.[15] We know that access to contraception and abortion increases birth spacing, improves birth outcomes, increases paternal involvement in child-rearing, and ultimately leads to healthier children and families.[16] Today, the public health goal of improving access to contraception so people can gain more control over whether and when to get pregnant is rarely contested outside of Catholic contexts because it turns out that having reproductive autonomy leads to better outcomes. Going further, reproductive autonomy, on balance, leads to beneficence, nonmaleficence, and justice in patient care.

Unfortunately, however, the Catholic directives for health care create an environment that is less safe than other medical settings. By restricting standard ob-gyn services and medical interventions, often without the patient's knowledge, the ERDs produce a health setting that functions as if it were resource-poor, when, in fact, the resources can and do exist. As in resource-poor health settings, clinicians in Catholic hospitals often move mountains to work around barriers to care, but they should not have to do so, and their efforts to overcome religious restrictions are hit and miss. Some patients get help; some do not. Some experience harm, or maleficence, specifically due to the religious limitations on medical treatment, what I term *doctrinal iatrogenesis*. This book shows how ERD-constrained care is both unsafe and unequal by virtue of allowing bishops to usurp medical authority. In Catholic hospitals, bishops—not doctors or patients—have the ultimate decision-making power over what can happen to the reproductive bodies inside their buildings.

Bishops and Bodies

Introduction

DOCTRINAL IATROGENESIS

Willa[1] was living in a small city[2] in the U.S. South with her husband and four children when we spoke. They had wanted to stop at three kids, but her doctor steered her away from sterilization, encouraging her, instead, to use some form of nonpermanent birth control such as an intrauterine device (IUD) or a contraceptive implant. Willa was uncomfortable with this advice. A white woman in her mid-twenties, she'd had side effects in the past with various birth control methods, but she agreed to think about it. Placing no blame on her doctor, Willa said, "And so I thought about it and I guess I thought about it too long, and I got pregnant again."

Her husband then agreed to get a vasectomy, but he canceled the appointment. She quipped, "He chickened out twelve hours prior." So, with a fourth child on the way, she began to plan for the sterilization procedure she wanted. Willa hoped to have a tubal ligation—in which the fallopian tubes are severed so that eggs cannot travel through them into the uterus—immediately following childbirth. It was during this planning process that she became aware that her husband's military medical insurance, Tricare, allowed her to deliver only at the nearby St. Mary's[3] Catholic hospital rather than the neighboring non-Catholic one. The problem, Willa's physician informed her, was that Catholic hospitals do not allow doctors to perform sterilizations.[4]

Willa had two options. The first involved transporting her the day after giving birth at St. Mary's to the non-Catholic facility for a tubal ligation procedure and then back to St. Mary's. Her insurance would cover this, and the arrangement would allow for an easier surgery, given the temporary anatomic shifts caused by pregnancy.[5] It also would enable her to recover in the hospital with support from the nursing staff. The second option was to wait until six weeks after the birth for a delayed tubal ligation, but this would require a more invasive surgery. Furthermore, because it is an outpatient procedure, she would return home to her infant and three other children to recover without the help of the nurses on the labor and delivery ward.

Willa dismissed the first option as "too emotional." She did not want to be separated from her newborn immediately after the birth. She recalled:

> So mentally for me I was like well if I can't get it done right after I give birth at the same area and I have to leave my newborn and I have to go somewhere else without my newborn, mentally I couldn't handle it . . . We decided on the six weeks, which in the end that still—in the end that hurt me too . . .
>
> [I had] to go through a whole new healing process . . . I couldn't really bend, I couldn't really walk . . . the nurse was like, "Okay, get in the car," and I actually fell out of the wheelchair to my car . . . I couldn't pick up my son because you have to twist and turn . . . and it's much harder to breastfeed.

Willa's recovery from the tubal ligation was more difficult than she had anticipated. It took her about two weeks to get back to normal, during which time she struggled to breastfeed her infant—let alone care for the other three children. Looking back, she regretted not having accepted the transport option: "I think pain-wise and healing-wise, I think it would have been the smarter choice instead of having pretty much the whole eight weeks in pain."

Why Willa had to make this decision at all gets at the heart of the issues explored in this book. Her experience was a direct consequence of the ever-expanding market share of Catholic hospitals within the American healthcare system. The Catholic Health Association of the United States (CHA), which is a professional association representing all medical facilities affiliated with the Catholic Church, reports a membership of 668 hospitals nationwide, of which approximately three-quarters are in urban and suburban areas and the remaining quarter in rural areas.[6] While nationwide approximately one-sixth of hospital care is provided by Catholic hospitals, in certain states, Catholic health systems are more predominant.

In Alaska, Iowa, South Dakota, Wisconsin, and Washington, over 40 percent of hospital beds are in Catholic hospitals; in Colorado, Illinois, Oregon, Missouri, and Nebraska, nearly one in three hospital beds is in a Catholic facility.[7] Historically associated with care for the poor, Catholic hospitals are now integrated into the rest of the American healthcare system, providing services through both public and private insurance. Some Catholic hospitals function as safety nets, whereas others function as high-end private facilities, and many lie in between. And, whether patients know it or not, all these facilities restrict care according to Catholic doctrine.

Catholic hospitals are an extension of Catholic ministry, and federal law protects the church's "institutional conscience rights" to restrict the care given within its ministry's walls.[8] Despite the fact that Catholic hospitals employ and treat people of all faiths, Catholic hospitals limit or prohibit a wide range of services related to reproductive and sexual health.[9] The CHA does not provide statistics on the religious composition of its patients, but other research shows that Catholics are no more likely than non-Catholics to seek out Catholic health care.[10] U.S. patients, even religious ones, rarely choose a hospital based on its religion. Instead, patients prioritize such factors as reputation for quality, geographic proximity, and physician

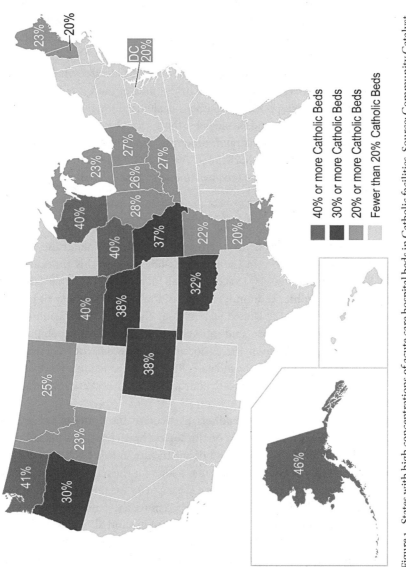

Figure 1. States with high concentrations of acute care hospital beds in Catholic facilities. Source: Community Catalyst, https://www.communitycatalyst.org/resou.rces/publications/document/2020-Cath-Hosp-Report-2020-31.pdf.

access. Commonly, as in the case of Willa, patients have no choice at all because their insurance determines where they can go.

Willa's story is not an aberration. Nearly half of American women ultimately turn to sterilization to end their childbearing years because it is safe, effective, and under their own (rather than their partner's) control.[11] Furthermore, most American women also think you can get sterilized in a Catholic hospital.[12] Americans know very little about how hospitals like St. Mary's restrict care, despite the fact that one in six American hospital patients is treated in hospitals governed by religious policies of the United States Conference of Catholic Bishops. The USCCB, an organization of active and retired male members of the Catholic hierarchy, holds religious authority over all matters within Catholic institutions in the United States. They devise and revise religious policies for Catholic health facilities in cooperation with the pope, Catholic ethicists, and theologians; the 2018 revision also listed Catholic healthcare providers and administrators among its contributors.[13] Bishops are confirmed by, and subject to, the authority of the Vatican, and they commonly use their organizational power to influence broader American policy as well.[14]

———

Over the past decade, I have conducted over a hundred in-depth qualitative interviews with physicians and patients around the United States about their experiences with reproductive care in Catholic hospitals. During this time, abortion was still legal—if not always easy to access—in all fifty states. Research participants reflected the geographic, economic, racial, and religious diversity of patients and physicians overall in the United States. Along the way, I also collaborated on nationally representative surveys and regional mixed-method studies on the topic. To date, I have co-authored more than a dozen peer-reviewed articles in the medical literature related to Catholic health care. Readers interested in a more detailed discussion of my methods and scholarly journey to this project are invited to read the appendix.

This book synthesizes my own findings, particularly the stories of patients and providers, with the research of others on this topic. I have chosen to generally refer to people who are on the receiving end of health care in this book as "patients." The gender neutrality of the term "patients" allows for the representation of nonbinary and transgender people who have the capacity for pregnancy. That said, the language in this book never could entirely remove the gendered lens because Catholic religious restrictions on health care are grounded in a devotion to a strict gender binary and the Church hierarchy's commitment to a world in which the different roles and rights of males and females are believed to be inherent and immutable from birth.

I acknowledge that using "patients" rather than "women" runs counter to decades of effort by feminist health pioneers to empower women by referring to them as "women," or even "clients," to emphasize their personhood and agency rather than their subjection to a medical system.[15] However, the people who participated in this research are very much subject to a medical system. The term "patients" lays bare the disempowerment of people navigating healthcare settings when institutional restrictions are not evident or transparent; when patients must depend on providers to explain why they cannot get what they need and what to do about it. Additionally, using pseudonyms, I identify particular patients by first name and particular physicians by "Dr." to further underscore their power differential. These language choices do not reflect how power dynamics should be but, rather, how they are: imbalanced.

Bishops and Bodies tells the story of what I have learned, exploring the tensions between patient autonomy, medical standards of care, and religious authority in Catholic hospitals. Altogether, this is a critical ethnography; it brings together the perspectives of patients, providers, and, to the extent it can, Catholic leadership with an "ethical responsibility to address processes of unfairness or injustice within a particular *lived* domain."[16] While religious policies center the beliefs of bishops, doctors do not follow them in the same way at each Catholic hospital, and some patients know more than others about how religion affects their care. This book will show how individual hospitals' compliance with the bishops' policies is erratic and opaque; some make case-by-case exceptions and still fail to alleviate the bioethical problem of denying patients standard care on a larger scale. In all this, patients' autonomy and bodily integrity are routine casualties.

DOCTRINAL IATROGENESIS

When religious restrictions compromise a hospital's ability to meet the standard of care, *doctrinal iatrogenesis* can result. Iatrogenesis refers to patient harm caused by medical treatment itself. I use the term "doctrinal iatrogenesis" to refer to the poor physical and mental health outcomes that result because religious policies limit medical treatment. Willa suffered from doctrinal iatrogenesis, yet she expresses little bitterness about having been denied a consequential medical procedure at the hospital where she gave birth. While not Catholic, she is a Christian who values the religious freedom of the clergy who run the hospital. Crucially, she had time to consider in advance how St. Mary's religious policies would affect her care.

Other patients are not so fortunate, like Amy, whose story I heard from Dr. Ana Altera, a high-risk obstetrician. Employed by an independent, nonprofit clinic system with no religious affiliation, Dr. Altera delivers her patients' babies at St. Vic's, a Catholic hospital, because it is the sole tertiary care provider to its rural area. Aside from St. Vic's, there is no high-risk obstetric care, and little highly specialized care of any sort, within a two-hour drive. When Dr. Altera first took the job, in the early aughts, she did not face opposition from the institution in performing sterilizations at St. Vic's. She simply filled out a form explaining why another pregnancy would be detrimental to the patient's health, and the religious authorities in the hospital would grant an exception to the official prohibition on sterilizations.

All this changed after a devout Catholic physician in her hospital informed the local bishop that the hospital was performing sterilizations. The bishop responded by cracking down on exceptions. Knowing how much their patients relied on sterilization, Dr. Altera and her colleagues partnered with lawyers and advocates to find a solution and landed on a model that some have called a "hospital within a hospital."[17] The bishop ultimately agreed to allow the clinic doctors to buy an operating room in the hospital for performing tubal ligations; it would be designated as not-Catholic, even though it resided inside St. Vic's. Doctors could perform sterilizations only on patients giving birth by C-section. (The bishop presumably allowed this because those patients were already having surgery right near the fallopian tubes.) The agreement could not help patients like Willa, who wanted a postpartum sterilization while hospitalized after a vaginal birth, but it was something. The bishop also prohibited the doctors from using any Catholic hospital personnel during any part of the procedure, from C-section through tubal ligation. To perform a sterilization, the operating room must be staffed by the clinic's on-call ambulatory surgery personnel. This restriction applied to medical assistants, nurses, and anesthetists.

Dr. Altera's ob-gyn colleague at the clinic, Dr. Sara Sherman, whom I also interviewed, explained the conditions of the agreement:

> You can't use any medications owned by [St. Vic's], you can't have hospital personnel, employees, involved in any aspect of their care. You can't use hospital electricity or oxygen, you can't use hospital instruments, you can't have hospital personnel clean the instruments, you can't dictate your operative report on a hospital dictation machine, you can't use the hospital tube system to send your specimens to pathology, you can't use a consent form that has the hospital name on it. And it goes on and on and on and on and on and on. And if there's any violation of any of these—in our situation, the [tubal] room has been sold to the clinic, by the hospital—but that's revocable at any time.[18]

The agreement was far from perfect. How electricity went unshared is unclear. But in practical terms, there were more glaring problems. In this rural area, staff often lived far away from the hospital, and the clinic could not finance the around-the-clock staffing needed to maintain a dedicated, twenty-four-hour operating room. If they knew the patient wanted a tubal ligation following a C-section in advance, they could schedule it during the workday. But if the person desiring a tubal ligation arrived for an emergency C-section after hours—in other words, not planned in advance—the doctors' ability to perform the sterilization depended on their ability to round up clinic staff. While many signed up, there were holes in the schedule. Despite the imperfections, these were the best terms they could get from the bishop.

One night, Amy, a rural white woman with very low income and multiple medical problems, came in to deliver her third child. She had been transferred unexpectedly into Dr. Altera's care from a small rural hospital because it had become clear she needed the higher level of specialty care (tertiary care) available at St. Vic's. Although she'd had two vaginal births and had expected a third, Amy's labor stalled after several hours at St. Vic's, and Dr. Altera realized she would need to perform a C-section for both the baby's and Amy's safety. In the calm of her stalled labor, while discussing the impending surgery, Amy told Dr. Altera she wanted a tubal ligation done at the same time. She indicated that the required consent paperwork should be in her chart, as she had completed it months earlier, during prenatal care. Dr. Altera recalled responding to her: "I said, 'Oh, I hadn't even known that that was something you'd wish for.' She goes, 'Oh, yeah, yeah. You know, [my primary care doctor], his nurses brought it up . . . So I signed the papers so I'm all set.' And I thought to myself, 'Oh, no.'"

Dr. Altera looked to see what staff she could bring in, but as she feared, that night no one had signed up. Being such a rural area, it was not easy to mobilize volunteer staff quickly in the middle of the night.

> So I went back in the room and I told her that and I said, you know, "I can't do your tubal ligation." And she's like, "What are you talking about? My abdomen's going to be wide open, right?" I said, "Yes." And she said, "Well, isn't it right there, I mean, isn't it all just right there? Isn't it like kind of easy at that point?" And I said, "Well yes." She goes, "So why can't you?"
>
> And I said, "Well, I can't because, you know, the hospital has certain rules and unless I can bring in a team of clinic employees, I can't bypass those rules." And she's like—you know, kept looking at me like "What are you talking about?"

Dr. Altera recalled pausing a moment as she tried to imagine the perspective of her patient who seemed to know little about the convolutions of hospital ownership or how religious institutions can restrict reproductive care in the United States. Amy had no reason to know, as this was her first experience coming to this facility.

Dr. Altera thought to herself, "Start from square one." And she explained: "I said, 'Well this is [St. Vic's] Hospital. It's a Catholic hospital.' I said, 'Are you aware of any restrictions placed on birth control by the Catholic Church?' And she goes, 'Well I'm not Catholic' She goes, 'I guess I sort of, I guess I know sort of what you mean, but what does that have to do with me? I'm not Catholic.' And you could sort of see it just went on from there. So I told her, you know, that the rule applies to every patient who's within the hospital . . .'"

Amy appeared upset and scared. Contraception had not worked well for her in the past and had given her health problems; she was overwhelmed at the idea of another pregnancy or doing the tubal ligation at a later time. Dr. Altera recalled that Amy pleaded: "'I can't go through another procedure. Look at me.' And I was, like, I couldn't have agreed with her more and I told her that. And I just kept apologizing. 'I am sorry we're in this situation. I don't know what to do.' And she finally looked at me and she said, 'Would you do it anyway?' She broke my heart.

Dr. Altera did not do it anyway. She had been warned that if the bishop found out about such a violation, the agreement would be voided. She feared that "any other woman going forward, who's planning her C-section and tubal ligation tomorrow or next week or next month, they'd all lose [that option] . . . that's been the threat."

After that difficult conversation with Amy, Dr. Altera and her team proceeded to the C-section. They closed her up without the sterilization. She felt horrible. She recalled:

> The morning after it happened, I contacted . . . the clinic president and the hospital president, sent an email to both of them. I said, "You need to know about an angry patient. Here's what happened. She's angry. She has every right to be angry." And I said to both of them in my email, "And it felt rotten to be the person who carried out this restriction, it felt rotten. I never thought my autonomy as a physician would be limited in this way, ever." And I believe I said to both of them, "If I were faced with taking this job today, now, with these restrictions, I would never have taken this job."[19]

When I interviewed Dr. Altera's colleague, Dr. Sherman, a year later, she told me Amy had become pregnant again shortly thereafter. Due to Amy's multiple medical problems, this was an extremely high-risk pregnancy that required multiple hospitalizations. Amy's doctors ultimately delivered the baby via C-section during one of her hospital admissions, not because they did not think they could keep her pregnant safely longer but because they were afraid she would go into labor in the middle of the night again and they would have to risk denying her the sterilization again because of the religious rules. They delivered the baby at thirty-two weeks, two months early, during the day, to ensure they had adequate external staff members on hand. The doctors had more faith that the baby would survive premature birth after a stay in the neonatal intensive care unit (NICU) than in whether Amy would survive another pregnancy. This false choice was created by the Catholic restrictions on care.

I asked Dr. Sherman whether she thought Amy would sue the hospital or speak out about what happened to her. Not getting the tubal ligation she wanted had significant consequences for her life; she now had an additional, premature child. Dr. Sherman surprised me when she said that, in the end, Amy was not angry at all. She felt incredibly well cared for (or at least, that is the impression she gave her medical team). All the specialists and staff who attended her knew her history and felt terrible about what had happened. According to Dr. Sherman: "People took care of her obsessively . . . she had eight hospitalizations and, you know, she saw cardiologists and endocrinologists." Dr. Sherman went on: "I think the reason, honestly, that she was not more upset was, I think she really bonded to some of the doctors and really felt like they were working very hard for her, which they were, and, you know, I think she felt quite close to some of the doctors." But even if Amy's stress was somewhat mitigated by the staff's devoted medical attention, the stress itself was entirely unnecessary, a product of doctrinal, not medical, policy.

Denying women control over reproductive decisions and access to standard obstetric care has consequences. In Willa's case, her delayed sterilization led to an unplanned child and a difficult recovery. Amy's case also produced an unplanned pregnancy, one that almost killed her. And while Willa had relatively more lead time to consider how religion would affect her and she could, potentially, make an alternative plan, she also was limited by her insurance. In the end, both Willa and

Amy were unable to avoid being negatively impacted by the religious restrictions. In reproductive medicine, the mundane can become morbid, or nearly so. The denial of a common, safe, and relatively noncontroversial procedure for religious reasons can be the cause of medical and emotional harm—that is, doctrinal iatrogenesis—and also the source of significant distress for providers who become implicated in those harms.

The Ethical and Religious Directives for Catholic Health Care Services

The USCCB embed Catholic doctrine into healthcare delivery via the policies laid out in the Ethical and Religious Directives for Catholic Health Care Services, a public document.[20] Hospitals must agree to follow the bishops' directives as hospital policy to be sponsored by the Roman Catholic Church. Nearly all Catholic hospitals become members of the Catholic Health Association of the United States because membership in the network offers them professional leadership and national advocacy.

The CHA is a separate entity from the USCCB, and they are not always of like mind. They sometimes clash publicly, most notably over the Affordable Care Act (ACA), which the bishops claimed would provide federal funds for abortion. In 2010, the cardinal leading the USCCB charged that, in supporting the ACA's passage, CEO and president of the CHA Sister Carol Keehan "weakened the moral voice of the bishops in the U.S."[21] Despite such tension, the CHA website still describes the bishops' ERDs as "the document that offers moral guidance, drawn from the Catholic Church's theological and moral teachings, on various aspects of health care delivery."[22] The CHA offers webinars on how to interpret and apply these directives in healthcare delivery. Thus, while the final authority over care in each hospital falls to the local bishop, the CHA provides members with practical support to navigate conflicts that can arise from religious policies. The CHA and USCCB dynamics parallel gender tensions in the Catholic Church generally, where nuns and sisters (women in religious orders) remain barred from formal power. They can be of service but not ordained. The modern CHA is led by sisters whose predecessors historically founded most Catholic hospitals and served as nurses, while the USCCB is led by male clergy at the rank of bishop or higher who hold firm to the reins of religious authority.[23]

The ERDs enumerate points of interactions between religious doctrine and medical practice in Catholic institutions, providing firm instructions for each. The first half of the seventy-seven directives address overarching social, spiritual, and professional obligations of Catholic healthcare organizations. The remaining half more specifically delineate how to deliver clinical services related to the beginning of life (sex and reproduction, Directives 38 through 54), the ending of life (from embryonic to geriatric death, Directives 55 through 66), and in partnering with affiliates that do not "operate in conformity with the Church's moral teaching" (Directives 67 through 77).

My interpretation of Catholic health doctrine is informed by what the ERDs say, what doctors have told me about how religious authorities in their hospitals interpret and enforce them (when, for example, ethics committees approve or deny physicians' appeals for exceptions), and what research in peer-reviewed medical journals report about how these directives ultimately affect practice. When, periodically, the religious policies have conflicted with how physicians report being directed by their ethics committees or leadership, I also have relied on Catholic scholars' writings for explanation.[24] I do not delve into theological analysis beyond this, as the many and varied potential interpretations of Catholic theology have limited relevance to the day-to-day operations of Catholic hospitals. For the purposes of this book, what matters is how the bishops have interpreted Catholic theology for healthcare delivery, and what those interpretations mean for those delivering or seeking care.

I will have more to say about particular directives that affect clinical services and how they do so in the remainder of this book. For now, the important point is, simply, that the ERDs represent an ambitious Church undertaking to accord medical practice with religious doctrine in Catholic facilities in the United States, whether or not their doctors are familiar with the document itself or why exactly their practice is restricted.

SPECIFIC CLINICAL CONFLICTS IN CATHOLIC MEDICINE

Catholic hospitals diverge most widely from their non-Catholic counterparts in the realm of reproductive care. Physicians in Catholic hospitals are prohibited from offering contraception or performing a sterilization because the official interpretation of Catholic doctrine opposes sex without the intent to reproduce. Sex, reproduction, and heterosexual marriage are inseparable within Catholic doctrine. Working from this religious tenet, the bishops do not allow Catholic health systems to support forms of reproduction that might occur outside of heterosexual sexual intercourse, including in vitro fertilization and surrogacy, two techniques commonly used by queer couples or people experiencing infertility. In more recent years, the bishops also have explicitly opposed surgeries that change sexual and reproductive functions, including gender-affirming surgery. Doctors who have tried to schedule hysterectomies for gender affirmation have found those surgeries cancelled.[25] Physicians who act outside the constraints of the ERDs risk being fired or losing privileges to work in the hospital if they are not employed by it.

The directives include a prohibition on abortion, which additionally limits care for pregnancy complications. Until the U.S. Supreme Court's 2022 decision in *Dobbs v. Jackson Women's Health Organization* struck down the right to abortion, these blanket restrictions on patient care were unique to Catholic hospitals. Within weeks of the decision, media outlets began reporting horrifying stories of medical providers withholding treatment from patients in the midst of obstetric complications and miscarriages.[26] Fearing legal repercussions, doctors in states without abortion protections began telling patients that their hands were tied until either the fetus died or the patient was close to death. This is no small risk. In 2012, Savita Halappanavar died in Ireland after complications stemming from delayed miscarriage management in accordance with the country's ban on abortion. Her death prompted protests that ultimately drove Ireland to liberalize its laws about pregnancy termination. But while the consequences of abortion restrictions may be news to most Americans, they are all too familiar to physicians who provide reproductive care in Catholic health systems.

To many physicians I interviewed, the fact that Catholic hospitals' abortion policies restrict miscarriage treatments seems cruel and absurd. If a miscarriage is clearly inevitable, why make a patient suffer longer or risk infection? Unfortunately, the ERDs' interpretation of Catholic doctrine, like blanket bans on abortion, forbids doctors from doing anything that facilitates the end of life of the fetus. Doctors have to wait.

One ob-gyn nurse I spoke with, a white woman I call Jennifer, worked in a Catholic hospital, the only hospital in her mid-size city in a Western state. A few years prior to our conversation, she was pregnant herself. One day in her first trimester, she began to bleed. Knowing quite a lot about pregnancy, she was sad but not scared. She bled steadily for about a week, thinking she would likely pass the pregnancy on her own. When she began exhibiting symptoms of anemia, she went to see her physician in his office. Her doctor agreed with her assessment that she was miscarrying, but he was hesitant to schedule a procedure to empty her uterus (a dilation and curettage, or D&C) in their Catholic hospital. She interpreted his resistance as him not wanting to attract the attention of the hospital's religious authorities.

She recalled: "I can see the factors that probably played into it. I think it was [him] not wanting to do a D&C, probably not wanting to open that particular can of worms about whether it was okay to do a D&C. Because a scheduled one is even harder to get done in that hospital than one in the ER . . . if there's a D&C on the schedule for a possibly viable pregnancy, then the Ethics Board gets involved."

Instead, her physician ordered her a transfusion to address her anemia and advised her to wait for the pregnancy to pass on its own. She continued to bleed heavily the next twelve hours after the transfusion. By now, she had given up any hope for saving the pregnancy and realized she needed medical intervention. At her Catholic hospital, the ER staff performed multiple ultrasounds to ensure the fetus was dead: "They did so many ultrasounds. They ended up doing, I think, three, although I may have missed one. And I remember telling them over and over again, 'This is not a viable pregnancy. I've been bleeding enough to need a transfusion for a week. This is not viable.' And they're like, 'Well, we just need to make sure.' And I'm like, 'Have you found any cardiac motion?' 'No. But we need to check again because maybe we missed it. It's very early in your pregnancy.'"

At this point, she just wanted it over with, but the staff decided to do another transfusion to address her anemia, which was worsening as they waited. Once the staff were finally convinced the fetus had passed, about seven hours after her arrival, the hospital allowed her physician to empty her uterus, and she went home.

The D&C solved Jennifer's immediate medical crisis. Unfortunately, her treatment led to additional medical problems. After enduring the emotionally challenging pregnancy loss, which she knew was unnecessarily prolonged and complicated by the hospital's religious rules, Jennifer found out during her next pregnancy that she had developed Kell antibodies in response to one of the two transfusions she received. This condition can lead to a potentially lethal fetal blood disorder in a future pregnancy, anti-Kell.[27] Jennifer's husband also happened to be Kell-positive, raising the likelihood that the baby would suffer this hemolytic disease. The high risk of a fetus or newborn developing this blood disorder haunted their next pregnancy and birth with the constant threat of sudden fetal demise.

Jennifer's is a stark case of doctrinal iatrogenesis. Both blood transfusions had been necessary only because of the religious policies that caused her doctor to avoid scheduling a D&C to stop the bleeding initially, and then later caused the hospital to delay the D&C once she was there. While the restrictions on Jennifer's care were a direct product of religious restrictions on miscarriage management, today one in four American women live in states whose abortion policies are equally likely to produce a medical crisis and emotional harm.[28] While Jennifer's subsequent child was born healthy, her family experienced a period of profound stress awaiting the birth. And although Jennifer had preferred to go through labor, her doctor scheduled an early C-section—a major surgery she might not have needed—out of an abundance of caution. As in the cases of both Willa and Amy, policies that place limits on reproductive care led to additional surgical and medical risks, as well as unintended negative health consequences.

WHY THE GROWTH OF CATHOLIC HEALTHCARE SYSTEMS MATTERS

If hospitals that followed the directives were transparent, rare, and just one of several patient choices, the existence of the ERDs would pose less of an ethical conflict for doctors working in Catholic healthcare systems. In this alternate universe, healthcare providers might feel assured that their patients had made an informed decision, based on their own religious commitments and preferences, unhindered by proximity, cost, or insurance network. In reality, even if a patient has multiple alternatives to Catholic providers nearby and their insurance permits them to choose, research shows it is difficult for people to discern that a hospital is Catholic or what that means.[29]

The size of the Catholic footprint in the U.S. health system amplifies already existing inequalities in people's reproductive freedom and wellbeing.[30] Since the 1990s, reproductive justice advocates have been shining a light on how the predominately white reproductive rights movement and political infrastructure has focused narrowly on preserving the right *not to* reproduce. Meanwhile, the inverse—the right *to* reproduce—is routinely devalued for women of color in the United States; some examples include sterilization abuse and glaring disparities between Black and white maternal mortality.

Religious restrictions on reproductive care have disparate racial impacts and further this injustice. One study showed that, in nineteen states, women of color are more likely to give birth at Catholic hospitals than white women.[31] Another study that analyzed Illinois Medicaid plans showed that Black and Hispanic women were enrolled in plans with a higher proportion of Catholic hospitals than their county overall.[32] A third study found that decreases in the availability of sterilization after hospitals were bought by Catholic systems in six states impacted Hispanic women more than others.[33] Taken together, this budding area of research shows that women of color are routinely overexposed to maternity care that lacks standard postpartum contraception, miscarriage management, and other reproductive care. This overexposure may cause or exacerbate persistent racial disparities in maternal morbidity and mortality.

On top of these inequities, physicians know that patients may not have the benefit of choice in an emergency situation. The experiences of Willa, Amy, and Jennifer parallel the narratives of health care I heard repeatedly from both patients and doctors. Their experiences reflect those of a wide variety of patients I interviewed or heard about through their physicians: patients with religious, racial, and sexual diversity who had private insurance, public insurance, and no insurance at all. Throughout the book, I will share stories of patients with a variety of backgrounds from urban and rural areas who were impacted by the Catholic directives. This book examines the consequences of the gap between patient autonomy and medical practice in the growing sector of Catholic health care in the United States, a problem intimately connected to the lack of universal health care and a policy context that supports massive, religiously restrictive health systems to fill that void. As such, these findings can help us understand how doctrinal iatrogenesis is not remotely limited to Catholic hospitals. State abortion restrictions grounded in religious beliefs, especially in the absence of a reproductive care safety net,[34] induce the same kind of patient harm.

Chapter 1 unpacks the legal, economic, and social changes that have driven the growth of the Catholic health sector. It shows how Catholic hospitals have evolved from mission-based, charity institutions to federally funded major players in American healthcare delivery. Catholic hospitals have responded to the same financial incentives as other hospitals in the United States, even as they have retained their unique relationship to religious authority. Chapter 2 takes a closer look at how religious policy and standards of care collide in healthcare delivery. By examining how specific religious directives compel care that is counter to expected treatments in the field of obstetrics and gynecology, we can see that the standard of care is contested because the goal is contested. Simply put, ob-gyns seek different outcomes for their patients than do the U.S. Conference of Catholic Bishops.

Chapter 3 examines the illusion of choice in American health care. As we shall see, however, patients expect a level of consumer choice in health care that they do not have, and even those who actively seek out Catholic care often are surprised by their experiences with religious restrictions. Chapter 4 explores the particular burdens of religious policies on three patients who went to a Catholic hospital for an obstetric emergency who did not know their hospital had a Catholic affiliation or did not know how it would impact their care.

Chapter 5 shows how physicians who wish to play by the hospital's rules (for one reason or another) work around them for many of their patients. Doctors who "play by the rules" often find themselves sending their patients elsewhere—even if "elsewhere" is a door down the hall. Chapter 6 shows how ob-gyns attempt to meet the needs of patients in less rule-abiding ways. As religious authorities increasingly limit physicians' above-board workarounds, doctors have tried different strategies, including what is, essentially, subterfuge. Finally, chapter 7 considers a harrowing episode in which a Catholic hospital was publicly disaffiliated by the local bishop for performing a life-saving abortion. An opportunity to expand ultimately brought the hospital and the Church back together.

––––––

We all need health care. Depending on where one lives or the kind of insurance one has, a Catholic health system may be the most attractive or even the only option for reproductive care. Today, Catholic hospitals have more secular names. The people working inside them may or may not be Catholic, Christian, or members of any faith community; many endeavor to work around or minimize the negative impacts of religious restrictions on patients' care. This book is, ultimately, about how a patriarchal stronghold, the Roman Catholic Church, maintains influence over Americans' reproductive lives; how patients experience the Church's imposition on their reproductive autonomy; and the challenges of practicing good medicine within theological constraints that few Americans, and, strikingly, even fewer Catholic Americans, support.[35]

CHAPTER 1

Growth

HOW CATHOLIC HEALTH CARE EXPANDED

Catholic hospitals and health systems now comprise about one-sixth of the U.S. healthcare sector. Over the past 200 years, they have evolved from small religious facilities staffed primarily by nuns to mega hospitals staffed by professionals and managed almost identically to their non-Catholic counterparts, with one major exception: the Ethical and Religious Directives for Catholic Health Care Services.

Today, Catholic health systems are more likely to bear names that sound vaguely mission-based, like Dignity and Providence, instead of words with explicit references to the Catholic Church. Indeed, the majority have undergone rebranding over the years. Looking at the website of OSF Healthcare, it is hard to figure out that the letters stand for Sisters of the Order of Saint Francis. Catholic Healthcare West became Dignity Health. The website of CHI Health—a recent rebranding of Catholic Health Initiatives—bears no mention of the word Catholic on the opening webpage. CHI now sits with Dignity Health under the umbrella of CommonSpirit. Hospitals associated with the Sisters of St. Mercy are now known simply as Mercy. Names like Mercy, Providence, Trinity, Essentia, and Ascension may sound religious to some who know and are looking for it, but most people, it turns out, do not. The names of South Hampton Memorial, Bob Wilson Memorial, Avera, and Natchitoches Regional Medical Center offer even fewer clues of their affiliation with the Church, yet they are the only hospital option in their regions. The care they provide conforms with the requirements set out by the United States Conference of Catholic Bishops.

The Catholic Health Association of the United States is aware of patients' possible confusion. In 2018, an article in the *New York Times* reported: "Father Bouchard of the Catholic Health Association acknowledged the gradual change in the look of many Catholic hospitals. 'Especially because of partnerships that we've developed with other entities in some cases, there might be a less prominent Catholic identity,' he said. 'But it is certainly not in an attempt to deceive anybody . . . We want to make everybody feel welcome,' he said. 'If a Catholic hospital maybe doesn't emphasize overtly Catholic identity as much as they used

to, it is not to trick anyone. It's simply to make people feel comfortable and welcome in an increasingly pluralistic society.'"[1]

While the sentiment is ostensibly welcoming, it also creates a bit of a smoke-
screen. Today, whether their patients know it or not, four of the ten largest health
systems in the United States are Catholic.

This chapter describes how and why these initially small religious hospitals
became such formidable competitors in the healthcare industry. Over the course
of the twentieth century, Catholic hospitals integrated into mainstream medicine
and helped ensure that a universal, governmental health system did not emerge to
supplant them. Catholic hospitals effectively joined forces to maximize the power
of Catholic health capital in a healthcare business that rewarded market share.
Together, Catholic hospitals fought for legal recognition of what they referred to
as institutional "conscience rights" as reproductive rights advocates increasingly
called the ethics of religious health care into question.

An Institution Transformed

Following the model of early European hospitals, early American hospitals, including Catholic ones, provided care to people who could not afford or access better
options. Catholic and other religious voluntary hospitals existed alongside a relatively smaller number of private and government-run municipal hospitals; none
provided the level of care a person would ideally seek.[2] In the eighteenth and nineteenth centuries, orders of Catholic sisters and brothers founded hospitals in population centers to care for the ill and dying who were not necessarily welcome in
non-Catholic hospitals, such as Italian and Irish immigrants. They also founded
mission hospitals where there were few Catholics or healthcare alternatives.

In addition to medical care, these early Catholic hospitals provided spiritual care
that ensured that dying Catholic patients would receive their last rites. It was important to the founders, as one historian wrote, "to institutionalize medical treatment
that infused standard medical practice with a Catholic perspective on life and
death."[3] Their mission was to care for the sick and poor in general, while incorporating the specific religious perspectives of their founders. Medical care at that time
was neither particularly sophisticated nor expensive, and the relatively uncompen-
sated labor of sisters as nurses made the enterprise both charitable and sustainable.

During this time, reproductive health care was not a source of distinction or
conflict for Catholic hospitals. There were no hormonal contraception methods to
dispense or withhold, and sterilization was uncommon for contraceptive purposes.
While abortions were common in the late nineteenth century, they were provided
mostly by midwives or physicians outside of the hospital.[4] Most reproductive care
and treatment remained within the home, performed by women.[5] Reproductive
care found its way into American hospitals in the late nineteenth and early twentieth centuries as part of the medical profession's broader campaign for social
and economic dominance of the healthcare market. Childbirth moved into the

hospital setting, as did the few legal abortions that physicians deemed medically necessary.[6]

As medical advances at the turn of the twentieth century opened new possibilities for patient care, including reproductive care, clergy soon found themselves in the position of regulating medical work. The nuns, too, saw it as their duty to make sure doctors followed the rules.[7] In particular, clergy, nurses, and doctors often clashed over the management of obstetric emergencies. New antiseptic techniques and advances in anesthesia made for safer surgeries, which meant doctors increasingly had the ability to save a mother whose life was threatened by pregnancy or labor. And yet, Catholic hospitals prohibited interventions that might kill the fetus, even to save a mother's life, as religious doctrine held fetal life on par with that of the mother.[8]

Doctrinal debates over emergency obstetric care nearly split the young Catholic Hospital Association, which had formed in 1915 to advocate for the shared interests of the growing number of Catholic hospitals. The most conservative Catholic leaders involved in health care questioned whether the mother's life should be saved *at all* during either a life-threatening pregnancy or delivery if it meant the loss of fetal life. At least for the short term, the organization resolved its internal differences through appeals to professionalization. In 1922, the CHA published a voluntary code of ethics that condemned both abortion and sterilization, but it also encouraged hospitals affiliated with the CHA to pursue the new medical standards being promoted by the American College of Surgeons (ACS).[9] This approach accommodated medical, administrative, and staffing practices not necessarily intrinsic to Catholic hospitals at the time, and it also created reams of paperwork that helped clergy and hospital administrators detect and investigate patterns of surgical practice that violated Catholic beliefs. Requirements for documenting preoperative diagnoses and retaining tissues after surgery would keep physicians honest if not faithful. Pathologists, for example, could be instrumental in determining whether hysterectomies really were performed for birth control instead of cancer treatment. Thus, the same structures used to ensure professional and scientific standards of medical practice could also help keep hospitals in line with Catholic doctrine.

Perhaps because these recordkeeping requirements advanced their own interests, Catholic hospitals outpaced non-Catholic hospitals in meeting minimum ACS standards. By 1929, over half of Catholic hospitals met ACS standards, compared to only a quarter of non-Catholic hospitals. During this period of institutional growth, CHA leaders carefully navigated a middle path, ultimately avoiding a binding code of ethics until after the most intractable conflicts in obstetric care had become moot. That is, by the 1950s, medicine had advanced such that women were more likely to survive difficult pregnancies; it was less common to have to destroy the fetus to save the mother's life. At the same time, medical opinion grew more publicly disdainful of abortion and judgmental of the women who needed them. With abortion increasingly stigmatized and Catholic hospitals' position strong and secure, the CHA leaders created a detailed Catholic code of medical ethics in 1948. The USCCB signed off on a revised version of the code in 1954, which became the first binding version of the Ethical and Religious Directives for Catholic Health Care Services. Thus, ultimately, American Catholic hospitals used standardization to protect both their religious purity and their market share. This pragmatic and strategic approach to leadership in Catholic health care would endure, balancing margin with mission for decades to come.[10]

By 1940, the United States was home to a large, growing, and complex system of hospital care. The majority of American hospitals were voluntary, nonprofit institutions. Church-affiliated nonprofit hospitals were providing 30 percent of hospital care as measured by admissions, with 40 percent provided by nonprofits not affiliated with a church, 19 percent by government institutions, and the remaining 11 percent by proprietary, for-profit hospitals owned by corporations or physician associations.[11] The medical profession, as a rule, opposed proposals for national health insurance during this time, but it welcomed the federal government's investment in capital improvements, including hospital facilities. The Hill-Burton Act of 1946 provided a generous source of funding for both private and public hospitals at the same time that it granted hospitals maximum autonomy. With ready access to capital funds, Catholic hospitals built larger facilities, expanded into new areas, and quadrupled the number of patients treated annually between 1945 and 1960.[12]

By the late twentieth century, Catholic hospitals had secured ongoing public funding, built a reputation for delivering quality health care, and had proliferated. As Catholic hospitals expanded, their staff professionalized. Sisters were gradually replaced by secular nurses. A study of the Catholic Hospital Association journal noted the trend with concern in the sixties.[13] Ethnographer Adam Reich wrote much later of the Catholic hospital he studied: "The last sister left Las Lomas in 2007. And while managers continued to speak of self-sacrifice and vocational devotion, this rhetoric came with a patina of spirituality over an increasingly businesslike core."[14] While Catholic hospitals still had names like St. Mary's or Sisters of St. Mercy, the care they delivered looked increasingly like that in secular hospitals. The one major exception to this, of course, was in reproductive care.[15]

Beginning in the late 1970s, Catholic health care experienced the same kinds of consolidation that was transforming the rest of the medical economy.[16] From 1979 to 1985, the number of Catholic hospital systems dropped from 124 to 91, even as the number of Catholic hospitals increased from 533 to 553.[17] Catholic hospitals had 17 hospital consolidations in 1996 and 1997 alone, outpacing consolidation in for-profit systems.[18] Time and time again, this growth pitted Catholic hospitals' mission against their margin. Growing Catholic health systems brought in huge profits in some years. For example, Catholic Healthcare West (CHW), which later would be renamed Dignity Health, had a net profit of $160 million in 1996, and an A+ bond rating by Standard and Poor.[19]

Starting in the 1990s, profitable Catholic healthcare systems increasingly merged with non-Catholic hospitals. More often than not, Catholic hospitals have been in the stronger negotiating position during mergers, thanks to their connection to a flourishing national system. They frequently have forced previously secular facilities to adhere to the ERDs as a condition of the merger.[20] In these cases, the newly acquired (or merged) hospital loses its ability to perform abortions, vasectomies, and tubal ligations, or to prescribe and insert contraception, without the approval of a Catholic ethics committee. And as smaller hospitals closed, Catholic hospitals obtained a greater percentage of market share.[21] From 2001 to 2020, the number of hospitals operating according to Catholic health restrictions grew by more than 29 percent, while the rest of the hospital industry shrunk by 14 percent.[22] The number of these that were the only hospital in their area increased from thirty in 2013 to fifty-two in 2020. Catholic systems have expanded to include urgent care centers (864), ambulatory surgery centers (385), and physician practices (274).[23] In 2021, the CHA posted that its 668 member hospitals admitted over 5 million patients. Combined with the other Catholic healthcare facilities, CHA member facilities had 107 million outpatient visits, 20 million emergency room visits, and 500,000 newborn deliveries that same year.[24]

Throughout the Catholic health sector's growth, the bishops held a hard line on reproductive care. Increasingly, they do so with the protection of the law. In the years immediately following the legalization of abortion, many abortion procedures were provided in hospitals. The Catholic hierarchy endeavored to ensure that their hospitals would *not* be among them.[25] The first conscience legislation, the Church Amendment, was ironically named not in relation to the Catholic or any other church but, rather, for its author Senator Frank Church in 1973. It was written in response to both *Roe v. Wade* and a legal decision about a Montana Catholic hospital's right to prohibit sterilization. The Church Amendment protects individuals and institutions from having to provide abortion and sterilization.[26] Several related conscience laws followed suit at the state and federal levels. One federal law, the Weldon Amendment, has effectively hamstrung local efforts to limit religious power over reproductive care. Included in HHS's annual spending bills since 2005 alongside the Hyde Amendment banning federal funding for abortion, the Weldon Amendment bars the U.S. Department of Health and Human Services from funding a federal agency or program, or state or local government, if it "subjects any institutional or individual healthcare entity to discrimination on the basis that the health care entity does not provide, pay for, provide coverage of, or refer for abortions,"[27] meaning that, if a state wants to compel access to full-spectrum reproductive health care in religious facilities, it has a lot to lose.

CARVE-OUTS AND CONTROVERSY

As the consequences of the growth of Catholic health care have become harder to miss, some communities have pushed back against new limitations on reproductive services. When I interviewed Lois Uttley in 2019, she told me the story of how she founded her organization MergerWatch, the primary source of data about the growth and funding of Catholic health care in the twenty-first century. In that role, Uttley has worked with local communities for more than twenty years to stop mergers, or at least mitigate the ensuing loss of reproductive services. Uttley had a background in journalism and then governmental public affairs for the New York State Department of Health when she became the communications director for Family Planning Advocates (FPA) in 1996, a political advocacy group representing family planning organizations statewide and the patients who depend on them.

As soon as Uttley began working at FPA, she learned that the organization had been receiving panicked calls from patients who had previously received contraceptive services from Leonard Hospital. Leonard had just merged with a nearby Catholic hospital, St. Mary's. Uttley explained:

> These women were all from a low-income housing project near Leonard [Hospital] [and] were saying "Now what do I do?"[28] They were not getting a referral somewhere else, they were just being told, "Sorry, we don't do that anymore." It was then we realized that all the lobbying we were doing in the state capital to keep abortion and contraception legal and accessible and well-funded was starting to be undermined by developments in the health industry that we had been paying no attention to.

Uttley's director, JoAnn Smith, asked her to see what she could do about it. The answer was to create MergerWatch, which later spun off as its own nonprofit organization. The Leonard Hospital case was ultimately settled by a judge who ruled that staff would have to hand out a piece of paper letting women know about family planning resources elsewhere. But unless the hospital was required to provide a way for the women to get to those facilities, Uttley observed: "It was one of those compromises that doesn't really help anyone."

Leonard turned out to be a bellwether. Catholic-dominated hospital acquisitions and mergers were producing especially dire consequences for women in communities without a non-Catholic provider. The experience motivated Uttley and her colleagues to think creatively about alternatives.

When MergerWatch was contacted by advocates in New York's Hudson Valley about a potential merger, they leapt into action. Three local hospitals—Kingston, Benedictine, and Northern Dutchess—were planning to merge to form Cross River Healthcare. Only Benedictine was Catholic. The two non-Catholic hospitals had, nonetheless, agreed to abide by the ERDs. They announced this with great fanfare, saying: "This will be really great, this will improve healthcare in the Hudson Valley." Local reproductive rights activists centered in the area's progressive communities, like Woodstock, disagreed. They reached out to Uttley for help and formed their own cleverly named community groups, Save Our Services (S.O.S.) and Preserve Medical Secularity (P.M.S.). In response to strong public criticism, the hospitals abandoned the merger.

At least for the time being. Soon after, a state healthcare commission mandated that the two hospitals nearest one another—Kingston and Benedictine—merge to reduce what was then perceived as an excess of hospital beds in the area. The merger happened, but MergerWatch and local advocates successfully lobbied the commission to require Kingston to continue offering reproductive services. They negotiated a "carve out," the first of many that Uttley's team helped negotiate across the United States. In the Kingston case, the hospitals agreed to create a separate, non-Catholic fiscal entity with its own board and staff. This new entity would build and manage a separate building in the parking lot that would provide abortion care, interval tubal ligations (six weeks or more postpartum), and other outpatient contraceptive services.

While the Kingston carve-out was on some level a success for reproductive rights, its placement in the parking lot was a concrete manifestation of the stigma of reproductive services. As a practical matter, the location made the clinic an easy target for anti-abortion protesters. The next time a community asked MergerWatch to help, the organization negotiated a fiscal carve-out integrated into the physical structure. Typically, a segment of the hospital, or even a floor, would be sold to a non-Catholic entity, and all ERD-restricted services would happen there, much as was the case in Dr. Altera's hospital, St. Vic's.

In her twenty years with MergerWatch, Uttley has always waited for the cases to find her, because the organization relies on local advocates to make it work. Her track record includes twelve mergers that were entirely undone, thirty-four that advocates stopped before the mergers went through, and about twenty that went ahead with a creative solution or carve-out. As we talked, she conjured memorable stories from her time in the trenches. "We worked on so many different methods of throwing obstacles in the path of these proposed mergers." She recalled one case in Batavia, New York, in which the hospital was incorporated as a membership organization with no fee, an uncommon practice among hospitals: "It meant that people could join as members and then at the annual meeting have a vote. So, we had this huge campaign to organize people in Batavia to become members of the hospital and then there became so many and they were all opposed to this merger that they killed it."

Other times, the merger opponents successfully used antitrust law, "raising concerns about the combined merger getting too big a market share." She also recalled cases in which activists convinced major donors to remind hospital CEOs and boards of directors that their charitable purpose was to provide care, not religious control over care. She explained that she and her colleagues typically explored all the potential leverage points, some of which were completely unrelated to reproductive rights.

While Lois Uttley's work may have particularly high national visibility, several other advocates also have identified creative ways to limit the loss of reproductive services occasioned by the growth of Catholic hospital systems. Susan Berke Fogel has been working on religious hospital mergers for decades. She was the head of women's health work at the California Women's Law Center in the 1990s when she got a call from an employee at Grass Valley's Sierra Nevada Memorial Hospital. The hospital was being acquired by CHW, and the employees wanted Fogel's help pushing back on the merger.[29] Fogel helped advocates organize a town hall meeting, attended by about 400 people who showed up in the rain. She remembered saving a chair for a representative from CHW, who was invited but did not show.

Community opposition to the merger was intense, but, ultimately, could not stop it. Instead, reproductive health advocates got CHW to allow Sierra Nevada to operate according to a then-new type of religious policy document, the somewhat presumptively named "Statement of Common Values" (SCV), in lieu of the more restrictive ERDs. The SCVs prohibit abortion, in vitro fertilization (IVF), and aid-in-dying, but not contraception or sterilization. Despite the fact that the SCVs have not been endorsed by the bishops, Catholic authorities have allowed several hospitals acquired by CHW to operate under the SCV framework. As Carol Bayley, CHW's director of ethics and justice education at the time, told a reporter: "What we have said to the bishops [is that] it's important that we have a relationship with these hospitals. We're not going to baptize them."[30] That is, CHW had an imperative to grow that she believed the bishops should value; that even if some of their hospitals were not purely Catholic (facetiously "baptized" or, in other words, following all ERDs), the growth imperative and business success of their Catholic system would be considered a high-enough Catholic priority for the bishops to approve the mergers—so long as there would be *no abortion*. Ultimately, it was.

While Fogel and her colleagues have never stopped a merger entirely, they successfully reduced the scope of the religious restrictions in new mergers from the ERDs to the SCVs in several cases. She recalled that in that period of time, both secular for-profit and religious systems were taking over numerous independent hospitals. Fogel and colleagues attempted to stave off subsequent losses of all kinds of healthcare services. Large health systems would buy smaller hospitals, either gutting or absorbing them, to reduce competition. If religious (usually Catholic), the parent health systems would impose the religious restrictions on the newly acquired facilities. "You had both of these things happening in the '90s, just an explosion of huge systems gobbling up independent hospitals" for market share and for mission expansion. After the Grass Valley case, Fogel said, her organization was "able to hold Catholic Healthcare West's feet to the fire on using the common values (SCVs) in all but one of the community hospitals they bought. And that was in Gilroy."[31]

The hospital in question was St. Louise, a historically Catholic hospital located in a central California farming region. Its only competitor, South Valley Hospital, a nonsectarian community hospital, was struggling economically and had closed. When CHW, which owned St. Louise, decided to move it from a small and outdated building into South Valley's facility, Fogel and other healthcare advocates pressured the Santa Clara County Board of Supervisors not to grant the $7 million bond funding required to make it happen unless St. Louise agreed to follow the SCVs instead of the more restrictive ERDs. But CHW threatened to close St. Louise if compelled to do so. The board, scared of losing its remaining hospital there, backed off.[32]

An article in the *Los Angeles Times* in 2000 led with the story of Zina Campos, who was denied a tubal ligation after giving birth to her ninth child: "For Campos and other Gilroy women who want their fallopian tubes tied, this fall's metamorphosis of their community hospital into St. Louise Regional means having the surgery at another hospital 45 minutes or more away. If they have transportation. If that hospital will accept their insurance. And if it is not also Catholic-owned. For their doctors, it means choosing between losing patients and traveling beyond the half-hour radius generally observed by obstetricians, whose patients can give birth at any moment."[33]

In the Gilroy case, Fogel recalled, the doctors played an active part in publicizing the consequences of having only this one hospital left in the area. She recalled their activism fondly: "They were tremendous, they were very willing to be outspoken." The doctors themselves came up with a policy proposal for the archdiocese. She explained: "If you had a patient who needed a tubal you could fill out a form and send it to the archdiocese [who] would sign off. You had to explain why your patient [needed it]. I've never seen anything like this before. I think they got a couple [signed off]." While the agreement did not liberalize the sterilization policy, by pushing it publicly, doctors at St. Louise brought more public attention than usual to the role of the bishops in healthcare decision making.

It is difficult to find documentation of how often many carve-outs or compromises exist in facilities operated by Catholic health systems across the United States. In general, they are not publicly or proudly advertised. The USCCB, however, has certainly noticed their existence. The 2018 version of the ERDs includes a new section, "Collaborative Arrangements with Other Health Care Organizations," that specifically targets carve-outs and other creative arrangements.[34] They wanted to more effectively "ensure that new collaborative arrangements—as well as those that already exist—abide by the principles governing cooperation, effectively address the risk of scandal, abide by canon law, and sustain the Church's witness to Christ and his saving message." Directive 74 states: "Whatever comes under the control of the Catholic institution—whether by acquisition, governance, or management—must be operated in full accord with the moral teaching of the Catholic Church, including these Directives." Directive 75 limits business arrangements with non-Catholic partners: "It is not permitted to establish another entity that would oversee, manage, or perform immoral procedures. Establishing such an entity includes actions such as drawing up the civil bylaws, policies, or procedures of the entity, establishing the finances of the entity, or legally incorporating the entity."

Finally, Directive 76 explicitly commands leaders of Catholic hospitals who sit on the boards of non-Catholic affiliates to use their power "to make their opposition to immoral procedures known and not give their consent to any decisions proximately connected with such procedures."

Speaking in 2018 as the president of the National Catholic Bioethics Center, John Haas called many carve-out arrangements a "ruse" that should never have been approved.[35] In the same news story, Bishop Robert McManus of Worcester, Massachusetts, commented: "Yes, local bishops will become more involved in scrutinizing partnership arrangements . . . Whatever types of partnerships evolve between Catholic and non-Catholic institutions, the protocols for incorporation have to be according to the moral teaching of the church. If that hasn't been the case, that might have to be revisited."

The new section of the ERDs emerged as a response to the work of Lois Uttley, Susan Berke Fogel, and the numerous healthcare advocates who have pushed back or negotiated compromises in desperate attempts to preserve access to reproductive care in the face of Catholic hospital mergers and expansion. To date, however, their work appears to have created a frustrating game of whack-a-mole. Advocates, doctors, and institutions devise workarounds and compromises to deliver the restricted care they deem indispensable, and the bishops create new policies to thwart them.

The Halo Effect

Catholic hospitals have had several strategies for protecting and even expanding their access to federal funds at the same time they reserve the right to restrict care. Conscience clauses may protect religious institutions legally when they restrict standard care, but it is the Catholic hospitals' explicit mission to care for the poor, stated in several ways in the ERDs, that in many ways has held them in good favor with the public.

Directive 3 codifies the commitment widely believed to set Catholic hospitals apart from their competitors: "In accord with its mission, Catholic health care should distinguish itself by service to and advocacy for those people whose social condition puts them at the margins of our society and makes them particularly vulnerable to discrimination: the poor; the uninsured and the underinsured; children and the unborn; single parents; the elderly; those with incurable diseases and chemical dependencies; racial minorities; immigrants and refugees."

Historically, it is true that Catholic hospitals served in many places as a facility of last resort for the poor. In some regions, it continues to be the case that Catholic hospitals treat more than their share of Medicaid and uninsured patients. On an aggregate level, however, national and statewide statistics show that Catholic hospitals actually serve *fewer* Medicaid and indigent patients than other types of hospitals. A 2020 watchdog report showed that Medicaid utilization in Catholic hospitals accounted for 7.2 percent of discharges and 8.0 percent of patient days. In comparison, other hospitals, including other nonprofit, for-profit, and public facilities, averaged together a Medicaid utilization of 9.2 percent of discharges and 9.7 percent of patient days. Charity care data tells a similar story. Catholic hospitals nationally provided 2.7 percent of their care for free, whereas most others provided more: nonprofit other religious provided 3.0 percent; secular nonprofit, 2.3 percent; for-profit, 3.8 percent; and public facilities, 4.2 percent. Catholic health systems receive $48 billion in federal funding for Medicaid and Medicare reimbursements each year, a number that has increased 76 percent since 2011 as their share of the overall market has increased.[36]

Additionally, in 2022, the Lown Institute Hospitals Index showed that Catholic health systems had five of the ten highest *fair share deficits*—meaning they spent less on charity care and community investment than the estimated value of their tax breaks. Providence St. Joseph's Health held first place with a fair share deficit of 705 million dollars, followed by Trinity Health (2nd), Catholic Health Initiatives (7th), Dignity Health (9th) and Ascension Health (10th).[37] Despite these statistics showing that Catholic hospitals are not more generous than others, politicians, healthcare executives, and other defenders of the Catholic Church have repeatedly cast them as saviors in a struggling medical system, accusing reproductive rights advocates who protest Catholic healthcare expansion as single-issue elitists who are out of touch with everyday people's problems accessing any health care.

In 2018, for example, the city of Chicago found itself in the midst of an explosive public battle over a subsidy then Mayor Rahm Emmanuel's office wanted to give Presence Health, a Catholic system, to support their expansion in Chicago's historically Black Southside.[38] Presence had already built its new hospital facilities, but the mayor wanted to give the system an additional $5.6 million to upgrade community centers in the neighborhood. Reproductive rights advocates and several members of city government opposed the plan, arguing that it was not appropriate to use taxpayer dollars to subsidize a health system that restricted abortion and other reproductive services. The city council vote might have gone against the subsidy had Mayor Emmanuel not shamed those objecting to the deal for bringing reproductive rights into a conversation about access to health care generally. Coverage in the *Chicago Tribune* reported: "Emanuel admonished those who opposed the deal for applying what he termed a sudden 'litmus test' on abortion."[39] An opponent on the council told the paper: "What I think the mayor and his team did successfully is that they muddled the debate and made it about, 'If you're against this, then you're against healthcare.'" Black elected officials from the Southside wanted the subsidy and questioned the motives of those opposing it, saying: "Women on the South and West sides are not dying from lack of access to abortions but rather lack of access to better health care." After the debate, the subsidy passed by a margin of two-to-one.

A similar dynamic has been playing out at the institution where I work, the University of California (UC). UC medical centers have affiliations with many external health facilities, including Catholic ones, to broaden their network for patient care, research, and medical training. The extent of ongoing and future planned partnerships that obligate UC doctors and students to provide care according to Catholic directives drew public interest in 2019, when University of California, San Francisco (UCSF) executives proposed a collaboration with four Dignity Health (formerly CHW) Bay Area hospitals. They proposed to rebrand them as Dignity/UCSF facilities. If the collaboration proceeded, the UCSF faculty, residents, and students would then see some of their patients within Catholic hospitals. Two of these hospitals followed the ERDs, while the other two followed the slightly less restrictive SCVs developed by Fogel's group.

In December 2018, UCSF Health executives pitched the idea to their governing board, the UC Regents, as a partnership motivated by strategic financial incentives.[40]

Dignity was offering a tremendous amount of immediate space at a time when UCSF hospitals were almost at capacity.[41] When public outcry from LGBTQ and reproductive justice advocates spotlighted what the changes would mean—namely that UCSF personnel would then have to treat UCSF patients according to Catholic doctrine while in those hospitals, including limiting their patients' contraception, gender affirming procedures, abortion, and other reproductive services—the executives reformulated their talking points to focus on expanding access to care. Opposition was strong and very public, state politicians began to weigh in,[42] and the proposal was withdrawn.

Soon after a rapid groundswell of opposition quashed the original four-hospital partnership, the UC Health executives unveiled a much more ambitious plan to affiliate UC medical centers across the state with Dignity facilities. Their press releases and other public statements shifted away from resolving issues of space shortages and cost-effectiveness and toward providing access to care. Their statements claimed (with little data) that the affiliations would create a safety net for low-income and uninsured people across California.[43] The greater motive appeared to be to broaden UC's health network, as all health systems have desperately endeavored to do to stay competitive. Dignity Health has a large primary care infrastructure, and the partnership would guarantee UC a source of specialty referrals, research subjects, training settings, and overflow beds with little upfront cost to UC. Becoming partners would enable fast and inexpensive growth. Faculty and students from all ten campuses, meanwhile, vocally opposed the idea, on principle, that providers and trainees associated with the country's largest public university system would be required to adhere to the Catholic Church's restrictions on transgender and reproductive health care.[44]

UC Health executives knew better than to defend the anti-abortion policies of Catholic institutions in California, the quintessential blue state. Instead, they argued that opponents of the affiliation wanted to sacrifice the poor of California, leaving them without a direct line to UC's premium physicians and technologies. Executives argued that, by affiliating, they could bring "UC-level care" into Dignity hospitals in underserved parts of the state. While it was pitched as a win-win, critics of the affiliations (including myself) pointed out the partnership would enlist public employees (UC clinicians) in discriminatory care as they would need to follow Catholic directives while working in Catholic facilities. Still, the system wanted the affiliations, as they would eliminate the need for UC specialists to compete with other specialists for the patients who are capable of travelling to UC medical centers. The affiliations, in other words, would provide a steady stream of new patients. As of 2022, UC has renewed and expanded multiple affiliation agreements with Catholic facilities throughout the state, despite continued opposition expressed in public meetings and major newspapers.[45] As with all health systems, growth is the name of the game.

Over and over again, this false choice—access to reproductive services or health care for the poor—recurs when Catholic systems are located in underserved areas. In Chicago, Mayor Emmanuel and his allies presented the Catholic health system subsidy as the only way to upgrade community resources in an underserved area. In California, the UC executives continue to argue that the affiliations can create a safety net for underserved Californians while ensuring the health system's long-term economic viability. In both cases, alternatives were not openly explored; reproductive autonomy and services were simply dispensable.

Catholic health systems are in the position to efficiently fill gaps in care in part because of their several hundred hospitals, outpatient clinics, and urgent care sites; they have the capital and national organizational support to leverage tremendous resources. Given the Church's larger economic crisis prompted by waning membership rolls and settlements related to decades' worth of sexual abuse, Catholic healthcare systems play an ever-larger role in bankrolling the Church's future in the United States, perhaps both literally and figuratively. Writing in the CHA's journal, *Health Progress*, Reverend David Nygren observed: "Catholic health care remains a most credible interface between church and society; some say it is the principal source of relevance for the church in the world today."[46] Indeed, governmental partnerships with Catholic systems to fill gaps in care has been expedient, convenient, and mutually beneficial in the short term, even as the pattern contributes to the long-term structural entrenchment of religious health care in the United States in place of universal health care.

Conclusion

Early Catholic hospitals in the United States served as an extension of the Catholic Church's religious and institutional mission. Their leadership deftly navigated growth alongside and within the U.S. healthcare system, ultimately gaining federal funding without losing the freedom to provide care according to Catholic doctrine. Catholic hospitals and healthcare systems invoked multiple and sometimes competing narratives to assert their value in society and justify their expansion. At times, they drew public support from their reputation as the safety-net resource to the poor. With the growth of a strong anti-abortion movement, Catholic hospitals' reputation for prohibiting abortion became an asset in some political climates. Ultimately, Catholic hospital systems have been able to expand and thrive despite the increasingly dense overlay of ideological conflict about reproductive politics and the ever-widening gap between Catholic doctrines about sexuality and the body, and standard, evidence-based reproductive care.

CHAPTER 2

Inferior

HOW CATHOLIC DIRECTIVES CONTRADICT
MEDICAL STANDARDS

"I was asked to please be present at the ethics committee meeting . . . just to lend support," began Dr. Jana Johnson, a high-risk obstetrician (perinatologist) working in a Catholic hospital in the Midwest. Her hospital was the only tertiary care center serving a large rural area. As she continued to speak, she recounted a case in which she clashed with her hospital's ethics committee over how the Ethical and Religious Directives for Catholic Health Care Services impacted the standard of care for pregnancy complications.

The case involved a patient who was between nineteen and twenty weeks pregnant—about a month prior to the baby having the capacity to survive in decent health if born early. The patient's water had broken, and the ultrasound showed no fluid around the baby. This, in part, meant that the amniotic sac membranes no longer protected her and the baby from harmful bacteria. The medical team could attempt to keep her pregnant for a few weeks longer with heavy medical intervention, such as continuous antibiotics and hospitalization, but eventually infection would most likely set in to the uterine lining or uterus and they would have to end the pregnancy anyway to save her life. The ultrasound also showed that the baby had a hypoplastic left heart, a severe birth defect in which the left ventricle does not form correctly.

Some infants born with this condition survive, although Dr. Johnson explained, "a lot of those kids end up with heart transplants." At best, it requires a major three-step surgery in the first year of the child's life. But as Dr. Johnson added: "Survival rates become very, very low if the baby's pre-term." With the patient admitted to the hospital, her ob-gyn and cardiologist reached out by phone to consult the pediatric cardiology team in a partner hospital a few hours away. They all met with the patient to discuss her case, the pediatric cardiologist joining by phone. They explained to the patient that the earliest survivor of this condition they were aware of had been born at thirty-two weeks, three months shy of where she was in her pregnancy. Dr. Johnson relayed how her colleagues reported that moment to her: "And [the patient] listened to that, and I think both physicians who were involved,

28

the ob-gyn and the pediatric cardiologist, said, 'You know, this is a very tough spot you're in, but it would be very reasonable for you to just say there's just almost a zero percent survival chance here, almost zero,' and therefore, she requested and received Pitocin." Pitocin is a drug commonly used to induce labor when it does not start on its own.

Dr. Johnson's colleagues' management of the case was textbook, per their specialty.[1] They assessed the prognosis of the pregnancy, discussed it with the patient, and allowed her to decide whether to forgo further and likely futile interventions. They also allowed her to decide when to begin treatment to end the pregnancy by inducing labor. They explained that the longer she waited the greater the risk of infection. With this information in hand, the patient made the difficult decision to terminate the pregnancy by inducing labor. She recovered, and, as expected, the fetus did not survive.

Because the fetus was still alive at the time of the ultrasound, one nurse who opposes abortion refused to assist in the case. Afterward, the hospital's ethics committee also objected to the team's management of the case, which is where Dr. Johnson enters the story. She had been away at a conference through all of this, but her ob-gyn colleague turned to her for help when the ethics committee decided to review the case.

Most hospitals are required to have an ethics committee, but those in Catholic settings have the unique charge of interpreting, applying, and enforcing the ERDs. Catholic hospital ethics committees typically have less than twenty members, about half of whom are clinical personnel and the other half a mix of religious, legal, and administrative members.[2] Ob-gyns I interviewed often turned to their ethics committees when they needed approval to offer reproductive care that the ERDs restricted. Physicians described their ethics committees as having a leader, typically a clergy member, who was available by phone when physicians needed approval urgently to use an ERD-restricted treatment. Thus, I heard about them most often when they functioned as gatekeepers—as opposed to consultants, for example, to aid clinicians and patients in shared decision-making about complex care.[3] Occasionally, physicians working in Catholic hospitals also discussed their ethics committees' surveillance and monitoring of medical practices, as in this case.

Dr. Johnson was a leader in their ob-gyn department, and, just as importantly, she had confronted this type of clinical scenario in the Catholic hospital before, so she agreed to accompany her colleague through the inquiry. Two members of the committee were quite angry. Dr. Johnson recalled:

> It went terribly, actually . . . It was a very hard experience for all of us, because the ethics committee is made up of many different people of different backgrounds. There are nurses, there are physicians, there are administrators, there's religious personnel, and there's probably twelve people sitting around the table, in addition to the three of us, who were presenting the case. And the majority, I believe, kind of—well, they didn't really say very much; they sort of nodded as

we discussed the case. But there were two members of the committee who were very vocally sort of accusing us of carrying out an elective abortion. And I said, you know, "There was nothing elective about this. This woman didn't choose to have her membranes rupture at nineteen weeks. She didn't choose to have a baby with the most severe form of congenital heart disease. There was nothing elective about this."

Dr. Johnson particularly objected to the committee members' use of the term "elective," which suggested the patient had some level of control over the situation, or perhaps even wanted to end her pregnancy. But while Dr. Johnson distinguished between "management of pregnancy loss" and "elective abortion" in such a case, the ethics committee did not:

> And the argument came back ... "We allow women with ruptured membranes to stay pregnant all the time at twenty weeks." And I said, "Yes, we do, but even that is not completely standard of care. Not completely standard of care, and this situation was unique in that the baby had almost zero chance of survival" ... and he said, "You don't know that. You can't be sure of that. This baby had a chance; you did an elective abortion." And then ... the religious personnel ... basically said the same thing, and we were sharply accused—with somewhat angry voices, we were sharply accused. And, you know, we stood our ground and did our best, but most of the people in the room really said nothing.

The ethics committee members asserted that more could have been done to save the pregnancy ("this baby had a chance!") even as the patient's medical team had already determined the fetus would not survive ("almost zero" percent).

The medical team and the ethics committee were not really arguing about the medical facts of the case. Rather, their disagreement represented one of the ways the United States Conference of Catholic Bishops' interpretation of Catholic doctrine shapes obstetric management in Catholic hospitals in the United States. The ERDs are clear on this point: physicians are not allowed to take action that hastens the end of life, even if death is inevitable. Only God can do that. In the case of a pregnancy, the doctor is permitted to hasten the death of a fetus only *after* a threat to the pregnant person's life is already present (for example, infection).[4] Even though Dr. Johnson's colleagues followed the professional standard of care for obstetric complications, they had transgressed religious policy by intervening before the mother's life was at stake.

Dr. Johnson found the accusation that her colleague had violated the prohibition on abortion extraordinarily unpleasant and disrespectful. It insinuated moral failure—but it also highlighted the limits of medical authority for physicians working in Catholic hospitals. Religious policies apply to a wider set of medical services and treatments than can typically be scheduled in advance, as with contraception, fertility, abortion, and transgender health care. The ERDs also can restrict emergent or urgent hospital care, creating distress for both doctors and patients. Ultimately, the incident forced Dr. Johnson to confront a key question she had previously managed to sidestep: Would she be able to offer women experiencing obstetric complications the standard of care recommended by her profession?

In this chapter, I survey the most common ways U.S. Catholic hospitals' religious policies conflict with medical best practices. This discussion is not meant to be a comprehensive list of all the ways medical standards and the Catholic Church collide; rather, I focus on issues that ob-gyns who practice within Catholic hospitals encounter time and time again.[5] I discuss four domains that are both conceptual and clinical in nature, in which reproductive medicine collides with the ERDs: *prevention*, *creation*, *evolution*, and *termination*. Before moving into the specifics, however, it is important to understand the different ways physicians and Catholic religious authorities understand the crucial yet contested phrase "standard of care."

The Standard is Contested because the Goal is Contested

If you have worked in medicine or even just spent much time around healthcare professionals, you have probably heard the phrase "standard of care." Most physicians I have interviewed echoed Dr. Johnson's confidence when referencing how following the "standard of care" is the best way to maximize patient safety. Other terms that medical educators, practitioners, researchers, and policymakers invoke in similar ways are *evidence-based care*, the *gold standard*, and *best practices*. All these terms signal professional consensus, supported by research and ethics, about the best way to practice medicine. Healthcare professionals rely on the concept of best practices to reduce subjectivity and arbitrariness in healthcare delivery. Most professional licensing organizations require practitioners to update their knowledge on evolving healthcare standards throughout their careers, thereby ensuring that patients benefit from the newest science. Yet, in reality, standards of care can be contentious, with social scientists, secular and religious ethicists, administrators, and medical professionals sometimes parting ways over values, politics, and the meaning of clinical evidence.[6]

When it comes to reproductive medicine, settling on one standard of care for common clinical scenarios is especially difficult: there can be two patients and, in some cases, that may mean a treatment is safer for one than the other. Deciding who should assume which risk in each situation is deeply personal and can depend on what side effects a patient can tolerate, how desperately a pregnancy is wanted, or, perhaps, whether a patient feels capable of caring for a child with substantial physical or cognitive challenges. This is why, outside of religiously restrictive settings, the standard of care is intimately linked—almost entirely inseparable from—the bioethical principle of patient autonomy. When a patient is pregnant or could become so, mainstream professional medical associations support the patient to decide between different medically acceptable courses and to choose treatment according to their own values, risk tolerance, and family preferences.[7]

What complicates discussion of reproductive freedom is that experts' support for contraception has not always been promoted to advance patient autonomy. At times, birth control advocates and medical authorities have used the language of "doctor knows best" to promote paternalistic and white supremacist beliefs about what is best for particular women or for society as a whole. Eugenically motivated forced sterilization programs date to 1907.[8] In one California program alone, at least 19,000 women confined to prison from the 1920s to the 1950s were sterilized without their consent.[9] In Puerto Rico, U.S. authorities pushed financial incentives for poor women to undergo hysterectomies as a way to slow population growth.[10] While subsequent legal protections should have ended such racist, eugenic programs long ago, abusive sterilization practices have been exposed in at least three prisons and immigrant detention centers in the past decade.[11]

Relatedly, journalists, scholars, and activists have increasingly shed light on how medical personnel have coerced women of color to accept methods of birth control that require a clinician to insert and remove them, diminishing their ability to just stop the method on their own when experiencing problems.[12] And yet, at the same time, low-income women and women of color who *want* to access reproductive services continue to face structural and institutional barriers, whether in obtaining birth control, getting an abortion, or paying for infertility treatments.[13] As the medical profession has begun to reckon with its eugenic history, in large part due to decades of advocacy by the reproductive justice movement,[14] leaders in the fields of family planning in particular have shifted away from pushing contraception and toward a greater respect for patients' reproductive preferences and self-determination.[15] Whether clinicians are particularly good at upholding patient autonomy without racial bias remains a tension in the field,[16] but autonomy remains the overt goal, nonetheless.

Catholic bishops are working toward a different goal than empowering the patient. In the realm of reproduction, a strict Catholic understanding of natural law holds that God, rather than clinicians or patients, wields ultimate authority over reproductive life.[17] As outlined in the ERDs, Catholic health systems must largely limit their reproductive healthcare services to facilitating healthy pregnancies and births achieved through heterosexual marriage, or at least heterosexual intercourse. In other words, the question of *who* should have children, *when* to have them, and *how many* is a divine matter rather than a medical one. It is between the couple and God. The medical or public health duty begins only once life has been created. Accordingly, Catholic leadership consistently opposes insurance coverage for contraception, infertility, and abortion but generously supports prenatal care and preconception health care.[18] Catholic doctrine as interpreted by the USCCB fundamentally opposes human intervention to usher out or usher in life in ways that do not transpire "naturally" or "as God intended." As such, patient autonomy is inherently undermined; not all standard reproductive or obstetric treatment options are even on the table for patients in Catholic hospitals. To take the analogy further, the patient may see only a small part of the menu.

Physicians working in Catholic hospitals are stuck between these conflicting goals of patient autonomy and God's authority via Catholic natural law. Research suggests that the majority of these physicians value patient autonomy more. For example, a national survey of primary care physicians asked them to prioritize four influences on medical decision making, and 55 percent gave "patients' expressed wishes and values" the highest possible weight, 18 percent ranked professional medical standards highest, 15 percent prioritized physician determination of what is in the patients' best interest, and, finally, only 5 percent held moral guidelines from religious traditions above all three.[19] Additionally, a national survey of ob-gyns showed that 52 percent of those working in Catholic hospitals replied yes to the question, "Have you ever had a conflict with that hospital/practice over religiously-based policies for patient care?" In comparison, only 9 percent of ob-gyn respondents experienced such conflict in Jewish hospitals, where religious institutional policies primarily surround Kosher laws about how to prepare food or accommodate Jewish holidays.[20] This large gap indicates that doctors generally do not oppose all religious institutional policies. One doctor I interviewed who worked in both Catholic and Jewish hospitals in major urban areas, painted a picture of how Jewish policies could be more confusing than medically consequential for those subject to them. He recalled watching an "African-American food server explain to the Latina patient why they don't serve cheeseburgers or she can't get a glass of milk with her chicken." Such modern-era confusion aside, he continued: "Otherwise, you know, there's no—I mean, it has no real impact. You know, the medical students have off for the Jewish holidays but that's about it . . . There's no limitations on, there's absolutely no limitations on reproductive health services."

In most hospital contexts, it is relatively undisputed that a patient should be able to choose between medically acceptable treatments according to their own goals. For example, a cardiologist may ask a patient to choose between two standard cardiac interventions if the treatments present different consequences for quality and quantity of life. The ERDs, nevertheless, remove choices related to reproductive care and gender identity. While not the focus of this research, perhaps a whole different book could be written about the way the ERDs impact care for people who are dying.[21] Ultimately, the directives aim to reduce medical autonomy of patients and the medical authority of clinicians; they are created to require medical staff and trainees to abide by religious commitments that are narrower than what is legally allowable, scientifically supported, or preferred by a majority of patients and physicians. The major medical associations and the USCCB have adopted different worldviews that aim toward distinct goals of care, patient autonomy versus divine will, making it a challenging terrain to navigate for those practicing with a foot in each world.

PREVENTION: CONTRACEPTION AND STERILIZATION

The Church's long-standing opposition to technologies, medications, and procedures for the purpose of pregnancy prevention is unpopular among Catholics and

non-Catholics alike. The advent and popularization of the birth control pill in the
1960s opened up novel debates about whether hormonal methods of contraception might be more acceptable to the Church than barrier methods, specifically
because they worked so differently.[22] However, in 1968, Pope Paul VI eliminated
any remaining ambiguity on the Church's position, issuing an encyclical, "Humanae Vitae," that described the use of artificial birth control as "intrinsically
wrong."[23] American Catholics greeted this announcement with deep disappointment; many left the Church.[24] By 1973, the vast majority of American women who
remained Roman Catholic had used contraceptives.[25] Today, only 8 percent of
American Catholics share the Church's view that contraception is morally wrong,
and even so, 98.6 percent of Catholic women between the ages of fifteen and
forty-four who have ever had sexual intercourse have used it.[26] Furthermore,
contemporary Catholics in the United States use sterilization to limit family size
at the same rate as other Americans,[27] all of which is to say that American Catholics use birth control with or without their priests' permission.

Catholic hospitals in the United States are, nonetheless, expected to stick to
Church doctrine. Directive 52 is quite clear on this point: "Catholic health institutions may not promote or condone contraceptive practices but should provide, for
married couples and the medical staff who counsel them, instruction both about
the Church's teaching on responsible parenthood and in methods of natural family
planning."

As used here, "natural family planning" (NFP) refers to a suite of techniques,
including the "rhythm method" and "fertility awareness," by which couples attempt
to control their reproduction by monitoring a woman's reproductive cycle. NFP
may involve temperature monitoring, checking vaginal mucus, calendar tracking,
and, of course, partner cooperation, as NFP requires abstinence from sex during
times of high fertility. Unfortunately, ample evidence exists showing that NFP is
not very effective, and most people are not very good at abstinence.[28] With *perfect
use* of NFP, as few as one to five women out of one hundred will get pregnant in a
year. In the first year of *typical use* of NFP, however, up to a quarter of women will
get pregnant. In comparison, user-controlled hormonal methods, including birth
control pills, the patch, and the ring, typically produce unintended pregnancies at
a rate of only four to seven per one hundred per year. Pregnancy rates for nonuser
controlled methods, such as the IUD, implant, and sterilization, are less than one
in one hundred.[29]

Directive 52 puts clinicians in a difficult position. The American College of
Obstetrics and Gynecology advises against NFP for patients who have medical con-
traindications for future pregnancy.[30] If the goal of contraception is to prevent
unwanted pregnancies, insisting that medical staff recommend only NFP defies
best medical practice.[31] To many physicians, the idea of offering ob-gyn care without contraception is absurd.[32] One physician recalled arguing with the hospital
lawyers when a Catholic health system bought the building in which his private
practice was located: "I said, 'This is ridiculous. I am a Board-certified OB/GYN

and I cannot do my job if I'm not allowed to discuss contraception and prescribe contraception.'"

No physician I interviewed felt *good* about restricting contraception. Even Dr. Terry Horn, who sought out a job within a Catholic hospital specifically because it offered a layer of protection from being asked to perform an abortion, explained how, for him, contraception was different: "My main thing is, personally, I personally am not a big advocate of abortion and I prefer not to perform them, which is one of the reasons I've always worked for a Catholic system. However, I am a big proponent of contraception and so that's where it's kind of a hard situation. I'm okay with tubals, I'm okay with all kinds of contraception and in fact I think that's probably a better solution, is to prevent unwanted pregnancy. And so that's a little frustrating at times."

Some physicians felt that refusing non-urgent services that were available at nearby family planning clinics (for example, routine birth control prescriptions) was a relatively minor breach of ob-gyn standards compared to denying more time-critical hospital care involving contraceptives. The directive on contraception, therefore, created additional conflict for physicians when patients needed it for excessive menstrual bleeding and rape treatment in the emergency department, or after giving birth. Visits to the emergency department for excessive menstrual bleeding, menorrhagia, are quite common.[33] Standard medical treatment for excessive menstrual bleeding is a regimen of three weeks of birth control pills or placement of a hormonal intrauterine device (IUD). If those do not work, a patient has surgical options, the most extreme being hysterectomy. While the ERDs do not mention this common clinical scenario, menorrhagia is a medical indication for contraception allowed by some Catholic health systems.[34] However, their pharmacies do not necessarily stock hormonal contraception because of the directives, thus creating barriers to emergency treatment that doctors I interviewed struggled with.[35]

Emergency contraception (EC), sometimes referred to as the "morning after pill" or by a brand name such as Plan B (levonorgestrel EC pills), can prevent pregnancy after unprotected sex.[36] EC pills primarily work by preventing ovulation.[37] EC pills also may impair the sperm's ability to get to the egg by thickening the cervical mucus. Alternatively, an IUD placed for emergency contraception can make the uterus less hospitable, decreasing the chance a fertilized ovum can implant. The medical field—while not offering spiritual definitions of life's beginning—defines pregnancy as starting after implantation, because it is common for a fertilized ovum to simply pass through and never implant.

Directive 36 allows medical personnel to offer EC pills, but not IUDs, to victims of sexual assault in Catholic hospitals as a means to "defend herself against a potential conception." Directive 36 continues: "If, after appropriate testing, there is no evidence that conception has occurred already, she may be treated with medications that would prevent ovulation, sperm capacitation, or fertilization. It is not permissible, however, to initiate or to recommend treatments that have as their purpose or direct effect the removal, destruction, or *interference with the implantation* of a fertilized ovum."

Medical personnel are instructed to confirm that a rape victim has not recently ovulated before providing EC and also that a pregnancy has not yet occurred with a pregnancy test, even though there is no evidence that pills like Plan B can harm a pregnancy. Despite the bishops' assertions otherwise, medical consensus is clear that levonorgestrel EC is not an abortifacient.[38]

Bishop Ignacio Carrasco de Paula, the president of the Vatican's Pontifical Academy for Life, explained to *America Magazine* that while "the church has accepted the possibility of preventing ovulation in a woman who has been raped via medication . . . the church does withdraw that option if there is a possibility that ovulation may have already occurred."[39] That is, at just the moment a person is most fertile it is not allowable; if she has already ovulated, there is a higher risk of pregnancy. Yet, Catholic doctrine regards the possibility of interfering with implantation of a fertilized ovum as intolerable and akin to abortion.

One of the most vexing areas of conflict between best practices and religious restrictions involves postpartum contraception. ACOG recommends assessing a patient's interest in contraception, discussing the various options, and providing the desired method in the course of prenatal care and delivery to ensure patients have timely access and insurance coverage.[40] During pregnancy care, the patient is within the health system, plain and simple. This means it is convenient timing for her; she will not require an additional appointment if she wants contraception after the delivery to prevent another pregnancy, and if on Medicaid, which nearly half of women delivering in the United States are, contraception and sterilization will still be covered.[41]

About 40 percent of patients do not come back for their six-week postpartum checkup, and Medicaid coverage expires in many states about two weeks thereafter. This makes the postpartum contraception backup plan to provide pill prescriptions, schedule the sterilization, or insert IUDs or implants at that time far less successful, especially given that 57 percent of women will resume sexual activity before six weeks postpartum.[42] Many people want to come back for contraception before doing so but simply do not or cannot before Medicaid coverage expires or they become pregnant. A clinician-initiated discussion of contraception during prenatal care and delivery certainly can feel paternalistic to some patients who do not want to discuss it then.[43] Nonetheless, it is a best practice to offer patients the option for all these reasons.

If a patient wants an IUD, ob-gyns in non-Catholic hospitals are increasingly trained and willing to insert it right after delivery; the procedure is less painful at that time since the cervix is still open. It is, additionally, more convenient for the patient since hospital staff can care for the baby during the insertion. Interestingly, for a period of time, many Catholic hospitals quietly allowed patients a different and also convenient postpartum contraceptive option: Depo-Provera injections. Depo-Provera is a progestin-only contraceptive that can protect patients from pregnancy for several months; and it is compatible with breastfeeding. Why this practice was quietly allowed and then ceased to be so is a bit of a mystery. After one Catholic hospital stopped allowing the injection, a study documented that their patients became pregnant again on average more quickly than their patients previously did.[44] A short interval between pregnancies has been associated with poorer health outcomes, whereas contraception buys parents much-needed time for economic and mental health needs.[45]

By the time they reach the age of thirty, sterilization has become American women's most popular method of contraception. After forty years of age, 39.1 percent of women rely on sterilization, far exceeding long-acting reversible contraceptives (LARC; 6.6 percent), pills (6.5 percent), and condoms (6.5 percent) in popularity.[46] Physiologically, if one is having a C-section, that is the easiest and safest time for her to have the sterilization because the abdomen is already open. But even if a patient has a vaginal birth, tubal ligation is also a less invasive procedure immediately afterward because the fallopian tubes remain pushed up close to the belly button for a little while before the uterus shrinks down to size. Depending on the timing of the surgery, the patient may still have an epidural in place from the birth, reducing the risks associated with another round of anesthesia. And, of course, childcare is so often an issue for new parents; conducting the procedure during a hospital stay for delivery means that nursing staff are available to care for the newborn. None of these benefits are allowable to patients giving birth in Catholic hospitals, because the ERDs prohibit sterilization as a form of contraception.

Once again, physicians do have a bit of wiggle room. While Directive 53 explicitly prohibits "direct sterilization," it also states that "procedures that induce sterility are permitted when their direct effect is the cure or alleviation of a present and serious pathology and a simpler treatment is not available." As we shall see, the changing interpretations of this directive between 2005 and 2010 have caused great consternation among ob-gyns. At baseline, however, the physicians I interviewed repeatedly asserted that the prohibition directly conflicts with least two major medical principles. First, never do two surgeries when you can more safely do one, because every surgery creates risks associated with anesthesia, infection, and recovery. Second, do the procedure the patient deems best for herself if at all possible. Many women deem sterilization the most acceptable and reliable way to avoid future pregnancy.[47]

There are, of course, additional reasons for physicians to prefer that sterilizations be conducted postpartum. Physicians mentioned concerns such as the wasted resources associated with scheduling an additional surgery six weeks later at another hospital, whether in the form of the patient's own time and money, private insurance dollars, or public tax dollars. Others charged religious hospitals with liability for future harm incurred by delaying a medical procedure (doctrinal iatrogenesis). If the deferred tubal procedure, or even an unintended pregnancy, were to have any medical complications, a reasonable person could attribute that liability to the hospital that denied the patient access to the earlier, easier, safer option. These sorts of financial, logistical, and legal considerations point to potential downstream consequences of denying standard care and represent the kinds of situations in which patients receiving care in Catholic facilities encounter a style of medical decision making that is different than in nonsectarian facilities.

CREATION: INFERTILITY TREATMENT

Six of the ERDs (38 through 42) address infertility treatment. A common theme of these directives is that procreation must not be separate from, as Directive 41 puts it, "the marital act." While Directive 38 allows "assistance," that assistance cannot "separate the unitive and procreative ends of the act and does not substitute for the marital act itself." In practice, this means that Catholic hospitals can provide *limited* fertility treatments, in *limited* circumstances, for *certain groups* of people.

Physicians may, for example, conduct surgical procedures to remove any physical impediments to the conception process, such as opening a blocked fallopian tube or removing a testicular cyst. Sperm testing also is allowed, but the sample cannot be obtained through masturbation, a practice the Church regards as dehumanizing and contrary to Catholic doctrine. Instead, the sperm must be collected through heterosexual, married intercourse using a condom (perforated to demonstrate that the intention is not to contracept).[48] The condom with the remaining semen can be brought in for sperm count testing. Similarly, the directives allow hormone injections to improve egg maturity and release more eggs, because this approach to fertility leaves the sexual act unchanged. This approach, nevertheless, carries risks for patients receiving treatment at Catholic facilities, as Directives 39 and 45 both forbid any destruction of embryos, implanted or not, thereby ruling out selective reduction of multiple pregnancies.[49]

Other directives limit the involvement of any sort of third party, whether an egg donor, a sperm donor, or a surrogate, on the theory that it "is contrary to the covenant of marriage, the unity of the spouses, and the dignity proper to parents and the child."[50] Directive 42 additionally cautions that surrogacy "denigrates the dignity of women" by commercializing the mother-child relationship. Collectively, these directives make it difficult for Catholic health systems to offer their patients infertility treatments. As a practical matter, however, this set of restrictions is rarely cause for concern among ob-gyns, as most infertility treatments happen in an outpatient setting with other specialists: reproductive endocrinologists. It is no accident, physicians told me, that most of these practices are located in buildings not owned by Catholic healthcare systems. For example, Dr. Tim Ward explained that, by the time a Catholic system bought his hospital, the in vitro fertilization practice had already moved offsite: "Several years before [they] took over, the IVF people moved their lab out of the hospital facility and they set up outside the hospital in their centers so that it didn't prevent IVFs from being conceived and they have no problem with them coming in there to deliver."

Perhaps more to the point, by the time a pregnant woman presents at a Catholic hospital for prenatal care or delivery, the origin of the pregnancy is no longer relevant to the care delivered within the hospital and surveilled by its ethics committee or bishop.[51]

EVOLUTION: TRANSGENDER CARE

Standards of care for gender affirmation for transgender patients are changing rapidly, but the standards do exist. An estimated 1.4 million people, 0.6 percent of the U.S. population, identify as transgender.[52] In 2019, the American Medical Association produced an issue brief that confidently asserted, "Every major medical association in the U.S. recognizes the medical necessity of transition-related care for improving the physical and mental health of transgender people and has called for health insurance coverage for treatment of gender dysphoria."[53]

The Catholic Medical Association is not among them. The Catholic Church has become increasingly vocal in its opposition to what its leaders have coined "gender ideology" and, sometimes, "gender theory."[54] Catholic leaders specifically oppose the understanding of gender as a social category, as opposed to one divinely and physically determined. They take issue with the aforementioned growing medical consensus that in some cases the distress caused by a mismatch between the body and its presumed gender category warrants surgically aligning the two. The ERDs contain no explicit mention of transgender health care, yet Catholic hospitals have repeatedly denied gender affirmation surgery, specifically hysterectomies.[55] And in discrimination lawsuits in which a gender confirming hysterectomy was denied, Catholic hospitals have used the prohibition on sterilization as their defense, saying it is not discrimination; they simply do not do sterilizations at all.

The catch is that sterilizations often *are* done in Catholic hospitals. An analysis by health economists showed that after hospitals are purchased by a Catholic system, there is a corresponding 31 percent decrease of sterilization procedures, but they are not eliminated.[56] Exceptions to sterilization prohibitions are made for various medical indications. Fundamentally, the Catholic leaders are taking a position against gender dysphoria as a valid medical indication.

While some Catholic ethicists working within Catholic health systems have argued that performing gender affirming surgery could be theologically justified,[57] more authoritative voices within Church hierarchy, including the USCCB and its bioethics arm, the National Catholic Bioethics Center, firmly disagree. Bishops writing on this topic have couched their objections in both theological and political terms. Theologically, interventions that change a person's gender identity from that assigned at birth are fundamentally against Roman Catholic natural law. The Bishop of Arlington captures this view of transgender health interventions:

> He or she has been created male or female, forever. Affirming a child's distorted self-perception or supporting a child's desire to "be" someone other than the person (male or female) God created, gravely misleads and confuses the child about "who" he or she is.
>
> In addition, "gender-affirming" medical or surgical interventions cause significant, even irreparable, bodily harm to children and adolescents. These include the use of puberty blockers (in effect, chemical castration) to arrest the natural psychological and physical development of a healthy child, cross-sex hormones

to induce the development of opposite-sex, secondary sex characteristics, and surgery to remove an adolescent's healthy breasts, organs, and/or genitals. These kinds of interventions involve serious mutilations of the human body, and are morally unacceptable.[58]

Engaging politically, the bishops have written public letters in objection to gender neutral bathroom requirements and other legal efforts to support the rights of transgender persons.[59] For the bishops, natural law supports a "distinct Catholic anthropology," namely, the belief that the body and soul are united completely and cannot be truly in conflict as those suffering gender dysphoria describe.[60] A National Catholic Bioethics Center (NCBC) position statement from 2020 asserts, "A person is the unity of soul and body, and 'soul' should be understood not as an immaterial self, but as that which makes the body be what it is, namely, a human person. We are either male or female persons, and nothing can change that."[61] Fundamentally, they see sex as both immutable and divinely fixed. In his essay on the topic, anthropologist Eric Plemons shows that "[Catholic] ethicists specifically name a refusal of transgender medicine as an important stand for Catholics in America and see the expansion of Catholic hospital systems (and the things they will not do) as an important tool for the defense of their beliefs."

Despite increased mobilization against the teaching of and very notion of gender fluidity within the upper ranks of the Catholic hierarchy,[62] the ERDs themselves never mention gender related health care at all. Until the ACA validated the need for care for gender transitions, making them a standard of care in the mainstream medical world, people seeking it had to pay out-of-pocket. That means gender related health care is a relatively "new" issue from the perspective of hospital administrators, and one that rarely came up in my conversations with physicians, most of which took place around 2012. Since the Affordable Care Act legislation recommended coverage of gender related health care in 2014 and 2016, twenty-three states, one territory, and Washington, DC, began to mandate its inclusion. But, reflecting state political divisions generally, that law has been interpreted to exclude it in ten states, with the remainder having no policy. With increased utilization of gender related health services, the USCCB will likely move toward formalizing their position within the ERDs in a future revision.[63]

TERMINATION: OBSTETRIC COMPLICATIONS, ECTOPIC PREGNANCY, AND ABORTION

The fourth realm where medical standards and religious policies collide involve activities that hasten an end to life. In reproductive medicine, conflicts arise when treatment for an obstetric emergency would facilitate the death of a fetus, as with Dr. Johnson's patient whose water had broken, or when a patient is experiencing a pregnancy that is stable but will not produce a viable fetus (for example, ectopic, anencephalic, molar pregnancies, or other fatal anomaly). That said, the ERDs do not compel staff in Catholic hospitals to engage in futile efforts to extend life. The

USCCB's interpretation of Catholic doctrine holds death to be a natural phenomenon that should be allowed to take its course—if that is the course it is taking.
Thus, the ERDs oppose a clinician facilitating death at any stage of humanity, from
embryo to one-hundred-year-old hospice patient. As such, the ERDs take a firm
stance against any practice perceived to be abortifacient.

Directive 45 states: "Abortion (that is, the directly intended termination of pregnancy before viability or the directly intended destruction of a viable fetus) is never
permitted. Every procedure whose sole immediate effect is the termination of pregnancy before viability is an abortion, which, in its moral context, includes the interval between conception and implantation of the embryo. Catholic healthcare
institutions are not to provide abortion services, even based on the principle of
material cooperation. In this context, Catholic healthcare institutions need to be
concerned about the danger of scandal in any association with abortion providers."

The final line about "scandal" can sound odd to the uninitiated. One theological dissertation on the topic defines scandal as concerning "not only the actions of
the 'bad person,' but how revealing these actions might affect others and the wider
community."[64] Concern about scandal and association with abortion predates the
Catholic Church's series of sexual abuse scandals. Nonetheless, those scandals may
have augmented the bishops' focus on cementing an image of moral purity in recent
years. Thus, not only is abortion completely prohibited but any relationship to
abortion providers—through any form of cooperation, shared resources, or even
referrals—is both prohibited and feared.

The abortion prohibition extends to pregnancies that are incompatible with life.
Healthcare providers in a Catholic hospital, for instance, cannot help a patient
abort a fetus that has no brain and will die soon after delivery. If a woman finds
out her baby has such a fatal anomaly—information that often arrives in the second trimester—she must continue the pregnancy another five months. She must
incur the greater medical risk and psychological cost gestating the doomed pregnancy all that time, even though the data show terminating earlier is safer.[65]

The physicians I spoke to—particularly the Catholic physicians—struggled to
reconcile these directives with recognized standards of care within their field.
Dr. Julia Konrad, a Catholic physician who had experience providing abortions in
her non-Catholic residency program, told me that she thinks the bishops are well-
intended but ill-informed:

> I still do identify myself as Catholic [but it does] not negate my ability to think
> for myself . . . if a lot of the people who were running the Catholic church truly
> understood the medicine behind a lot of the things that we do that they don't
> agree with, I think they would agree with what I do . . .
> I think people forget a lot of times that pregnancy is not a benign state for a
> woman and that a hundred years ago the maternal death rate was like one in
> six . . . if a woman has a baby with a lethal anomaly and the Catholic church says
> she should just carry it and deliver it and let the baby, and the baby will pass
> when the baby passes. But that's—for the woman, you know—what if she has a

post-partum hemorrhage? What if she develops severe preeclampsia? She's potentially compromising her life for a life that has no chance and that's not worth it. So, I don't think they understand that.

Even as Catholic hospitals downplay the physical risks of carrying a nonviable pregnancy to term, they do acknowledge that the practice carries psychic burdens. When an ob-gyn at a Catholic hospital has a patient with a nonviable pregnancy, she is encouraged to refer the patient to a perinatal hospice support program for spiritual and emotional support rather than abortion services.[66] Meanwhile, the patient continues to gestate a pregnancy that she will inevitably lose.[67]

The bishops' stance on abortion has additional implications for other aspects of prenatal care, including genetic counseling. Directives 50 and 54 do allow genetic counseling, but only for the purpose of preparing parents to cope with a child with special needs. Directive 50 makes this explicit: "Prenatal diagnosis is not permitted when undertaken with the intention of aborting an unborn child with a serious defect." How the clinician is to evaluate and adjudicate when or how to withhold a test is not spelled out.

Contemporary Catholic doctrine on pregnancy loss has improved considerably since the early twentieth century, when physicians were prohibited from intervening to save a pregnant woman's life in what theologians considered a natural process, even if deadly, such as an ectopic pregnancy or labor gone awry.[68] The ERDs, nevertheless, require that medical staff must demonstrate a threat to the woman's life *before* treatment begins, as spelled out in Directive 47: "Operations, treatments, and medications that have as their direct purpose the cure of a proportionately serious pathological condition of a pregnant woman are permitted when they cannot be safely postponed until the unborn child is viable, even if they will result in the death of the unborn child."

This directive puts physicians in Catholic hospitals in a particularly murky area if a patient is miscarrying a fetus before it can survive outside the womb. In such cases, ACOG practice guidelines strongly emphasize patient autonomy over treatment, assuming she is medically stable. ACOG states that the patient "should be counseled regarding the risks and benefits of expectant management vs. immediate delivery. Counseling should include a realistic appraisal of neonatal outcomes." If she is not experiencing infection or other life-threatening circumstances, ACOG advises that patients should be offered a choice of all three standard treatments during pregnancy loss: "Immediate delivery (termination of pregnancy by induction of labor or dilation and evacuation) and expectant management should be offered."[69] If the patient chooses expectant management, which is simply watching and waiting, ACOG gives detailed guidance about how to keep her safe and when intervention is critical. In and of itself, Directive 47 violates ACOG's emphasis on patient autonomy. In these circumstances, doctors are prohibited from offering patients all the possible options, and they are barred from carrying out the preferences of patients who know their options.

In practice, physicians recounted employing methods that worked around Directives 45 and 47, in both relatively above-board and more subversive ways, to reduce doctrinal iatrogenesis (see chapters 5 and 6), because most of them saw strict adherence as requiring substandard care. When not using workarounds, some used antibiotics to protect the woman from systemic infection while awaiting the inevitable fetal death during miscarriage. Dr. Jim Schmidt explained: "If there were a fetal heart[beat], we would just temporize . . . Wait and see, yeah, until the fetal cardiac activity stopped or she passed whatever products of conception spontaneously." If she became infected, they would, "treat the infection" until her fever spiked worrisomely, requiring a life-saving D&C.

Dr. Akshun Patel explained how he typically tells his ethics committee that he can wait no longer to intervene once she is infected: "When those symptoms are there, then the medical doctor takes over essentially and says, 'Look, you know, this is a no go. Sister, it is absolutely necessary that I save the life of my patient,' and then it becomes a different story altogether." Some physicians like Dr. Patel find this risk bearable, or at least manageable. Others do not, preferring to send their patients elsewhere for care (a practice less feasible in states that have since enacted abortion bans). With infection completely foreseeable, physicians must balance Catholic governance with their patient's wellbeing.

Dr. Ward is not willing to tolerate that level of risk because he fears bad outcomes for patients' future fertility: "All the obstetricians know that once an infection sets in inside the uterus, you're behind the clock in terms of trying to get the baby out, and if you've got a situation where you don't want the mother to be so infected that it compromises her fertility in the future. And if we wait until they have a high fever and they're really sick, you risk the woman's health and potential fertility."

Similarly, Dr. Lisa Kim sees Directive 47 as a direct violation of the standard of care when the patient's water has broken before there is a realistic chance of survival, and because of that, she tries to transfer patients out of the hospital quickly: "You'd offer most patients if they would like to terminate. But being at a Catholic hospital, we're not allowed to do that. We have to wait until the mother's life is in danger . . . We often tell patients that we can't do anything in the hospital but watch you get infected, and we often ask them if they would like to be transferred to a hospital that would go ahead and get them delivered before they get infected."

In theory, the act of even recommending they go elsewhere is, technically speaking, a violation of the ERDs that prohibit abortion referral, but it is a violation that many of the doctors I spoke with were eager to commit to ensure patients receive the standard of care and avoid harm.

The medical exemption in Directive 47 could technically apply to ectopic pregnancy; however, the directives do not state it that way. An ectopic pregnancy is one that implants outside the uterus, typically in the fallopian tube, and can be very dangerous. ACOG practice guidelines say: "Most cases of tubal ectopic pregnancy that are detected early can be treated successfully either with minimally invasive surgery or with medical management using methotrexate. However, tubal ectopic pregnancy in an unstable patient is a medical emergency that requires prompt surgical intervention."[70]

An ectopic pregnancy is extrauterine, meaning it is a pregnancy that is both nonviable and inherently life threatening to the mother; termination of ectopic pregnancies should be noncontroversial, even at Catholic hospitals. Directive 48, nevertheless, states: "In case of extrauterine pregnancy, no intervention is morally licit which constitutes a direct abortion." With this directive, the bishops insist that the medical standard of care, which preserves fertility and preserves the mother's health with minimum risk, is not permissible because it directly and intentionally ends an embryo's life. Instead, Catholic hospital ethics committees are directed by the bishops to instruct doctors to remove the entire fallopian tube as a theologically justifiable alternative.[71] This way, the doctor can address the pathology (a tube that might burst and kill the woman) without directly touching the embryo in the process, even though it will surely die after removal and the woman's fertility may decrease. This reasoning draws on the principle of double effect, which holds, in brief, that it is ethically permissible to cause a prohibited harm as a foreseeable side effect of bringing about a good result.[72]

Researchers have shown evidence of doctors in Catholic hospitals practicing this way at least as late as the 1990s, and several physicians I spoke with had heard horror stories of women harmed, or mentioned being taught the practice in the past. For example, as Dr. Katie Weber recalled: "One of the hospitals where I did my residency, if you have an ectopic pregnancy, as long as you took out the fallopian tubes you were okay, but you can't do a salpingostomy and take the embryo out of the fallopian tube. That's an abortion. But taking out the whole tube with the pregnancy in it is okay . . . I'm old, that was pre-methotrexate."

Furthermore, a survey fielded in 2008 found that 5.5 percent of physicians in Catholic hospitals were, indeed, limited in how they could manage ectopic pregnancy by religious restrictions (compared with 2.9 percent of physicians in non-Catholic hospitals).[73] That said, the practice is considered so out-of-step with modern medicine that not a single doctor I interviewed had been restricted in how they treated ectopic pregnancies in recent years, either inside or out of a Catholic hospital. Most were surprised when I asked. Frankly, ectopic pregnancy is a clear situation of life or death. The doctors and hospitals do not seem willing to interpret or implement Directive 48 in a life-threatening way. Whereas the other out-of-step directives may exacerbate patient suffering or risk more ambiguously, Directive 48 prescribes malpractice too egregious to survive a court challenge.

CONCLUSION

Bishops and doctors are talking past each other when it comes to "providing the best care possible for the patient." Doctors are thinking through a medical framework designed to present patients with safe choices informed by science, and the bishops appear to view the same clinical moment through a theological framework designed to override or remove those choices in favor of their beliefs about God's will. While both perspectives offer the potential for conflict with patient autonomy, the medical profession consistently endorses patient autonomy when it has been shown to improve public health outcomes (for instance, contraception), and at least gives lip service to the principle of autonomy, even though incidents of coercion, bias, and abuse in reproductive health care continue to surface. Autonomy is simply not as compelling within a religious framework that ultimately asks it adherents, and those inhabiting its spaces, to honor hierarchical authority.

This leaves patients stuck in the middle, albeit often unknowingly. Some devout Catholics share the Church's viewpoints—this is, presumably, why some portion of the devout seek care in Catholic hospitals, to make sure they are abiding by the strictures of their faith. In these cases, issues of patient autonomy are, arguably, somewhat different, as these patients have *chosen* to limit their options to those endorsed by the Church. Most lay people, however, have only a limited understanding of what this means in terms of medical practice. In the next chapter, we turn to the experiences of patients who sought reproductive care in Catholic hospitals. Catholic facilities attract patients for a variety of reasons, even though knowledge of how reproductive care differs in Catholic and non-Catholic hospitals and what that means for their lives remains elusive.

CHAPTER 3

Consumer Medicine?

PATIENTS AND THE ILLUSION OF CHOICE

"I think that any business is not going to lead off with what they don't do," Charles Bouchard, senior director of theology and ethics at The Catholic Health Association, said in response to the Times *analysis.[1] "They are always going to talk about what they do do. And that goes for contractors and car salesmen. They are not going to start off by saying, 'We don't sell this model,' or 'We don't do this kind of work.'"*
    —New York Times, 8/10/18, quoting Fr. Charles Bouchard in,
    "As Catholic Hospitals Expand, So Do Limits on Some Procedures"

Father Bouchard's statement to a reporter from the *New York Times* captures how deeply embedded financial and marketing pressures are within all health systems in the United States. It also suggests that Catholic hospitals are disincentivized to be transparent about the religious constraints imposed on care in their facilities. The reporter, Katie Hafner, asked him to respond to her Catholic hospital website analysis that showed, similar to an academic study,[2] that only about one-quarter of Catholic hospital websites mention the Ethical and Religious Directives for Catholic Health Care Services or explained in any way how care is restricted. Bouchard acknowledged in response, somewhat obliquely, that patients might not choose a Catholic hospital if they knew that their healthcare providers operate under restrictions that diverge from medical standards of care and limit patient autonomy. Instead, Catholic hospitals, like contractors and car salesmen, emphasize what services they *do* provide. And for patients who have choices over their care and who choose to go to Catholic facilities, those perceived benefits may be attractive.

So, what is it that Catholic hospitals *do* sell? As they play down the Catholicism of their hospitals, many Catholic health systems play up an image of high-quality care with an intangible something-extra. Advertising taglines hint at it vaguely but differ little from nonreligious health system taglines. For example, Dignity Health's tagline "Hello humankindness," or Providence's "Health for a better world," are similar to the caring image advertised by nonreligious hospital systems, as in Sutter Health's "We Plus You" and Kaiser Health's "Together we thrive." If the advertising campaigns do not meaningfully distinguish religious from nonreligious health care, sometimes religious symbols on hospitals are visible to passersby, and some churches and community organizations have connections to them through fundraising and charity work. Despite the near complete disappearance of clergy from a Catholic hospital studied by sociologist Adam Reich, he found a spiritual image was projected in various ways, even if superficially. He wrote that the institution's history and the religious images on the walls still lent a "patina of spirituality," even as it marketed itself to the privately insured patients in the area and funneled indigent patients away. Nonetheless, some continue to embrace the idea that Catholic hospitals care more about patients and are more trustworthy due to their religious roots.[3]

Of course, many Catholic hospitals are, in fact, good hospitals, and patients of all faiths choose them for the same reasons they choose other hospitals, such as quality of care, insurance coverage, and location, while perhaps not understanding the restrictions. A well-run cancer center, stroke center, or labor and delivery ward will draw patients through their good reputations. Doctors might be drawn to do their procedures at a particular hospital because of its robotic surgery unit, radiology scanning equipment, or a particular referral network. These strengths can exist in any health system, and when studied on a national level, patient satisfaction and health outcomes in religious and nonreligious or Catholic and non-Catholic facilities are, ultimately, similar.[4]

Locally, however, each hospital is unique to some degree, and Americans like to consider themselves informed consumers of health care. We have seen Americans chafe against the decrease of consumer power in medicine since the 1980s; their opposition to healthcare reform is so often fueled by the idea that "socialized medicine" will take away our ability to choose our own doctor. When they have the option—particularly for non-emergency care—patients prefer to be active participants in selecting their healthcare providers, clinics, and hospitals, whether or not they have meaningful choices, which begs the question: Do more Catholic people ultimately choose Catholic hospitals and clinics for care?

A national survey my team conducted shows they do not.[5] In fact, they are slightly more likely to seek out a hospital specifically because it is not Catholic. However, there is a correlation between having a high degree of religiosity, among Christian and Catholic women, and seeking out a Catholic provider. Because of this, I intentionally wanted to interview people who feel religion is important in their lives to hear about their healthcare experiences and to find out how they felt about religious policies that affected their care. I made a deliberate decision to recruit heavily from geographic areas saturated with Catholic hospitals in parts of the country that were more religiously conservative.[6] Relatedly, more than half the patients interviewed for this study were morally opposed to abortion in some way, with an overrepresentation of Southern and Midwestern patients living outside of major metropolitan areas.

I specifically wanted to hear from a lot of women who identify as religious and who opposed abortion because, at least theoretically, some of the religious restrictions would be better aligned with their beliefs and interests. I wanted to know if they embraced them, and if so, how, and why. It turns out that many of them got more than they bargained for. I found that religious women, even Catholic ones, followed comments demonstrating a deep respect for religious freedom with disappointment at the ways specific Catholic directives affected their reproductive care. The interviews were peppered with big and little surprises, destroying my assumptions about ideological concordance and defying stereotypes abundant in our divided nation.

Even as my respondents surprised me, their answers returned to a common refrain: "Choice." Not the same "choice" Americans use as a euphemism for abortion but, rather, a vision of health care as an unregulated free market in which both patients and providers are unconstrained and uncoerced by the government, religious leaders, and healthcare systems. Of course, it is a fantasy that anyone in the United States navigates health care as a free market. American medicine has been regulated and constrained by financial interests, resource shortages, and safety considerations for over a century. Nonetheless, most of my respondents voiced a desire for free will in matters of health care, including and beyond abortion, even as they deferred to hypothetical constraints on that free will in the name of religious authority. This chapter is, ultimately, about how and why patients end up getting care in Catholic facilities, their feelings about how that care is delivered, and the experience of not having any choices at all.

ROSEMARY: INFORMED CONSUMER

Rosemary is a white woman who lives in a Southern city. She spoke with pride about her stable family life, telling me in the same breath about the three miscarriages she and her husband experienced: "I've had one husband and we've been together for twenty-three years and we have three children together. And we lost three." She then noted that the miscarriages explained a significant age gap that existed between her two youngest children.

Rosemary grew up Baptist but agreed to raise the children in her husband's preferred Methodist church. When asked how often they attend church, she replied with levity: "When we're good, on Sundays." Rosemary believes in the value of contraception. She joked: "Oh, I believe. I've got a twenty-year-old son. I believe strongly in contraception. *[Laughs]*." She nonetheless describes herself as a moral conservative. She explained, for example, that she draws a line between contraception for high schoolers versus college students: "I would say I am a little more probably morally conservative ... Like I saw a post last week that there's an RA in one of the dorms that leaves a box of condoms outside of the dorm for kids to freely come and pick up. So, I think that's great. I've also seen at a high-school level that they pass them out before prom. I don't really like that. I don't know. I just feel like high school, that's too young and I don't know. I have a moral problem with that, but not at college."

Rosemary opposes abortion: "I'm prolife ... And that's really just my religious background. That's how I interpret the bible, and so I'm a pro-lifer." She is not, however, an absolutist. She explained: "I would say that when the fetus is not going to be viable, I understand that." She has had friends who have had abortions, and a good friend of hers is an ob-gyn who has talked with her in detail about some cases where she has performed them. Still, she told me: "Personally, it's not something I would ever choose . . . I also don't really push my beliefs on everybody. I'm more to myself and I support what my friends and family would do . . . I'm not a judgmental person but for me, and my daughters . . . I would just guide them to deliver that baby and we would find another option."

In keeping with Rosemary's pro-life orientation, she referred to her early miscarriages as babies. There were no medical complications with these miscarriages. She summarized: "I had a D&C on one, so that was just a quick in and out. And then the other two I did not need a D&C." Going into a bit more detail, she explained that, for the first one: "I was fourteen weeks, but that baby hadn't been thriving in there and so that's why I needed the D&C." An ultrasound found no heartbeat, which did not come as a great shock since she hadn't been having the usual morning sickness. The second miscarriage happened quickly, like a period, shortly after an early pregnancy test showed she was pregnant. For the third, she went to a Catholic hospital, where the staff sent her home with the hope that she would not miscarry.

I asked her to tell me a little more about that third miscarriage, the one that involved care at a Catholic hospital. From her narration, it is not clear whether the staff's hands were tied by the ERDs or whether she would have wanted intervention in any case: "I started bleeding and so I went to the hospital and it was still a thriving pregnancy so I went home—I think I maybe did another hospital visit. It was over a couple of days. And again, they did the ultrasound. The heartbeat, everything looked good, but then I passed that one at home, and I knew when I did . . . [going through] it is just a huge loss and disappointment. And the other symptoms, it was fine. I mean, it was a heavy period is what it was."

Her ob-gyn had performed the dilation and curettage (D&C) for the first miscarriage at Metropolitan hospital, a non-Catholic institution, although he also worked at St. Elizabeth's hospital at the time. Thinking back, she struggled to remember why she went to Metropolitan versus St. Elizabeth, thinking it might have had something to do with her original plan to have a tubal ligation at the time of delivery: "I think he delivered in both places, I want to say, because he delivered at the Catholic hospital. You couldn't deliver there if you were going to have your tubes tied because they didn't allow that. So, you would deliver at another hospital."

Her doctor told her about this policy when she expressed her preference for sterilization after the birth: "In my [prenatal] appointment—this was with the first baby that we lost—I said, 'Three and we're done. I want my tubes tied.' And he said, 'Well we're not delivering at [St. Elizabeth's]. We'll be delivering somewhere else.' I had no idea you couldn't do that. I guess I had never thought about it. I knew it was a Catholic hospital but I hadn't—I didn't realize they weren't allowed to do tubals there."

When she was able to stay pregnant with her third and youngest child—after the three miscarriages—she hoped to deliver at Metropolitan so she could get the tubal ligation done at the same time. It was close to her home, and the hospital had a good reputation. But by then, her doctor had an exclusive appointment at St. Elizabeth's: "I [ended up delivering at St. Elizabeth's] because that other option closed down, I think. If I recall correctly, the other hospital ended up closing or maybe he just no longer had his privileges there.[7] So with my doctor—and I wasn't going to change mid-pregnancy—I had to deliver at [St. Elizabeth's] then. And so I said okay, then we can't have a tubal. And my husband said, 'I'll just get a vasectomy.'"

For Rosemary, this solution was a small price to pay to stay with a physician she trusted. "It was inconvenient, but I was okay with that. I mean, I respected my doctor. I wasn't going to change doctors. I really liked him."

When I followed up with Rosemary to see how her husband felt about getting the vasectomy, she joked lightly: "He was fine with it until the actual day. [Laughs] But yeah, he was okay with it." Given that Rosemary was not delivering by C-section, her husband's vasectomy actually presented less overall risk to the two of them, but this argument is not usually compelling enough to persuade male partners to undergo sterilization.[8] The rate of tubal ligation is over three times that of vasectomy.[9] Perhaps even more to the point, many women do not trust their partners to follow through; for some, a tubal ligation immediately after delivery provides security when male partners do not assume comparable responsibility for contraception.[10]

Rosemary seemed unbothered by this situation. In her telling, she just accepted the limitations and never really pressed her doctor about it: "So, whenever we had first talked about it, it wasn't a big deal at all because I had another option, delivering at the other place. But then I lost those babies and we tried for a year, so by the time I delivered I just knew it wasn't even an option . . ."

The hospital's limitations on her care were acceptable to her, both for her own situation and in principle. She did not find the idea of religiously restricted care problematic, at least in this context.

When I asked how she would feel about being denied something she needed or wanted because of a doctor's personal conscientious objection or a hospital's policies, Rosemary responded in classic consumerist fashion: "If I needed something that a doctor is not willing to do, I would find another doctor and do it." Essentially, Rosemary would shop elsewhere to get what she needed. Her answer displayed a confidence, or some might call it a false consciousness, that alternate healthcare options reliably exist. On the specific topic of abortion, she said: "Well if it's a religious-based hospital, I understand, I understand why there's restrictions on life." To Rosemary, it was understandable that hospitals imposed restrictions on patient care; in her own college educated and middle-income experience, such restrictions were entirely navigable. In many ways, Rosemary's views encapsulate the neoliberal perspective that views health care as a business and patients as consumers. Her reaction to encountering a religious constraint was to assume responsibility to find a solution that preserved the hospital's religious freedom.

Her answers changed somewhat when we returned to the topic of miscarriage management. I asked her how she would feel if her physician steered her toward a nonreligious hospital to maximize her options for care during a miscarriage. She demonstrated a type of confusion and concern not uncommon in the interviews:

> LORI: So if you were early in pregnancy and you were at the doctor getting prenatal care and let's just say you didn't have three children already and no experience with miscarriage, and you're sort of new to this. And the doctor says, "This is a healthy pregnancy, but I tell all my patients if something unexpected happens like bleeding or leaking fluid, go to this nonreligious hospital to have all the options for care." What is your reaction to hearing that?
>
> ROSEMARY: Honestly, I don't know that I would understand that, why my doctor is telling me that, when he has just said I have a healthy pregnancy. So, a), I would be worried, okay, but beyond that, I would wonder why my doctor is still going to be affiliated with that hospital when he's saying if there's trouble, I need you to go somewhere else or consider going somewhere else. . . . I want my doctor to be able to take care of me no matter what and advise. I think a doctor needs to be able to advise you to your best health no matter what. I really don't think a hospital should be able to restrict you in that.

In this scenario, as with several other respondents, her first reaction was to fear for her own pregnancy. Yet, her response quickly shifts to questioning why her doctor would risk abandoning her in her time of need. In the same way Rosemary says you should stick with your doctor, she also believes a doctor should stick with their patient. A doctor should not abandon the patient because of foreseeable institutional constraints on care. Rather, the doctor should do everything within their power to protect the patient's best interests.

I asked her how she would advise a loved one about this dilemma. She imagined telling her own daughter to shop elsewhere for reproductive care, for fear of a bad outcome: "I'm going to guide her away from the Catholic hospital so that—because when it comes to my kids, I want what I believe is the best option to best healthcare available to them. And if I don't believe they can get it all at a hospital because of religious reasons, I'm going to guide them away. . . . I would worry really about something like infection setting in, where it would be life-threatening to my daughter or my family member. And so I would just let them know: 'This isn't going to be an option . . . [if you go elsewhere] you can stay with your doctor through the entire pregnancy, no matter what happens.'"

It is worth noticing what Rosemary does not comment on. Having had some degree of choice in her own health care, Rosemary does not contemplate a situation in which alternate hospitals do not exist within a reasonable distance, or that regulators might not approve a non-Catholic competitor opening up in a well-served area, or that an insurance company might limit coverage to only the hospital with religious restrictions. Rather, Rosemary, a woman who values her own ability to make choices that reflect her own beliefs and preferences, assumes the invisible hand of capitalism will correct the problem of choice-limiting health systems.

Rosemary's comments on the doctor-patient relationship harken back to the ideal of medicine as a calling based on an altruistic desire to serve and heal rather than a profession that also exists within the relations of capitalism.

Several other respondents spoke more directly to the tension between medicine as a business and a calling, for instance, summoning the image of the wronged consumer.[11] These respondents described shopping for a better doctor, hospital, or insurance plan in retaliation for not having their needs met. For example, when asked what she would do if she could not get the reproductive care she sought due to religious restrictions, one interviewee said: "I would be aggravated that I wasted my time. I would probably like leave them like a negative review or something so other people don't go see them." Others expressed anger that reflected some degree of violated intimacy, as if a jilted lover: "I would just find a new doctor . . . Yeah. I mean, if that's the way that they want to run their practice, then that's their choice, but then I won't be their patient."

These responses were, however, unusual. Most of the women I spoke with took the responsibility for being denied care back onto themselves.[12] They blamed themselves for not having researched their options more thoroughly, or for not having planned for contingencies, saying, for example, "I was upset but I mean, I also understood that I didn't do my research either before I picked an ob-gyn." And, "I could've gotten angry and write really bad reviews about this hospital, but I chose not to 'cause I knew [it was Catholic] coming in," even though she did not know how it being Catholic would affect her. And Nadia, while angry at the hospital for not being transparent about their policies, ultimately also blamed herself for not anticipating them.

NADIA: IN SEARCH OF AUTONOMY

Nadia is a Pentecostal, Puerto Rican woman in her mid-thirties. She lives in the Southeast with her husband, her ten-year-old daughter, and, at the time of the interview, her grandmother, a hurricane refugee. Religion is important to Nadia and her extended family. They attend church and Bible study weekly. For work, Nadia staffs the front desk of several medical offices within a large health system that does not appear to have a Catholic affiliation. The system, nevertheless, has come to own many hospitals that are Catholic. She gave birth in one of them to her daughter when she was twenty-three years old.

She remembers the care at the hospital fondly. She had a scheduled C-section because of the baby's positioning. The hospital declined her request for a sterilization although, in her memory, staff did not emphasize the religious reasons. She explained: "I wanted them to tie my tubes, but they didn't believe in that so they didn't do that there. And plus, I was young and only had one kid so they wouldn't do it, but I knew I only wanted one kid. But they're like, 'Oh you're going to change your mind.' And it's ten years later and I still haven't changed my mind."

I asked a few more questions to clarify this story. Ideally, women discuss their plans for postpartum contraception or sterilization with their doctors as part of their prenatal care. I tried to understand if her desire for a tubal ligation had been discussed at any point prior to the delivery. Nadia said, "I don't remember 'cause my whole pregnancy was such a blur 'cause I didn't have a really good pregnancy." But regardless of whether she explicitly requested the tubal ligation beforehand, she could not recall any discussion or helpful education during her prenatal care that would help her know in advance that the sterilization option would not be available to her for whatever reason:

> I didn't find out until later that that was the case, so I didn't really have a choice but to, you know, keep the same doctor and go through with it. I didn't know the hospital itself did not tie women's tubes after they gave birth. That part I didn't know. I didn't find out until I went in to check into the hospital. I was talking to the lady and I'm like, "By the way, do I have to tell anybody I want my tubes tied?" And that's when they told me . . . They told me that even if they could do it, they wouldn't do it because I was too young and I only had one child. If I had more than two kids, then if I was at a place where they could tie my tubes they would.

In Nadia's telling, it is unclear whether she perceived her age or the hospital's religious policies as the more significant barrier to her care. And, in fact, she was not entirely sure it was a Catholic hospital (it was), telling me, "I think it was a Baptist hospital . . . Yeah. And I think that religion doesn't—they don't believe in that or something like that." (For the record, Baptist hospitals in the United States do not prohibit sterilization.[13]) What she did know, with great certainty, was that she always wanted only one child. Nadia felt a duty to become a mom because she was physically able to do so, whereas "some people don't get the opportunity." She wanted the experience of becoming pregnant and giving birth—that is, once. Nadia confessed: "I don't really like kids. I was going to love mine, but I knew that I didn't want, you know, I didn't want to have more than one."

Looking back at what she might have done differently, Nadia said: "I wouldn't have even got pregnant . . . I don't know why people choose to have kids, especially more than one." Her tone was facetious, but she was dead serious that she wanted only one child. Even ten years after the fact, Nadia resented a paternalistic policy that left her at risk for pregnancy. In the years after the birth, she remained upset about being denied the sterilization, and it weighed heavily on her until she had a Mirena intrauterine device (IUD) inserted. "It was something I had to constantly think about and not forget to do because I didn't want any more kids . . . and we don't believe in abortion so if I did end up pregnant accidentally, I'd have to keep it."

Given Nadia's religious beliefs and her opposition to abortion, I wondered if she resented the influence of the hospital's religion on her care. Her response was adamantly pro-choice in the consumer-not-abortion sense. She argued that, as the patient, she should be able to choose what happens to her body. She simultaneously faulted her twenty-three-year-old self for not asking the right questions and making informed choices:

I found it odd because when you go to a hospital you want them to do what you want them to do. You should be in charge of your own medical care and not their beliefs. But I guess we can also choose the hospitals we go to . . . my ob-gyn happened to be in the same women's hospital, so it was convenience rather than anything else . . .

I was upset that they didn't do it. I was kind of upset too that they didn't tell me beforehand, like a pamphlet or something, like if you choose to have your baby here, this is how it's supposed to go and these are the rules or whatever or this is what we believe in, what we don't believe in, you know. But they didn't and it was my fault 'cause I didn't ask either. So for me it is what it is. I'll just have to, you know, just deal with it.

Like so many patients in the study, Nadia blamed herself for not overcoming the barrier, for not asking questions she had no reason to know she needed to ask. I would have thought her frustration might have dissipated by now, with the IUD, which is a contraceptive method that has mostly satisfied users.[14] But to Nadia, even the small failure rate associated with an IUD seems like too much of a risk. That insecurity and the disrespect for her clearly articulated preferences nagged at her:

We should be able to make our own decisions, whether we have one kid or we have six. You know, 'cause there are people like me who know for sure that they only want one kid and that's it. You're not letting them dictate their own care, you're not letting them dictate their future, because then, you know, contraceptive [sic] is never 100 percent for sure either . . . So now here I am pregnant and I did everything I had to do to take care of it, but because they didn't feel like doing it at the hospital, now I'm dealing with another pregnancy. I just feel we can avoid a lot of stuff.

Nadia felt the permanence of tubal ligation would put her mind at ease, and she would consider it for the future. In theory, she could have scheduled the procedure and had it done at some other time, but her IUD worked well enough for her that she did not feel compelled to undergo a surgical procedure anymore. Still, she said: "If I did by some stupid reason end up pregnant again . . . I wouldn't pick [the Catholic hospital] because I would want a sterilization right now, for sure."

Nadia's distaste for the paternalism that limited her reproductive choices held true for other religious restrictions as well. If a doctor objected to providing her with contraception, she would find another doctor. She wishes doctors and hospitals were forced to disclose their religious views on a website. Still, her account assumes that the onus is on the patient to learn what is and isn't allowed and plan accordingly:

I guess everybody's entitled to their opinion and you have to pick and choose wisely who you want your doctor to be for those reasons exactly. Although I've never come across that situation, I think it would suck though because when you're looking for a doctor, you can go online but it doesn't really say "this doctor does not believe in" blah, blah, blah. You don't find that out until you actually get to the appointment. And by then it's too late 'cause now you have to find another doctor . . . It should be on their website or—you know, 'cause everybody Googles people and doctors. People Google them all the time and I think it should be disclosed so you can make, you know, a wise decision.

Likewise, Nadia thinks women suffering miscarriage should avoid Catholic hospitals if they do not want their care constrained by Catholic doctrine. Assuming they have other healthcare options, she urges, "If you want your choices and you want your say in it, then don't go to a hospital that's going to limit that . . . they're going to tell you, 'No, we're going to have to, you know, wait it out and see,' and if that's not what the pregnant person wants to do, then don't go there."

I was a little surprised at how adamant Nadia was on this point, given that she herself opposed abortion. I pushed to clarify how she felt personally about the idea of intervening before the fetus had died during miscarriage:

> LORI: Okay. And as somebody that, like you said, is very opposed to abortion, do you feel conflicted at all about treating a miscarriage before you know for sure that the fetus is dead? . . .
>
> NADIA: Yeah. No, I would definitely—I would wait until there are no signs that my baby can survive . . . I would wait it out 'cause my God is a great God and he's capable of doing anything and turning every situation around . . .
>
> I'm very open on how people want to treat their pregnancy, their lives, what they believe in. I respect all of that . . . [but] if it was my sister, my best friend, anybody in my close circle, I would definitely give them my advice to—you know: God can do anything. So until they don't find a heartbeat and then until they say he has passed, and for your health we have to take it out, then that's what my advice would be. I would never advise someone to just—yeah, "Oh, they told you that it might die? Oh, go ahead and have the abortion." I would never say that.

Nadia, in other words, largely agreed with the Catholic bishops' prescription for treatment. Personally, she would choose to wait until she miscarried on her own or the fetus had conclusively passed, even when the miscarriage is inevitable. But she departs from the bishops on one key point: The choice should be the patient's to make.

ZIA: SHOPPING ELSEWHERE

Zia lives in the Southwest. She is white and Latina. She owns her own home, which she shares with her father, her sister, and her sister's children. Zia works as a records clerk in a governmental setting. She and her sister share caretaking of their disabled father. "When I started taking care of my father, I worked full time and I had to go to part time to take care of him . . . my sister takes care of him while I'm at work and then she goes to work." Zia's mom was Catholic and her dad is Christian, so she and her sister grew up attending both kinds of church services. She does not have a strong religious preference now and attends church only once a year or so.

I asked her if she had children. She told me, "No, but my sister is actually carrying a baby for me right now." Zia had a long history of infertility, including several miscarriages during her previous marriage. A childhood disease had reduced her ability to carry a child to term: "I was told that I probably wouldn't be able to have kids. So over the last few years, me and my going-to-be ex-husband were trying to like conceive. . . . I did get pregnant a few times but every time like resulted in miscarriage . . . that's why we went with like my sister to carry the baby for us . . . [but] our marriage didn't wind up working out."

At the time of our interview, Zia and her husband were in the process of divorcing as a result of domestic abuse. She had decided to end the marriage only shortly before the interview, and she did not have a clear idea of what would happen in the long term. Issues like custody had not been decided yet: "[The eggs] were mine and then it was like my husband's sperm . . . we haven't really—me and him haven't been split up for that long. We had some issues in our marriage and some of it turned like to—like domestic and—you know, some things happened towards the end of our marriage, I wound up just kicking him out and I'm not going to put up with something like that."

She was not daunted by the idea of raising a child on her own. She continued: "My sister and her kids live with me so—and I have like 10 nieces and nephews—so, raising a baby is a piece of cake for me . . . But the other changes, you know, *that*, I have no idea about, like divorce or like trying to like share custody. *That's crazy.* I have no idea about any of that."

In the midst of all of this change, Zia and her sister have to figure out where the baby will be delivered. She took her sister on a labor and delivery tour at St. Peter's Catholic hospital because it is known to have a good labor and delivery service: "I wanted to have my child at [St. Peter's] just because their care is very good. It wasn't because of like the religion or anything. It's just because they provide like excellent care. And so when I was talking to one of the doctors from there, I had mentioned that, you know, that my sister was carrying my child for me because of like all my miscarriages and everything, and [the doctor] told me that I couldn't."

Taken aback, I asked, "What did he mean she couldn't?" I knew that Directive 42 of the ERDs condemns and forbids surrogacy, but it had never come up in my discussions with physicians. The doctors I spoke with told me that, if anything, hospital ethics committees generally did not ask a lot of questions about *how* a pregnant woman got pregnant once a pregnancy had been established. Until speaking to Zia, I could not quite imagine a situation in which the surrogacy directive would be actively policed and enforced. I wondered what exactly the doctor meant and if she could she recall the conversation.

She told me:

He wasn't like rude about it or anything. He was just like, you know, like we thought that you were having the baby. I was like "No, my sister's—" and I explained, you know, my sister is carrying my child for me because I've had so many miscarriages . . . my body can't carry. And he's like, well—he's like that's not really what our hospital like supports . . . our situation wasn't something that they would support. So, I got a little offended and that's why I decided to go to a different hospital. . . .

The hospital wasn't refusing to let Zia's sister deliver the baby there. They were refusing to recognize the surrogacy. In practical terms, this could mean that the hospital would refer to Zia's sister, not Zia, as the mother throughout the birth process, including in filling out the birth certificate information: "My little sister was there with me. And so I was just like, you know, okay—you know, thank you for your time and it was—I just got up and walked away. I didn't want to hear anything else that he had to say."

Hurt and discouraged, she left, and that was the end of her contact with St. Peter's. Zia found a new hospital. She is a low-income woman, doing something controversial in a conservative state. She had little power at her disposal to push back and little desire to draw attention to herself in that way. Later, she asked her Catholic grandmother, who is fairly religious, whether she had heard anything about Catholic beliefs against surrogacy. "Even my grandma was like, I've never heard of that. Because my grandma 100 percent like supports, you know, what's going on, you know, like with my child."

Zia and her sister made alternative plans to deliver in a non-Catholic medical center when the time comes. Zia was disappointed to not have been able to take advantage of the best her area had to offer. While research on patient satisfaction shows that Catholic hospitals fare no better or worse nationally on average than other types of hospitals, Zia had heard otherwise.[15] She embraced the belief of those around her who told her care was better at Catholic hospitals generally, even though she had a close friend who suffered emotionally and physically after being turned away from one during a miscarriage. She understood the limitations, but she still believed they provided superior care for childbirth: "I do believe that Catholic hospitals do have better care. They really do. But not when it comes to miscarriages or anything else because it's not in their belief to—even if you're having a miscarriage and the baby is still alive—to end that child's life. You know, they don't believe in abortion and they don't believe in anything like that . . . In the event of like you're having a miscarriage or something, I personally would not go there . . . [if] your child is still alive that is not the place you want to go." In line with Rosemary's consumer choice perspective, Zia encourages hypothetical women with hypothetical choices to shop elsewhere.

Zia respects Catholic hospitals' position on elective abortion, but she, nevertheless, thinks their position on miscarriage, surrogacy, and sterilization go too far. She sees religion as declining in importance to younger people, and she thinks the hospitals should take note: "My grandma, she's very religious and she was completely against me having a D&C [for my miscarriage]. But I—in today's world religion isn't such a big thing anymore and I have my own beliefs . . . if somebody doesn't agree with me, well, I really don't care because that's how I feel. You know, I don't want to offend anybody and I don't want to, like, hurt anyone. But I wouldn't want to go through what my friend went through."

While Zia feels the hospital restrictions on abortion are reasonable, she doesn't see the value in suffering for a religious policy: "When it comes to abortion like if they don't—if they don't do it, you know, like I understand, you know. But when you're having a miscarriage like the medication for a D&C, you know, they should change that so you don't have to suffer." And regarding sterilization, she also hopes for a policy change: "It's a woman's body and if you don't want to have any more children then you should be able to make that decision, not a hospital or somebody else kind of make that decision for you." However, when asked if she can imagine them ever changing, she simply replied, "No, I don't think that's ever going to happen."

KAYDEN: HIS MOTHER'S OB-GYN

I first heard Kayden's story from Dr. Ward (introduced in chapter 2), who had agreed to stay in touch after our initial interview in 2012. Dr. Ward had experienced several conflicts between the ERDs and patient care after a Catholic health-care system bought his urban, non-Catholic hospital. Dr. Ward, an ob-gyn, had been treating Kayden's mother for years and had watched Kayden and his sister grow up. Kayden had been assigned female at birth, but he began transitioning in his late teens with support from a pediatrician at the local children's hospital. In 2013, Kayden and his mother came to see Dr. Ward about having Kayden's ovaries removed. Dr. Ward scheduled the surgery over Kayden's school break.

What happened next came as a shock to Dr. Ward:

> I scheduled it here at [Mercy], just taking out ovaries and not technically a sterilization procedure, and I had it scheduled on a Wednesday and I booked it about six, seven weeks·in advance. And the Monday prior to the surgery, forty-eight hours before, we got a call from the surgery scheduler that it's not permitted here. And we said you've got to be kidding, you know. Such short notice and the kid's on his college break and blah, blah, blah. Long story short: "No, and there's nothing you can do about it. We've taken it off the books" . . . I explained the whole scenario [to Kayden] . . . they didn't even notify him.

Mercy Hospital cancelled Kayden's surgery shortly before news of Catholic hospitals cancelling gender affirmation surgeries (and the subsequent lawsuits) had begun to surface around the country.[16] Dr. Ward's previous conflicts with Catholic governance had surrounded women and pregnancy; he did not anticipate any problems with Kayden's case. Kayden was a man who had no intention of bearing children. Dr. Ward surmised, "I'm not sure in the medical bylaws where that falls 'cause it's not really a sterilization procedure, and I think it was just their sense of discomfort with somebody transgender having their ovaries removed."

Thanks to some nimble rescheduling, Dr. Ward was able to perform Kayden's procedure at his alternate hospital site, a smaller and older facility much farther away. The event was upsetting to everyone involved—especially Kayden. Dr. Ward put the two of us in touch.

Still a college student in a Western city at the time we spoke, Kayden wanted to tell me his story, but he had no interest in going public. He did not feel the desire to come out to the new people he had met at college and, besides, he told me, "It's kind of hard to get to a personal level with my friends over there." At home, it is different. "I've been surrounded by people who have known me from before, so it's been kind of easier and more comfortable for me." This was striking to me, as it is far from obvious that someone going through a gender transition would feel more comfortable in their home community. But Kayden appreciated his parents' support. At college, he felt more vulnerable, and he preferred not to draw attention to his gender transition.

Looking back, Kayden wonders if he should have transitioned sooner. He missed out on the potential benefit of puberty blockers:

> I think for me it was more of like I was in denial for most of my childhood. I didn't want to think that I was any different than everybody else and I wasn't quite sure how my parents would react to it just 'cause I know that, you know, at the time they grew up in [a country with traditional ideas about gender] they had no knowledge of what transgender even is. So, it was really hard for me to sort of come out. So, I went through the whole like depression phase and everything. And then I finally just told myself that I think it was time to be honest, not just to everybody but to myself as well.

He started the process with counseling and hormone replacement therapy. About a year later, he underwent surgery to have his breasts removed. A couple years later, he needed additional surgery to meet the sterilization requirement to change the gender on his citizenship documents in his mother's birth country,[17] where he also held citizenship. After the surgery, they would need to travel there to complete the necessary paperwork.

It was at that point Kayden and his mother reached out to Dr. Ward. When Kayden's mother had had ovarian cysts, Dr. Ward performed her hysterectomy. His mother liked and trusted Dr. Ward and took some comfort in his familiar presence as she ventured into entirely uncharted territory with her son. They did not seek out a Catholic hospital. They simply wanted to go to Dr. Ward, who had always done his surgeries there, long before it was Catholic. Mercy was across the street from his office.

While Kayden might, if given the option, have preferred to work with a physician with more experience in transgender care, he was anxious to get the surgery scheduled, and he wanted to stay within his mother's comfort zone: "I definitely wanted to just go through all the surgeries that I could get through early in time so I didn't have to worry about it later. And I knew that I was prepared for it. So, for me it was more of like a—I was actually grateful for my mom to allow me to go through it."

I asked Kayden if anyone mentioned that Dr. Ward's hospital was Catholic, or if that was a concern in anyway, but he said no. Kayden himself had not even reflected on the hospital's vaguely Catholic-sounding name. Had he had more information about religious restrictions governing care in Catholic hospitals, he certainly would not have chosen it. It was not an informed choice.

Kayden learned that there would be a problem only when, as he put it, "Dr. Ward called me to let me know that the nuns at the hospital had rejected my procedure." The call came shortly after his preoperative surgery phone call with a nurse who seemed to him inappropriately interested in his reasons for wanting the procedure:

> It actually first started with me getting a call from one of the nurses at the hospital, giving me kind of like a preoperative talk, I guess, letting me know what I needed to do before surgery and things like that. And I noticed that the questions were very personal, like she would ask me what I was getting, and then I told her what I was getting, which was a hysterectomy[18] and whatever, and then she sort of was like, "Why?"
>
> And it was just sort of a very personal—like I didn't understand why she needed to ask me that. So, I kind of assumed she had the paperwork in front of her. So, I briefly just answered, "Oh, I'm undergoing a gender reassignment change," you know, and she was like, "Why?" Like she kept asking why and then I basically sort of—I kept answering very briefly. I didn't give her a full-length answer.
>
> And then after she was done with all that stuff, I think a day after that was when Dr. Ward called me and I distinctly remember he was like, "We have a problem." And my heart just sank. I was like, "Oh, no, I have to get this done now" and everything. And then he basically told me that the nuns of the hospital had called him and said that he was not allowed to do my procedure because it was unethical. And he said that he was going to look for another place where I could do my surgery on the same day at the same time because he knew that I needed to get it done.

That Dr. Ward told him the verdict came down from nuns was notable, although Dr. Ward had not mentioned it to me. It lent a distinctly religious and less bureaucratic flavor compared with other episodes of permission-denied by "ethics committees," which all hospitals have in one form or another, even if they function less as gatekeepers in non-Catholic settings. Dr. Ward pledged to come through on Kayden's timeline, but Kayden remained shocked and hurt by the rejection: "I never thought that I would be a victim of like medical discrimination based off my situation. So, it was more of like a shock to me. And then that's when I started getting upset . . . I went upstairs to tell my mom, and she got really mad . . . we had already booked a flight to [our home country] and everything. So for my mom, it was more of like a time thing. She was just worried about whether or not I was going to be able to recover fully before flying . . ."

While Kayden's mother remained focused on logistics, his girlfriend was angry at the hospital. He told me: "She actually works at that hospital. And so she was just like, you know, really angry about it." Yet even she had had no inkling that the ERDs would be a problem for Kayden's care. It had never come up in her department—which was not, for the record, obstetrics and gynecology.

No one ever told Kayden a specific reason the procedure was cancelled. He surmised it came down to the hospital's discomfort with transgender care as well as the Catholic Church's well-known prohibitions on sterilization: "I think it's my whole situation in general and then just the whole process of removing something that, you know, should be in your body kind of thing. And like I think that they just thought that it was unethical to remove something that could like potentially give, you know, life."

Kayden's deduction reflects both a truth about the Catholic position against gender confirming surgeries as well as a lot of guessing. As discussed in the prior chapter, the current version of the ERDs do not explicitly prohibit transgender care, but statements from prominent Catholic theologians suggest a more formal ban is coming.

I asked Kayden if he was tempted to speak out about his negative experience. He responded: "I definitely wanted to. I was just afraid that my name would be used or something, just because I'm very, very stealth. So, no one knows that I'm transgender and everything [at school], and I prefer to keep it that way. So, I think for me I really did want to kind of let people know what happened to me, but I was just afraid."

At this point in Kayden's life, he hoped that, by telling me his story, he might publicize an issue few people realize is a problem. For people like Kayden who seek care at a Catholic hospital because they trust the doctor who works there, they may have even less reason to "do the research" about whether a hospital might have a religious affiliation and/or institutional religious policies might affect them. In Kayden's case, even Dr. Ward did not know and, therefore, could not help him avoid the demoralizing experience. Unlike Rosemary and Zia, both Dr. Ward and Kayden blamed the hospital and not themselves in this instance. Neither supported the hospital's right to refuse this care and both found the policy wholly unethical. Kayden felt betrayed, not as a consumer but as a human being.

DESIREE: ON NOT HAVING CHOICES

Desiree is a survivor of child abuse, sexual assault, drug addiction, and the post-traumatic stress disorder (PTSD) related to these experiences. When I talked with her, she was in her mid-forties and had been sober for a long time. "I live alone, and I've lived at my current residence for thirteen years," she explained, "and I've been struggling to try to get the many degrees that I want." She hoped to be an obstetric nurse but had been stuck on the program's waiting list: "Waiting on the waiting list for four years. Now [I] changed my major to psychology and I'm having some emotional problems but, you know, I'm still hanging in there . . . hopefully in September I'll be back in school for psychology and I'll be able to do what I want and that is help other people with mental illnesses."

She is a Black woman who grew up in the South in what she described as "a religious cult and, you know, it was a very distinctive one." It was there that she experienced violent sexual assault and ongoing child abuse. She gave birth to two children who were then handed over to her family to raise. Eventually, she fled the area on her own. The sexual abuse had left Desiree with permanent injuries, and she was diligent about seeing a gynecologist in her new city, while simultaneously navigating drug addiction. Her choices for care were limited by being on Medicaid, a situation that has improved since the passage of the Affordable Care Act in 2010. Looking back at that earlier time, she remembered: "There was no medical transportation so you just kind of like—I was in my twenties—you just kind of like [do] what works . . . Medicaid wasn't widely accepted back then." She mostly received care at a clinic in a Catholic hospital: "I went there for a GYN exam because, you know, some things happened to me when I was young, you know, and I was like split down to my anus. So, I have like a lot of infections and stuff, and the abuser gave me herpes, so I like always want to keep up with my GYN health and . . . just to try to make sure I'm okay, checking up on everything."

Desiree found out she was pregnant for the third time during a routine gynecological visit at the Catholic hospital's clinic. She made clear she did not want to go through with the pregnancy, in part because she was troubled by the potential impact of her drug use on the fetus, but the hospital staff would not discuss abortion as an option:

> When you're in a religious hospital, they don't want to talk about [it]. They want you to keep the baby whether it has—I was on drugs . . . they were like not really concerned about the health of the baby. They were just more like, "Get off drugs and, you know, if you don't want the baby, give the baby up for adoption . . ."
>
> I just don't even see how they would say go through that traumatic experience and continue with this care. It just was not in my best interest . . . But they weren't like really interested in what I wanted to do. They were more interested in, you know, their I guess doctrines or edicts of their hospital. It was a Catholic hospital.

Desiree herself is not Catholic, and she resented how the hospital's policies trumped her own desires. Desiree had no choice about where to go for care. Unlike Rosemary, Nadia, Zia, or Kayden, Desiree had no reason to seek treatment at a Catholic facility other than it was the only one she could reach and would take her. She had no existing relationship with a doctor she trusted, no cultural connection to a familiar space. Instead, she obtained care at the only facility she could—and she was only too aware of how that facility restricted her options. Showing that she valued the notion of consumer medicine but felt excluded from it at the time, she told me: "I was very frustrated, I was very frustrated because I felt like if you're a hospital, you know, I'm the patient and I thought patient-centered care [was] what it was about. But not there."

Desiree considers herself a nondenominational Christian. "I believe in God. I don't consider myself religious . . . I don't go to church or anything. I just call

myself a Christian because I believe that, you know, Christ died for our sins."
She is among the slim majority of American Christians who support the right to
abortion.[19] Now, she wanted an abortion herself, and she resented the hospital
staff for refusing to provide one. Right or wrong, she felt her drug addiction was
harming the baby[20]: "I was ashamed to be on drugs, but I didn't want to have a
drug-addicted baby . . . I didn't want the baby to be addicted to drugs . . . When
I was at [St. Mary's] they were like, 'Well the Lord wants you to . . . you're on
drugs. You know, that's not good, you know.' Like, 'I'm an everyday drug user,
all day and all night. Why would you want me to have this baby?' . . . I was absolutely clear."

Desiree was worried about the baby's health, and she neither wanted to nor
felt capable of caring for a child. Nor did she want this baby handed over to her abusive family. The clock kept ticking. Once she was too far along to get an abortion,
the diocese and a state agency set up an adoption. She explained, "It was too late
to have an abortion and they came and—knowing that I use drugs—and they
helped me, and I had the baby, and they came to get the baby."

She became pregnant two more times during this period of heavy drug use and
was able to obtain abortions. Showing herself some compassion, she said: "I was
just basically trying to survive. I mean, I lived in [a southern state] you know, under
severe abuse and then I was just thrown in the city and I just did the best that I
could." This time, she knew not to look for help at her regular clinic. A Planned
Parenthood clinic provided the first abortion, and an independent abortion clinic
outside the state provided the second, at a later gestation. Both clinics provided
her with three months' worth of birth control pills, which was not enough but was
better than nothing. She learned to use the rhythm and barrier methods during
the gaps.

Desiree also recalled the violence toward abortion clinics in those days:

> Planned Parenthood was being attacked heavily. You couldn't really get what you
> wanted, and it was on a sliding scale, and Medicaid really didn't cover every-
> thing that you needed to cover for abortions and birth control.
>
> So, I went there, and I got like—I think they gave us like ninety days for free,
> and then I just used the rhythm method 'cause I—yeah, I didn't want any kids . . .
> I counted my days and, you know, I'm educated. By that time I was educated. I
> counted my days and the only time I had sex, just wear condoms and foam.

For Desiree, birth control pills offered a less-than-ideal solution. They required fre-
quent trips for refills to clinics that were under constant attack. At one point,
Desiree tried using a Mirena IUD, but the device caused her pain. Once she decided
she could no longer tolerate the pain, she had a hard time convincing a doctor to
take it out: "It hurt and I had them to remove it. She said that it was psychosomatic,
but it wasn't. It hurt." The physician ignored Desiree's description of pain—an experience all too common among Black women.[21] When the doctor eventually agreed
to remove the IUD, the pain disappeared. That the physician's dismissiveness was

both paternalistic and racist was obvious to Desiree, who had substantial experience carefully managing her reproductive health during the period of her drug addiction. Throughout this time, she continued to receive her routine gynecological care at the Catholic hospital clinic, because it remained the most accessible Medicaid provider.

In her mid-thirties, Desiree gained control over her drug addiction. "I stopped using drugs 'cause I've learned other ways to deal with the PTSD. I mean, I didn't even know I had PTSD." She connected with a counselor who, she said, knew how to help her; specifically, the counselor effectively helped her understand the connections between the experiences of childhood trauma and her drug-addictive behavior. Around the time she was forty, she became pregnant a sixth time—and this time, she hoped to keep the baby. Tragically however, the fetus had a fatal genetic anomaly that was potentially a risk to her own health.[22] She was devastated: "They had to take it. It had a genetic defect and it would've killed me and the baby . . . I was forty years old. That was the first time I wanted to be pregnant, but, you know, it was a genetic mutation. But at no other time I wanted to be pregnant, none."

Desiree aborted that pregnancy in a non-Catholic hospital. The loss left her devastated, and she told me she had not spoken to anyone about the experience before.

Desiree's beliefs about abortion were rooted in her own history in quite specific ways. The experience of reuniting with the two children she had given up when she was young helped her recognize and name her feelings. She told me:

> I didn't know what was my belief until I told them. If you don't know what you're doing—you know what I mean—I believe that you should use a condom and the foam, condom for sexually transmitted diseases, foam for pregnancy, and count your days. I believe that you should try your best not to get pregnant because an unwanted child is the worst thing that you can do. So, I do believe if someone wants to have an abortion, then, you know, go ahead. I believe in all of it, and I do feel strongly . . . I was an unwanted child so yeah, I feel very strongly about people's right to contraceptive[s] and if need be, abortion and adoption.

Given her Christianity, I wondered if there was some part of her that supported Catholic hospital restrictions. She had grown up with the same absolutism in her family as the Catholic Church, believing that abortion was wrong even for, as in her case, rape. So I asked where she drew the line, if at all. She considered gestational limits and their equity implications, positing an idea that seemed to come to her in that moment. She proposed that only women with limited resources, like her, should be allowed to abort later in pregnancy:

> I don't suggest that you wait twenty-four weeks. But with the system being the way that it is, you may be twenty-four weeks before you can get the care that you need. If you're poor, you don't go into the doctor's office and say, "Hey, I need this." If you're poor, then you have to wait until the doctors for the poor people

show up. There are doctors for people who have regular insurance and there are doctors for people who have Medicaid, and sometimes it may take that long in care . . . for people who can't get the care that they need, twenty-four weeks, yeah, *because I lived there, I lived there, and I know that you can't get what you need.*

But if you have money, you shouldn't be able to wait to twenty-four weeks. You should just go ahead and get it over with because that's what I think every woman wants to do.

And I have a lot of experience of sitting six hours waiting for an abortion, talking to all the people in the lobby. Nobody wanted to wait. We wanted it done as soon as we found out. Like a D&C would've been great. But they just—medical care's not going to let you have what you want when you have Medicaid . . . I wouldn't take that [twenty-four-week] law off the books, because everything is slow.

While her equity-driven policy would likely be difficult to operationalize in practice, her sentiment was poignant. After a lifetime of battling for her own sexual and reproductive rights, she saw no need to provide leeway to those with few barriers to health care.

While healthcare options for low-income women remain limited, access has improved somewhat under the ACA. I asked Desiree how she would feel these days if a doctor told her that they or their hospital, opposed the care she was seeking on religious or moral grounds. She replied: "That would make me feel less angry than I felt before, because now I know I have options. I would say, 'Thank you and have a nice day.' I would leave immediately." She demonstrated some respect for Catholic hospitals' desire to operate according to their own principles, so long as other options for care remained available. She returned to equity concerns, citing the situation she was in when she was young:

They can have religious policies. That's fine. But I just think when it comes to people who have Medicaid and—they should have other options besides the Catholic hospitals . . . if there's a life-threatening thing going on and it's against their religion, then that's infringing on my rights, you know . . . I just don't want them to be clustered, that if there's a 9-1-1 call and my baby is half out of me—or it's in me or something, where they will have to perform an abortion.

I just don't think three religious hospitals should be in my zone. I think maybe one religious hospital and one not religious hospital, you know. I just think it should be even so a person can have a choice.

Desiree's way of speaking about having choices melds consumer rights with religious freedom. I asked Desiree what advice she would have for women needing pregnancy care, given religious constraints at many hospitals. She was concerned that patients might not know about the implications of a Catholic affiliation. She recommended that Catholic hospitals serve only Catholic people to avoid problems but recognized that would not solve all problems: "I would say, 'If you're not religious, you should go to a nonreligious hospital. If you're religious, you should go to a religious hospital. . . . Because some people are going to go to church once or twice a year and not really fully understand, you know, Catholicism . . . if you don't fully understand Catholicism, then you should go to another doctor.' And that should be like in their brochure somewhere, where they're advertising themselves. And I have nothing against Catholicism or religion or anything. It's just I'm not that way."

CONCLUSION

People get reproductive care in Catholic hospitals for diverse reasons that rarely hinge on the religion itself. For Rosemary, physician continuity was paramount; she prioritized trust and comfort with her doctor over most other factors. The inconvenience of not being able to get her desired sterilization after delivery was minimal since her husband was willing and able to get a vasectomy in an outpatient, non-Catholic setting instead. Zia wanted to deliver at her Catholic hospital for its quality labor and delivery service but was blocked at the entry, being told her surrogacy agreement would not be honored there before she ever became a patient. Nadia did not intentionally seek out a Catholic hospital, even though she was a highly religious Christian with abortion beliefs in line with Catholicism. She thought her hospital was Baptist. She lived begrudgingly with the consequences of her sterilization denial. Kayden wound up in a Catholic hospital motivated by his mother's trust and comfort with Dr. Ward, who did procedures there routinely. He sensed going to his mother's doctor made his mother more supportive of his gender affirmation surgery, but the decision ultimately led to an unanticipated encounter with discrimination and rejection when the Catholic hospital abruptly cancelled his long-awaited procedure. Finally, Desiree made painfully clear that as a Medicaid patient in her city she had no real choice of health care before the ACA. This meant her primary source of reproductive care was her Catholic hospital, and, thus, during her period of drug addiction, she went to term with one unwanted pregnancy and eventually found abortion care elsewhere for the next two. Her need for abortion care was directly abetted by the Catholic hospital denying her contraception when she needed it.

The illusion that Americans are healthcare consumers who can freely choose between a variety of doctors, clinics, and hospitals permeated many interviews, even though, in reality, many could not freely choose, or at least they could not do so in a meaningful and informed way. Almost all the patients with whom I spoke blamed themselves in some way for not being able to access the care they had anticipated. They said they "should have done their research" or that they "knew what they were getting into." Even those who wished they had known better did not necessarily oppose hospitals' legal right to restrict care per religion; they opposed the fact that they did not know about them and that they did not have meaningful and timely healthcare alternatives in general. Many told me that doctors should be required to disclose any religious restrictions early on, to enable patients to make better choices about care. Even then, some continued to support the religious rights of healthcare providers to restrict it, with the exception of Desiree, who knew, better than the other patients I spoke with, the real limits of consumer choice.

One of the things I found most remarkable about these conversations is that even the patients who personally opposed abortion, whether they identified as Christian or Catholic, did not want Catholic hospitals restricting their care; they wanted their providers to be *able* to provide full spectrum care even if they were individually *unwilling*. Furthermore, some felt compelled to warn others to help increase public awareness about a phenomenon potential patients may not understand. They wanted to help people become more informed healthcare consumers with little hope for larger structural changes that would alleviate the restrictions in the first place.

Notably, all the patients in this chapter sought care for non-emergencies. Even if they blamed themselves for "not doing enough research," they were describing situations in which one could, in theory, do research as opposed to medical emergencies, when advance planning is less likely. The next chapter looks at what can happen when patients end up in Catholic hospitals seeking urgent and emergency care that is restricted by the ERDs.

CHAPTER 4

Emergencies

PATIENT LOSS AND SUFFERING

Health care can be mysterious, even in the best of circumstances. Medicine is complex. Healthcare systems and insurance plans are highly inconsistent in how they deliver care and what services they cover. Nurses, administrators, and doctors must translate medicine to the uninitiated daily, and they never have enough time. Regardless of one's level of education, it is a lot to navigate. The politics and stigma of health care involving reproduction only exacerbate the problem, creating barriers between healthcare providers and patients and within communities and families. Moreover, during medical emergencies, patients rarely have time or capacity to access even the limited information available—even if one has choices of where to go, even if one knows how to research. Leaving patients in the dark about standard treatment options during pregnancy loss can deny them the fundamental dignity of choosing how to physically experience that loss.

Lack of information is different from uncertainty. Medical sociologists have long studied the challenge of practicing medicine when medical knowledge is uncertain.[1] Uncertainty in medicine never ceases to fascinate because, on balance, mounting medical knowledge seems to make certitude even more elusive; new answers just breed more questions.[2] When scholars refer to medical uncertainty, they are referring to the reality that some aspects of medical science and clinical care are truly unknowable. But the way that doctrine affects care in a Catholic hospital is all too knowable to those with access to the information. Patients lack knowledge not because it is unknowable but because it is not widely shared in a timely way. When it comes to patient awareness of hospital religious policies, not knowing has more to do with how and why relevant information is shared—or not—than with science.

In the last chapter, we considered the stories of patients who, for one reason or another, sought care at Catholic hospitals. As we have seen, these individuals encountered unanticipated obstacles to health care, even as they mostly blamed themselves for not "doing their research." Yet their ignorance is not at all anomalous. Over one-third of American women who go to a Catholic hospital for care related to reproduction do not know it is Catholic.[3] Furthermore, as discussed earlier, they have incorrect expectations about what is allowed in Catholic hospitals—the vast majority believing that tubal sterilization and contraception will be available and almost half thinking abortion would be allowed for a lethal fetal anomaly despite policies against all of these services.[4] There may be good rea son for this confusion, as hospitals follow religious policies unevenly and some-times make exceptions (see chapters 5 and 6), meaning that some people know someone else who got a birth control prescription or a tubal ligation at a Catholic hospital, making it hard for the average consumer to correctly guess what services are typically available.[5]

Interestingly, our research found that Catholic women were just as likely as non-Catholic women not to know about Catholic restrictions on reproductive health care. Those women who self-identified as highly religious appear to be slightly more aware of the policies, at least concerning abortion. Catholic women who attend reli-gious services weekly were statistically more likely than other respondents to know Catholic hospitals do not provide abortions, even for fetal anomalies.[6] How-ever, very few women, Catholic or not, know how abortion prohibitions can affect miscarriage management and obstetric emergencies. This is a complex matter that on rare occasions surfaces in the news when a patient is harmed, like Tamesha Means in Michigan, or even dies, like Savita Halappanavar in Ireland,[7] but it is not widely understood.

In this chapter, I put these findings into narrative context by examining what three patients do and do not seem to understand about what transpired with their own obstetric emergencies and what they wish they had known before seeking care. This chapter focuses on how patient knowledge about religious restrictions is medi-ated by those who know and have the power to disclose such information. I focus on the stories of three women who identify as religious: Jaelyn, Samantha, and Eliz-abeth. All had miscarriages in their local Catholic hospital, and all suffered vari-ous forms of doctrinal iatrogenesis. The stories in this chapter show us that, religious or not, Catholic or not, patients lack timely information about how Church affili-ation shapes their reproductive care.

Suffering Loss

Jaelyn, a Christian business consultant in a Northeastern city, was thirty years old when she became pregnant for the first time. She recalled: "It was very much planned, I'm a planner, I plan everything. So, I was definitely excited, I got preg-nant right away after getting off birth control. And I found out the day we came back from my dream vacation." But soon after, her excitement shifted into nerves. Looking back, she sees that feeling as a foreboding sign. Jaelyn's cervix had been compromised from a colposcopy a few years earlier, done to remove tissue grow-ing at an alarming rate. She and her doctor planned to monitor the situation closely as part of her prenatal care.

As a Black woman, Jaelyn had put great care into her choice of doctor: "I chose her because she was female and a Black woman. And I wanted to—I know how disparity works in that regard. And I wanted somebody who at least I thought would see me." I knew what she was referring to. News stories and academic research have provided ample documentation for something many Black women already know; namely, that Black women suffer worse pregnancy outcomes and die at higher rates from childbirth in the United States than other women. This is a reality driven by racism, not race.[8] I probed to get Jaelyn to say more about her specific concerns. She elaborated, mentioning a key source of the phenomenon: "Black women are seen to be able to sort of take more pain . . . so I chose a Black woman for my comfort . . . I wanted someone who would be an advocate for me and see me as wholly human."

Jaelyn had been with this doctor since she was twenty-two, so it seemed only natural that she should continue to see her when she became pregnant: "I wasn't thinking about having a baby, or any of that stuff when I started seeing her. And even when I was pregnant, I never even thought about how she had practiced at a Catholic hospital. And she never mentioned it to me . . . I feel like it was all brand new to me when the event happened."

One night in Jaelyn's second trimester, she began to cramp, and then the cramps became rhythmic. She determined she was in labor and headed with her husband to the hospital where she had planned to deliver. She said: "[My doctor] had not talked to me about 'if there's an emergency, let's do this, this is the protocol.' So, I just went to the emergency room."

Once there, Jaelyn faced a long wait before seeing a doctor. She recalled the receptionist feeling badly for her, but there were many other emergencies competing for the staff's attention. She was eventually wheeled up to the labor and delivery unit, only to be told she did not yet qualify to be there:

> I was in so much pain, and you know I was screaming, "Please help me. I do not want to lose my baby." And so somebody took me up to labor and delivery and they were like, "no." They asked me how many weeks I was, and I was like, "I'm nineteen and five days," and they were like, "[you] have to be at least twenty weeks to come up here."
>
> So they sent me back downstairs, and the person just left me, whoever wheeled me up just kinda left me, and then finally I guess I was through the triage portion of it, and the [ER] doctor saw me and was basically like, "Yep, you are in labor and your cervix is open and so your bag is coming out and you know, we're going to send you up to labor and delivery."

With frustration and a touch of sarcasm in her voice, she continued: "So guess what, I end up in labor and delivery to deliver a baby where they, two hours earlier, sent me back from because I was not twenty weeks."

Once upstairs, the on-call ob-gyn confirmed that the amniotic sac was visible and protruding from the cervix. She recalled being told: "There's nothing we can do, because if we try to push it back in, it's very likely you're going to get an infection. And the baby will die. And it puts you at risk too. So, we have to see this thing through." Jaelyn was devastated at the loss, but having already spent two to three hours in the emergency room, she also desperately wanted the physical pain and emotional crisis to end. Instead, the doctor let her know this was just the beginning. She recalled asking: "Can we just get it over with," and they were like, 'No 'cause we're a Catholic hospital and we cannot assist in it, we have to wait until the baby's heart stops.' So they hooked me up to a machine where we got to see and hear the baby's heart for like eight or nine hours, I don't know, it was something crazy."

As explained earlier, medical standards of practice for patients in Jaelyn's situation focus on allowing the patient to choose between three options for miscarriage management: inducing labor with medication, dilating the cervix to remove the fetus and tissue (a dilation and evacuation, or D&E), or expectant management (no intervention while stable). In a hospital unconstrained by religious restrictions, a patient like Jaelyn would typically be invited to discuss the pros and cons of three choices, none of which are clearly superior in terms of physical safety.[9] People make their choices based upon a variety of medical circumstances and personal preferences. The key, however, is that they are *able to choose*.[10]

By requesting to "get it over with," Jaelyn made clear that she preferred a procedure, a D&E, to speed along the inevitable. That she was allowed only expectant management was how Jaelyn became aware that her chosen hospital followed Catholic doctrine. She vaguely knew the hospital was Catholic, but she had not thought about what this might mean prior to this moment, nor had her doctor mentioned the issue. She might have guessed that a Catholic hospital would not provide abortions, but she had no intention of seeking an abortion when she chose the doctor or the hospital. In the midst of losing a pregnancy she had very much hoped to keep, she simply longed for an end to her pain and suffering. But as Jaelyn would soon learn, Catholic hospitals place a spiritual value on suffering that she did not share. Directive 61 states: "Patients experiencing suffering that *cannot be* alleviated should be helped to appreciate the Christian understanding of redemptive suffering."[11] Jaelyn did not value her suffering at that moment, nor did she in retrospect. She knew her suffering *could be* alleviated, which is why she asked for intervention.[12]

I asked Jaelyn about how the staff responded to her desire to "get it over with," because I knew the staff would see this as a request for an abortion. She responded that she could not recall anyone expressing regrets about not being able to surgically or medically end the pregnancy; instead, everyone repeatedly expressed sympathy for her loss and offered pain control for her forthcoming delivery: "They apologized [saying], 'We know this is hard,' and that kind of thing. And they basically told me, his heart will stop and he'll either come out, or you'll push, or something along those lines. They asked me if I wanted an epidural, and initially I didn't, but then probably about six or seven hours [in] I decided, 'Yeah, let's do this, 'cause I don't know how long this is going to go on.'"

Having to listen to and watch the heart monitor for hours distressed Jaelyn. I asked her if they ever offered to turn the heart monitor off, or if she asked for that. She couldn't recall. She said: "Maybe they turned [the volume] down, but they still had the monitor up, so I don't know if the hearing of it was psychological, but I could see it. They were watching it and waiting until it stopped so they could move forward with the process."

It took twelve hours. At that point, the doctor let Jaelyn know she could "take him out now." She does not recall the doctors performing any kind of procedure other than rupturing the amniotic sac, which, in theory, could have happened many hours earlier had they not waited for his heart to stop. "She just bust the bag—'cause it was already hanging out—so she ruptured the bag and he came sliding right out."

The nursing staff told Jaelyn they would clean him up, take pictures, and bring him back so she could hold him. Jaelyn's voice lowered to an almost inaudible whisper when she recounted her response: "I don't want to hold him." She could not relate to the measures the staff took to offer her the opportunity to connect and say goodbye to him. It seemed to her as if they did not understand her state of shock and trauma. She continued: "[They asked] 'Are you sure?' And I was like [again, low and quiet] 'No. Can't do that.'" At this point, we took a slight pause in our conversation. This was a viscerally remembered exchange that revealed both the grief she felt about losing him and how profoundly misunderstood she felt by the hospital staff. They were following the protocol scripted for perinatal loss patients, which includes the period between twenty-two weeks gestation and seven days after birth,[13] but the protocol did not feel appropriate or meaningful to her.

Jaelyn continued: "They took him into some room—'cause I know my parents saw him, and maybe my husband. I can't remember. But I never went to see him. And they brought me a box with a little bear that they had with him with the pictures, and a blanket and hat they had on him, with a few pictures in a box. And they were like, you can go home."

When she got home, her ob-gyn called to check on her. She asked why Jaelyn hadn't called her, to which she could only reply: "I didn't know to call you."

Jaelyn recalled spending the following weeks immersed in grief. She was constantly weepy and spent a lot of energy asking other medical professionals whether more could have been done to save the pregnancy: "I got second opinions about what happened and whether it had to go down like that." She learned that a cerclage, which is a procedure to literally bind the cervix shut, might have helped earlier in the pregnancy, or even possibly if applied very early in her trip to the emergency room, but she could never be certain that a cerclage would have staved off the loss.

When she finally went to see her doctor for a follow-up visit one or two weeks later, she felt her doctor failed to "see her" as she had hoped, and it stung:

> I was still very emotional, and she was concerned at the level of emotion I was still experiencing. And I was befuddled [small chuckle] at why that would have surprised her so. I mean, any loss is a loss. But given the fact that I was halfway through my pregnancy—I was very much showing . . . Everybody knew I was pregnant—This just happens out of nowhere; three days after I found out the sex, we were all excited, we shared it with everybody . . . At that point I could feel him move and all those things and when you really start to plan your life . . .

So yeah, that was very difficult. And her response to me: "I'm really concerned with how upset you are . . ." I didn't even respond to her, I wasn't saying I was going to kill myself, I was just crying, nonstop, like crying.

Jaelyn's doctor gave her a referral to a therapist, but she did not use it. She felt her grief was proportionate to and appropriate for the events that had transpired. Jaelyn did not blame her doctor directly for what had happened, but she noted that the doctor had not helped before, during, or after the trauma, and her lack of understanding left a bad taste. And, critically, Jaelyn's doctor had omitted information about the hospital's religious restrictions, leaving her in the dark about her options in case of a medical emergency. She decided to look for a new ob-gyn.

I asked her what she would have preferred to have happened, looking back. Her response focused on two issues: the delay in getting seen by the obstetrics unit and the delay in getting treatment. She did not dwell on her wait in the ER, perhaps because ERs are known to have unpredictable flow. In contrast, she found the delay in being sent to labor and delivery because she was two days shy of twenty weeks infuriating. She zeroed in on what she called "the hypocrisy" of the hospital's being both unwilling to work to save the baby and unwilling to help her end her own suffering during the miscarriage. She said:

> You know, they weren't treating the baby like a life when I came up at nineteen weeks and five days, they were treating it like disposable, I don't want to say disposable, but yeah, [like] it wasn't that serious . . . but now it's a life and we can't touch it and it's got to run the course.
>
> It was very hypocritical. So I would have liked to, one, have been seen right away and hopefully have my child saved, but if that wasn't an option I would have liked the choice to get myself out of physical and mental anguish as quickly as possible.

In juxtaposing the words "life" and "disposable," Jaelyn's comments hint at how abortion politics infused the clinical experience. She would have preferred to have been offered medicine or a procedure to end the traumatic episode sooner, an approach that would have implicitly demonstrated that *her* life and suffering mattered: "To force somebody to continue to be in that state when the result is going to be more pain anyway. Like, 'Preserve *MY* life right now—you already told me you can't preserve this life—so, like, preserve mine!' And part of that is limiting my trauma."

Jaelyn and I spoke toward the end of the summer of 2020, a moment when the combined force of the COVID-19 pandemic and sustained Black Lives Matter protests offered daily reminders of how racism shortens Black life expectancy in the United States. All summer, people wearing masks marched in most major and many smaller U.S. cities, and "Black Lives Matter" was being painted into enormous street murals throughout the world. Jaelyn's imploring and urgent tone ("preserve *MY* life") seemed to echo the movement's imperative when she questioned the hospital's concern for her life. That night, she endured a lengthy and embodied experience of neglect that brought her no spiritual solace.

Jaelyn could not have been clearer. Waiting for her baby's heart to stop on its own was not emotionally or spiritually comforting for her then, and neither the passage of time nor the delivery of a healthy child a few years later have done anything to change her feelings. Jaelyn was exceptionally aware of how Catholic doctrine affected her miscarriage management in comparison with most women I interviewed. At the same time, she shows exactly how so many women do not know about religious restrictions until they are directly affected.

THE CHALLENGE OF ANTICIPATORY GUIDANCE

Let's pause for a moment to consider how things might have gone differently for Jaelyn. Most obviously, would she have chosen a different hospital had she known more about the Catholic policies? Would having information about this conflict in religious obstetrics in advance have made a difference? When asked, Jaelyn immediately responded that disclosure should be "part of the onboarding process" with a doctor in the first prenatal appointment: "I think there is an obligation to share certain things [like], 'If there is an emergency, or if you or the baby are in distress, here's what we will and won't do because we are a Catholic hospital as opposed to a [non-Catholic] hospital.'" Jaelyn cautioned, however, that doctors might need to ask the patient directly about whether they want to discuss pregnancy contingency plans. "I think it depends on the woman because some people want all the details and all the scary parts . . . and then others want to live in their bubble and deal with stuff as it comes up."

Jaelyn's sense that people vary in their preferences about receiving this kind of information is accurate, which complicates the question of whether it is practical or even possible for doctors to provide anticipatory guidance for their patients. While the vast majority of women want to know about a hospital's religious restrictions on care before seeking care there, how to best inform patients in advance is not obvious.[14] It is important to acknowledge that disclosure and guidance about the Ethical and Religious Directives for Catholic Health Care Services is likely not enough to mitigate the ethical problem of denying standard obstetric interventions. Yet, in the absence of a better solution anytime soon, I asked all patients about what kind of information they would want in the interim, how it should be communicated, and at what point in their care.[15] Basically, I asked what individual-level changes in clinical practice might support patients until the law can effectively address the overstepping of religious power in health care.

Regarding miscarriage specifically, about two-thirds of patients I interviewed supported the idea of receiving a detailed explanation of the religious restrictions on treatment early in prenatal care, when they could still change hospitals and/or doctors. They thought it was not only necessary but empowering. However, a minority did not support routine disclosure. Two respondents agreed with the Catholic hospitals' religious policies and considered their routine disclosure unnecessary and undesirable. One-quarter of the women interviewed felt the issue of miscarriage management would be too upsetting for pregnant patients to discuss; disclosure was not worth the potential anxieties it might generate.

Seven years out from the event, Jaelyn wishes her doctor had been more forthcoming. She says: "I'm like a really straight shooter, just give it to me. So, I might not be saying the right thing for the woman who needs the hand holding and the back stroking and the fantasyland version of everything. I'm not that person, I want to know, like tell me stuff so I can have a plan in mind. We all know we can lose our child. We all know miscarriage is a risk." For her, not knowing how care differed at her Catholic hospital contributed to her suffering, and ultimately, her experience of being harmed.

Here is where things get tricky. Demonstrating exactly why disclosure is not an adequate solution, Jaelyn told me that having had this information would not have changed her behavior, only her response to the situation. After reflecting on the question, she told me that she probably would have perceived the discussion as a medical formality, like any consent process of risks and benefits.[16] She said: "Nobody thinks that is going to happen to them. You are like, OK, you're hearing it and processing it as these are the steps that need to happen. She has to do this part, this is not going to happen to me." If, on the other hand, she had heard a similar story from a friend, she believes she might have taken the (hypothetical) conversation to heart. As she explained: "I had not heard of this kind of situation. Probably if I had, prior to me getting pregnant, I would have been like 'I'm not having a baby in a Catholic hospital, you hear what happened to such and such?' . . . it wouldn't have had to happen to me for me to think about what hospital, what doctor? You know, that sort of thing. But in the absence of knowing about these situations at all. . . . [it's just] 'they just have to say stuff like this, precautions.'"

The patients I spoke with who had heard such stories from their friends were notably more cognizant and concerned about the implications of Catholic doctrine for miscarriage. For example, when I asked Zia (from the previous chapter) if she had heard about religious policies that could affect miscarriage management—a question late in the interview that for most others drew a blank—she immediately said: "Yeah. I've heard about that." I asked her to say more, and she launched into a story much like Jaelyn's:

> One of my friends actually had gone to another Catholic hospital [in the region] called [Mercy] and she was having a miscarriage and the baby—there wasn't anything that they could do and the baby was still alive. And so, she was asking for help because she didn't want to have to suffer, you know, through that. That's really—that's something that's really emotional, you know. Like I know firsthand how emotional it is, and they told her that they wouldn't help her end the child's life . . . They said that it's against the Catholic religion.
>
> She was really, really upset and she's like very—she is very religious. She's Catholic, you know, and she understands. So, she was very upset about it and she wound up just going, you know, through and just waiting until the baby

passed and everything, which made everything so much harder. I just remember that. She wasn't—she wasn't right, like after that, for months.

I asked Zia whether she believed her friend was suffering because of the loss of the
baby itself or because of the trauma associated with denied treatment. Zia replied:
"I think—well, the loss, obviously, was like a big part of it because when you lose
a child—you know, a baby is always a blessing and, you know, her and her husband were very, very happy about it and then that happened. But then knowing
that she had to go home and then, you know, wait, I think that's what hurt her."
    The fact that Zia's friend shared her story of loss with Zia increased Zia's own
awareness of the range of possible pregnancy outcomes. Yet, people do not always
share these stories.[17] Reproduction is both prized and stigmatized for women, and
the stigma associated with having an unsuccessful pregnancy can increase the
harm associated with Catholic hospitals' restrictions. Not only do hospitals make
it difficult for patients to learn how their care is restricted, but even if they do learn,
they do not necessarily know what to do with that information or that it could apply
to them. This transparency problem is compounded for Black women, who have
every reason to fear not having their medical concerns taken seriously and suffering
a bad outcome due to racism.[18] Unfortunately, bad pregnancy outcomes do happen
to lots of people, and the ERDs only make things worse by denying patients autonomy over how to go through the sometimes lengthy and physically arduous process.

CONFUSION

Samantha is a white woman who was living in the Northeast with her husband
and four daughters at the time of our interview. A member of the Church of Jesus
Christ of Latter-Day Saints, she considers herself very religious. She grew up in the
faith and attends services or events about six times per week. She explained her
views about contraception and abortion, which were relatively more flexible than
I expected given her religious background: "There isn't necessarily like a church
policy about whether or not contraception is, you know, allowed or a moral type
of a thing. But we do believe that we've been commanded of God to multiply and
to have families, to raise children. So the idea is you want to have children but how
many you have is kind of a personal—you know—between you and your husband
and God, and you can decide what's right for your family."
    Relatedly, Samantha explained, she is grateful for contraception in her life
because it has allowed her to pace her physical and emotional readiness for each
child:

I like contraception because I think it helps me to feel prepared to have a baby.
I mean, historically, my pregnancies aren't the worst in the world, but I do get
kind of sick. So, I feel like I—having a little bit of say about when I'm going to
have a baby or when I feel ready to be pregnant for nine months, you know, that
has been really great. And I think it's also really helped our relationship so that

we can have intimacy and have fun getting to know each other and not like, "Oh, but this means we're going to have another baby."

Samantha values the control, the time, and the ability to have non-procreative sex with her husband; she seemed to be comfortable talking about these contraceptive benefits.

Samantha's first two children were born in a hospital in Utah with no religious affiliation. She fondly recalled how the hospital was able to meet her and her husband's religious needs during the birth: "They had some missionaries from the church that would come . . . they came by and they said, 'Hey, would you like to take the sacrament because it's a Sunday.' It was like Easter Sunday or something, so it was actually really cool because they came in and my husband was able to help bless the sacrament and we had the sacrament while I was getting ready to have the baby."

An effective hospital chaplaincy enabled these missionaries to access patients of their faith. She appreciated this, saying: "I felt like my needs were completely met, even though it wasn't like the hospital's priority to be religious. I still felt like my needs were met when I was there."

By the time of Samantha's next pregnancy, she and her family had moved to a city in the eastern part of the United States. She had not yet picked an ob-gyn when she started cramping and bleeding, around eleven or twelve weeks. She and her husband headed to the nearest emergency room for care, which was in a Catholic hospital. From her telling, it appears to have been a small hospital that lacked a labor and delivery service: "We didn't know where anything was in the area. So we just went to the closest hospital, and they were actually not equipped to have a maternity unit. So, when I went to the ER there, you know, it felt kind of alien to them to have this, 'Oh, we have a woman here who's having a miscarriage,' like, 'Why didn't she go to a different hospital?' you know. And they had everything they needed to take care of me, but it was an awkward and really emotional experience . . . it was just a difficult, tension-filled ER."

Samantha's emotional experience of her treatment there ("alien, awkward, and tension-filled") dominated her description. The staff did not seem to be prepared for someone experiencing pregnancy complications even though this is a common occurrence in emergency departments.[19] The Catholic hospitals' religious restrictions on reproductive care never came up in her account, though, based on her experience, I suspect they came into play in her treatment in a way that was not made clear to her. She perceived the hospital staff only as unprepared and haphazard: "It was a very old hospital and so I think the way that they had had to build and rebuild, it was like kind of a joke, like a maze, you know. And so at one point like this IV that they'd put in fell out and so there was blood and this isn't really my thing. I don't like seeing my own blood, and it was like the experience, the worst possible that I could have, you know, I guess aside from like dying or whatever. It was a pretty rough day."

She recalls that the staff eventually told her she needed an ultrasound, without explaining much about what they saw. "The tech didn't say anything. He was just—he did the ultrasound but wouldn't really talk to me. So, I was like okay, well I know something's wrong because you're not talking to me, but . . . You know, it was just things like that, where I'm like, 'This is strange and I'm uncomfortable . . .'"

It took a "number of hours" for the medical staff to formulate a treatment plan. She recalled: "I think I suspected it [was a miscarriage], but I wasn't aware of the process 'cause I'd not had one before."

Listening to her story, I gleaned that what seemed to Samantha like poor communication actually may have been intentional withholding of information. Given the religious policies and other accounts of miscarriage management in Catholic hospitals akin to Jennifer's in the introduction of the book, the medical staff was likely buying time to discern how to treat the miscarriage given the constraints of the ERDs. To me, it seemed they were stalling and awaiting fetal death, not rushing to the ultrasound, concerned that a heartbeat might foreclose other treatment options.

Eventually, however, they did move forward. "So when they told me, 'When we looked at the ultrasound, there was no fetal, you know, heartbeat or anything so we think that, you know, the fetus has died and you're miscarrying and we need to help you, you know, expedite the process. So you need to eat this pill.' And I was like wait, seriously?"

While Samantha had never heard of using medication to expedite a miscarriage, she was glad to eventually have been offered the misoprostol to help the end come more quickly. After she took it in the ER, they sent her home with nausea medication to help with the side effects. She, nevertheless, would have preferred more information about how the treatment would affect her once she left the hospital: "I was surprised. I didn't realize. I actually assumed they'd just be like, 'Well just go home and it'll run its course,' but I am glad that they gave me the pill 'cause it probably would've taken longer if they hadn't. But they also didn't really prep me, [or] be like, 'Hey, this is going to feel kind of like a delivery. You're going to be in a lot of pain.' So there was a lot that I just kind of had to struggle through after I got home."

When asked if she would have preferred to have been offered an aspiration procedure to empty her uterus (dilation and curettage, or D&C) right there in the ER, Samantha said yes. That said, she wasn't sure she would have known then how comforting it might have been to have left the hospital with an empty uterus rather than wondering for months whether it had emptied itself. "I might have wanted it, because after the fact, I did wonder and had questions like, 'Did everything—like is my body ready to go again? Like am I good to go?' So that was kind of difficult a couple months later, when I was actually kind of unsure, you know. Like well am I okay? Like I don't really know. So I wish they had offered more, I guess, or maybe educated me more. So I don't know."

To be sure, miscarriage management is a weak spot in emergency medicine generally. Researchers fault the physical environment, inadequacies in clinician training, and insensitivity to patients' emotional experience of the event.[20] There are numerous possible explanations for why Samantha was not offered a D&C at the ER, but best practices, nevertheless, emphasize informing a patient of all available options. Whatever the cause, it is clear that no one informed Samantha of the standard three choices of how to manage miscarriage (medication, procedure, or expectant), or even spent much time educating her on what to expect next.

In hope of gaining a clearer understanding of Samantha's experience, I attempted to confirm that her miscarriage took place at a Catholic hospital. I later confirmed that it was, but as we were speaking, Samantha was not sure: "I believe it was Catholic. I would need to double-check but they did have—I mean, it was a saint someone hospital. So I assume they were Catholic. A lot of—that was a very Catholic area . . . I wasn't thinking oh, this hospital has a religious affiliation or anything. I just wanted to be seen and get some help. I don't think anyone mentioned anything. There may have been some religious art on the walls, but I'm not certain about that."

Samantha's reaction is consistent with that of many people who do not know, or particularly care, whether a hospital is Catholic. It often is hard to tell, even if you are looking for it. In our national survey, only one in three women initially said it was somewhat or very important to know a hospital's religious affiliation before seeking care. But when the survey subsequently informed them that "*some hospitals restrict some ob-gyn and reproductive procedures because of the religion*," the level of interest changed dramatically. With that information in hand, four out of five women told us that it was important or very important to know a hospital's religious policies for care. In other words, most women do not know that a hospital *can* impose religious restrictions on care. Once made aware of that fact, they care very much.

Doctors working in Catholic hospitals rarely discuss the ERDs unless they specifically limit a service requested by a patient. But Samantha, of course, did not know what she should want or need, never having experienced a miscarriage before. Part of what I found so notable about Samantha's story is that she still does not know whether the hospital's policies affected her care, even after the fact. However, given what she shared, I came to believe the poor quality of care, delays, and disinterest in offering her surgical management related to the Catholic ownership. I share her story specifically to show how murky it can be for patients navigating new reproductive experiences with little disclosure of religious limitations on care.

Samantha is a person of deep faith, but her faith does not inspire her to want to regulate other bodies. She does not endorse blanket restrictions on abortions. In her words, a woman's decision to have an abortion "should be between her and God and her doctor." And while she supports an individual physician's rights to decline to provide certain care, she remains concerned about patient autonomy in the context of institutional restrictions, especially if the patient does not have access to other facilities. She explained: "It's one thing to have, you know, a provider, a doctor, say, 'I'm not comfortable with that but my colleague over here is. So, if you're okay, you can just see that person,' you know. That would be different. But to have the hospital say, 'We don't offer that procedure,' when maybe your insurance says you're only allowed to go to this hospital, that's a denial of healthcare that I don't think is fair."

The circumstances of real life mean that sometimes patients find themselves in hospitals they do not know much about. While Samantha's care for her miscarriage was confusing and neglectful, she ultimately received treatment, though not necessarily the one she might have chosen given more information. It is hard to imagine that she would have sought care elsewhere if the ERDs had been disclosed to her when she entered the ER, because she did not know enough about miscarriage management to have perceived it as problematic at the time. Disclosure simply is not enough. Still, had she known more about the religious restrictions, she might have had, at least, a greater sense of control that can come from simply understanding what is happening to one's body. The Emergency Medical Treatment and Active Labor Act requires emergency departments to treat people who show up in an unstable condition, including anyone who arrives in labor or miscarrying and needing help. Samantha's ER did take her in, but between religious restrictions and a general lack of preparedness, her care was certainly substandard.

REGRET

Like Samantha, Elizabeth is highly religious. She is a white Catholic woman living in a small Western town located about forty-five minutes outside a major city. She does not attend services often, but her Catholicism is very important to her:

> I do have a solid belief in God, but I have kind of taken myself away from my church, just because I don't—I think that The Church has gotten too politicized, and I think the community aspect is just—it's definitely a social status thing, and I'm just not finding it rewarding . . .
>
> I joined a mother's group in the church and I just really got weighted down with, you know, who spends the most money, fits in the best. And it just kind of ruined the experience for me, and I just kind of got to the point where I don't need to go to a church in order to have a relationship with God.

Elizabeth has a high school education. She belongs to a small subset of Catholic people (8 percent)[21] whose beliefs about contraception and sterilization are well-aligned with those of the Church. "I'm a married woman and so no, I probably wouldn't use birth control . . . And I also am aware of my cycles and how to prevent pregnancy naturally without using any other tools or devices." At the time we spoke, she had five children and had experienced one ectopic pregnancy and three miscarriages, which she sums up as four losses.

Elizabeth firmly opposes abortion in all instances. She wants more children, but her miscarriage experiences were traumatic. Each time, she hemorrhaged to the point of unconsciousness and retained the placenta, which required further medical intervention. Understandably, she has some fear about getting pregnant again: "I just think emotionally I'm not up for it anymore." She told me: "I've been contemplating [sterilization] in the last couple months, just because I just don't think I can go through another loss. But at the same time, I just feel like I would be devastated to know that my body could no longer have babies."

Elizabeth had primarily sought care at Catholic hospitals, but not because of their religious affiliation. She said: "For me personally, when making the choice, I usually go by who is closest to—what hospital's closest to me." As it happens, Elizabeth lives in an area dominated by Catholic hospitals, so she'd had more visits to them than she could count, including for her first loss, the ectopic pregnancy. She recalled the experience from several years earlier: "I went to the emergency room once because I had started spotting. And they did an ultrasound and told me that they didn't see anything and, with as far along as I was, they should have. And then they sent me home. And then a couple days later I went back because I was in excruciating pain, and at that time I was admitted and treated for ectopic . . . I was given methotrexate."

As mentioned in chapter 2, doctors often use methotrexate, a cancer drug, to stop the growth of the embryonic cells in the fallopian tube, after which the body reabsorbs the tissue. This prevents the tube from bursting and potentially killing the pregnant person. Since ectopic pregnancies clearly threaten the life of the mother, methotrexate is the common course of treatment. Nevertheless, Directive 48 prohibits "direct abortion," in the case of extrauterine (ectopic) pregnancy, which for years meant that Catholic medical ethicists counseled physicians to remove the whole fallopian tube without touching the pregnancy directly per the principle of double effect.[22] Today, it seems Catholic hospitals quietly allow methotrexate. But Elizabeth became deeply upset once she learned about the bishops' prohibition on methotrexate, and she felt somewhat betrayed by the hospital. Her providers there had encouraged her to participate in what she considered a grave sin, despite the hospital's religious affiliation.

The hospital's approach to treating her ectopic pregnancy, while standard, safe, and the best way to preserve her fertility, made Elizabeth question the religious adherence and spiritual quality of the hospital. In essence, it was not Catholic enough for her.

I guess I put too much emphasis on the fact that it's a Catholic church—[I mean] hospital. And so when I kind of researched the church's views on—because, you know, technically the treatment for an ectopic pregnancy is an abortion, and methotrexate isn't exactly one of the things that the church wants you to use to resolve it.

And I didn't know that, and I kind of felt like the hospital should have, you know, informed me better about that. I just assumed, because they are a Catholic hospital they would have . . . Because I always list my religion as Catholic on my paperwork, so I kind of felt like I did something wrong afterwards.

I asked if she would have preferred for the doctors to explain that methotrexate would destroy her pregnancy. But Elizabeth was not looking for medical clarification. Rather, she longed for a spiritually authoritative discussion that would have helped her see it as the right thing to do, as the path of action the Church would have wanted.

ELIZABETH: Well no, I knew that it would [end the pregnancy]. I just wish I would have known that the church didn't prefer that method . . . I just kind

> of felt like that I'd done something wrong that I wasn't supposed to and I
> should have resolved it another way. I mean, obviously you can't *not* treat it
> because I would die, but you know . . .
> LORI: What would—do you—after having read about it, do you have a sense of
> what you would have preferred?
> ELIZABETH: I don't think I would have wanted to lose my tubes, just because I
> wanted to have more children. So I think I would have ended up choosing that
> anyway . . . I think I would have felt so torn either way, but I don't know. I think
> it was just—I just felt like I had done something wrong all the way around.

She had assumed, because the hospital was Catholic and knew that she was Catholic, some sort of religious authority would ensure her care conformed to Catholic doctrine. She assumed that any matters involving doctrinal ambiguity would not be left up to her and her doctor. After all, she had heard of people needing special permission from clergy to get a tubal ligation:

> You just kind of assume that they would have Catholic priorities, because the
> church is pretty strict about that. If the Catholic church's name is affiliated,
> they're pretty strict about that with most things. And so I think it was just an
> assumption that they would be more strict about guidelines of care. I did know
> that several people that I knew that wanted to have tubal ligations needed permission from—as they said—the nuns to do that. So I just always assumed that
> the Catholic church kind of instigated their beliefs in the treatment of care, you
> know, how they handled patient care.

I asked Elizabeth if speaking to a Catholic advisor would have helped her. It turned out that she was, indeed, offered the opportunity to talk with a priest after the treatment, but she had declined. While she regretted that decision, she was more upset that no one had informed her that she was agreeing to a form of abortion *before* beginning treatment. She explained:

> I wasn't in the emotional state to talk to a, you know, a stranger or whatever about
> it. So it was later, afterward, when I had read that, you know, how the Catholic
> Church viewed ectopic pregnancy and the treatment of it . . . And so technically
> the treatment for ectopic is elective abortion, even though if you don't do it, you're
> going to die. So that terminology—and to me abortion is somebody making a
> choice to, you know, kill their baby—that's abortion, in my opinion.
> And so not having a choice in the matter of my losses, but the word abortion
> being used, was just as traumatic as my loss . . . knowing that the church viewed
> my lack of a choice as an abortion. Because, you know, no—I don't know very
> many women out there who had an ectopic viewed as you have any other choice.

Elizabeth was the first and only person I spoke with who genuinely felt her health care did not conform closely enough to Catholic doctrine. She was deeply unsettled to have been given a treatment that the bishops equate to abortion in the

ERDs. Yet, as we have seen, the bishops' preferred standard (default removal of a portion of the fallopian tube) is so far afield from the medical standard that physicians and hospital leadership routinely ignored the directive.[23] None of the doctors I spoke to could recall having to consult the ethics committee to treat ectopic pregnancies the way they had to for miscarriage, and it seems unlikely that hospitals' lawyers could win the infertility or wrongful death lawsuits that could result from this approach. Perhaps this is why the Catholic Health Association states on its website that administering methotrexate is morally acceptable, even while Catholic theologians and the bishops continue to write as if it is not.[24]

Elizabeth had trusted that a Catholic hospital would protect her from abortion and other spiritual transgressions. The fact that it did not filled her with disappointment and regret. Even with her relatively advanced knowledge of both Catholic doctrine and obstetrics, she had not realized that the ERDs sometimes conflict with medical standards of care. Once she learned of the existence of such conflicts, she argued that Catholic hospitals have a responsibility to alert their patients, particularly their Catholic patients, to both the spiritual and medical risks. The opportunity to speak with a priest *after* the treatment could not repair what Elizabeth considered the spiritual and moral threat of a therapeutic abortion.

Technically speaking, Elizabeth experienced not one, but four abortions, albeit three of them spontaneous and one of them therapeutic. For Elizabeth, the knowledge that medical staff referred to her miscarriages as "spontaneous abortions" was an additional source of anguish. She was very tearful at moments in the interview; she remained quite devastated by her losses. The stigma of abortion seemed to cling to her experiences of miscarriage despite her sophisticated understanding of their medical inevitability. She was terribly sensitive to the insinuation that she might have had a choice in the matter.

Elizabeth still remembers the insensitivity of the ER staff and the ambulance drivers who responded to the two miscarriages after the ectopic pregnancy. She recalls vividly how the ambulance driver for the second miscarriage referred to it as "spontaneous abortion":

> The ambulance driver or whoever was in charge kept saying, "Well, this looks like a spontaneous abortion," and he repeated that over and over and over again . . . *[Crying through her words:]* It wasn't an abortion to me, so you know, that was hard. I mean it felt, you know, it just felt wrong for him to keep saying that to me, you know, because I wasn't having an abortion. I was having a miscarriage. It wasn't a choice. So the terminology used, you know, in early pregnancy loss, you know, I mean you're already going through a whole lot emotionally, and I think using terms like that is just, to me it's inhumane to tell a woman who wanted her baby that *[more tears]*.

Years later, Elizabeth remained angry and hurt that medical and Church authorities alike used the word "abortion" to describe an ending to a pregnancy that a woman did not bring about by her own choice.

Her third miscarriage took place a bit further along than the other two—sixteen weeks. While devastating in its own way, the hospital experience was much more positive and emotionally sensitive than the previous two occasions. She explained:

> I just started having the bleeding . . . I went to bed and the next morning I got up and the bleeding had subsided, but I had—my water broke. So I went to the ER. This time, rather than staying in the ER they sent me up to labor and delivery. Once I got up there, they did a test to see if my water did actually break, and my doctor came in and ordered an ultrasound. And in fact I had no water left and the baby's foot had actually come down through the cervix. And so she ordered the misoprostol to kind of let the cervix open so the baby could pass.

Elizabeth did not mention the potential conflict with the ERDs or frame the use of a medication to end her miscarriage as problematic. Either she did not know or, equally as likely, no one knew. For the sake of the research project, I could have asked Elizabeth if there were heart tones, but I did not. She was crying, precisely because of her guilt and distress about the loss and the related stigma, and I could not rub salt in the wound simply for the sake of a scholarly clarification. But whether Elizabeth was aware of it or not, my conversations with other doctors and patients have made abundantly clear that Catholic hospitals frequently resist offering misoprostol before twenty weeks if the fetus is still alive. Why, in this case, was this course of treatment allowed?

One possibility is that the doctor simply decided, based on Elizabeth's prior history of hemorrhaging, not to check, so as to not complicate an already charged situation. Here's what Elizabeth told me:

> And after the baby passed my placenta didn't come, so lots of heavy bleeding and she had to call in [the doctor] to come in and do a D&C . . . [Crying, we paused, she continued:] Still not over it . . . It's hard not to cry about it . . . And I felt better this time because I was in with my doctor—like I said, I was in the labor and delivery area and I just felt more personalized, you know? Like I didn't feel like I was treated like a triage situation, you know, like her life was valued [more tears, pause].
>
> So this time because I was so far along I had to figure out funeral arrangements, which was hard . . . They would have taken the baby if I didn't want to do anything like that, but it was something that had always bothered me with my past miscarriages that I didn't choose to contact the church or have anything like that. But I think, you know, I just wanted it over so I could move on.
>
> So, we had her cremated. They helped with all of that. And they took pictures of her and her footprints and her handprints. They gave me a box with mementos and stuff . . . Just the difference of being up [on labor and delivery] and they let me stay as long as I wanted to hold her. They didn't rush me to leave so they could have the room. So, I just felt that, you know, that time compared to my others [in the ER] was just handled so much more compassionately.

While her care went much better this time around, Elizabeth's appraisal of her Catholic hospital experience overall was mixed. What is most relevant here, however, is that even Elizabeth was disappointed at the hospital's lack of transparency about how its religious policies dovetail with medical practice. Particularly with her experience with ectopic pregnancy, Elizabeth ended up feeling spiritually abandoned, caught between the bishops who authoritatively issue unsafe ectopic guidelines and the Catholic health systems that supposedly follow them, but know better in this case, if they want to stay in business. While Elizabeth was unique in not wanting more reproductive autonomy and, therefore, a bit of an outlier, I include her story to show how even the Catholic faithful can be harmed by the doctrine and by the lack of clear information about how directives affect care.

Conclusion

Pregnancy loss can be enormously difficult. Patients suffer physically and emotionally. Many experience self-doubt, guilt, and trauma. The stigma associated with miscarriage and abortion add weight to all of it. Even under the best of circumstances, patients struggle to navigate the deluge of information associated with modern medical care. Patients should not be *expected* to do extensive consumer research before going to a hospital if, say, their water breaks at eighteen weeks when they are traveling.

Catholic hospitals' lack of transparency regarding their religious policies exacerbates the difficulty of obstetric emergencies, making it challenging for people to know where to seek care, or how to interpret their experiences once they are there. Jaelyn, who considers herself a "planner," nonetheless found herself subjected to hours of physical and emotional suffering that was not medically necessary. Samantha still struggles to understand why her experience of miscarriage care was so muddled, alienating, and delayed. Even Elizabeth, who wanted Church-circumscribed care, felt spiritually harmed by the lack of clarity about when hospitals decide not to follow the bishops' rules and when, exactly, Catholic medicine becomes unsafe. She felt shame for inadvertently accepting life-saving treatment.

These three women are unique, yet they all suffered from the same fundamental problem. First, Catholic health care is bound by directives that run counter to the safest and most patient-centered care for pregnancy loss, and, second, being transparent about the conflict is not good for hospital business. ERDs may be on a website, but who knows to look? Few would think to do so in the midst of a medical emergency. And what do the ERDs actually mean, given that they are sometimes stretched or unevenly applied? The lack of clarity is by design, because religious restrictions do not attract patients. Most women do not want someone else making these decisions for them or usurping their physicians' authority, and especially not the U.S. Conference of Catholic Bishops.

As we will see in the following chapters, many physicians work hard to obscure, reduce, or remove the impact of the religious policies on patient care out of genuine concern for patient health and wellbeing. In some cases, patients can see the workarounds, but in many cases they cannot. When medical care functions in this way—with restrictions, workarounds, and obscured policies—it maintains a pattern of keeping patients in the dark. While patient outcomes may ultimately be better than if the physicians applied the restrictions rigidly and uniformly, both transparency and patient autonomy slip further out of reach as Catholic hospital networks expand and eliminate alternatives.

CHAPTER 5

Mostly Above-Board Workarounds

I think we pretty much all know what [the Directives] are and we just kind of, you know, we tell new partners about them and what you have to do to get around them.

—Dr. Nowara

Strictly orthodox Catholicism and modern women's health care are incompatible and sometimes you just have to choose between one and the other.

—Dr. Murphy

By now, readers may be wondering: If the Ethical and Religious Directives for Catholic Healthcare Services mandate substandard and unethical reproductive care leading to doctrinal iatrogenesis, how have Catholic health systems, and in particular their providers of reproductive care, continued to attract and retain patients? How have they avoided reputational disaster and malpractice-driven bankruptcies? Or, put more simply, why don't things go wrong more often?

The very short answer to that question is: Workarounds. In the field of obstetrics and gynecology, where religious restrictions affect reproductive care with regularity, clinicians in Catholic hospitals have found ways to meet many—though certainly not all—of their patients' reproductive needs. Some physicians employ workarounds that follow the religious rules, while others interpret them more creatively. This chapter focuses on the above-board ways physicians work to provide reproductive care for their patients, whether that care involves treating obstetric complications, offering contraception, performing sterilizations, or treating infertility. Sometimes, physicians take professional risks to minimize the negative impact of religious directives on their patients' health. Nearly all respondents, even those who disapproved of abortion, characterized religious restrictions as impediments to patient-centered and quality ob-gyn care—and so they worked around them.

In medicine, the term "workaround" refers to the diverse strategies clinicians use to overcome barriers to delivering patient care. Barriers often involve resource limitations, insurance requirements, legislative burdens, or obstructive bureau-cracy. A workaround is a "goal-driven adaptation" that allows a worker to "over-come, bypass, or minimize the impact" of a variety of constraints on achieving the work goal.[1] In the context of ob-gyn care in Catholic hospitals, the barriers to be worked around are the bishops' ERDs. Religious policies cause the resource lim-itations and barriers to health care.

Workarounds can be a means of diffusing the moral distress employees feel when institutional constraints make it impossible to "do the right thing."[2] In the context of health care, moral distress can and often does arise for medical workers when they cannot provide their patients with standard and timely treatment. Research about workarounds in other environments shows that workers feel par-ticularly compelled to employ workarounds to avoid or overcome conflicts in health care when there are no structural or policy solutions in sight, a situation that could not be more true in the context of Catholic hospitals.[3] Such moral distress is par-ticularly acute if clinicians feel they have failed in their professional commitment to *do no harm*.

In Catholic hospitals, as elsewhere in American health care, workarounds are a stopgap solution to a much larger problem. Not every doctor at every Catholic hospital uses workarounds, and even those who do are unlikely to use them for every patient. Workarounds can be idiosyncratic and informal, a characteristic that helps them go undetected. But they also can be faulty. The possibility of discretion raises serious concerns about racial disparities and other forms of provider bias in reproductive health. And, sometimes, familiar workarounds no longer work, espe-cially when certain clergy catch wind of them.[4]

Focusing on the practices that mostly follow the letter of the directives, even if they sometimes violate their spirit, I explore in this chapter the ways doctors in Catholic hospitals commonly work around religious restrictions. I leave for the next chapter an examination of the more creative workarounds, some of which might be described as quietly subversive and others as straight-up rebellious. Both the rule-abiding and more subversive workarounds fill out a larger picture of how Catholic health facilities continue to function in the secular world. Yet, as health-care systems grow and insurance networks consolidate, physicians are having a harder time implementing these workarounds, foreshadowing the increased pre-carity of reproductive rights both inside and outside of religious institutions post-*Roe*.

Not If but When

A gastroenterologist might not notice much difference between working in a Cath-olic hospital and in a nonreligious facility. For providers of obstetric and gyneco-logical care, it is a different story. Most know going into the job in a Catholic hospital that religious restrictions will override clinical judgment and patients' preferences for reproductive care on occasion. Physicians working in Catholic hospitals gen-erally understand that conflict with the ethics board can arise directly, in the form of a denied sterilization request, for example, or indirectly, such as from the looming threat of investigation into the management of an obstetric complication. In some environments, less overt tension about policing and enforcement of the directives exists and occasionally workarounds are so well established they seem like fully sanctioned practices.

Not a single physician I interviewed took seriously the idea that they would be required to implement medical care in full accordance with the ERDs, as written. As we have seen, even the CHA itself rejects the most extreme of the directives, such as those prohibiting "direct abortion" for ectopic pregnancy. Multiple physicians told me that the ERDs directly challenge their obligations to serve the patient's best interest. Dr. Karen Bari, a Muslim doctor working in a Northeastern Catholic hospital, saw workarounds as a viable way to "do your job," as long as the hospital administration could be counted on not to police the ob-gyn practice too closely. When asked what advice she would give to an ob-gyn colleague considering a job in a Catholic hospital, Dr. Bari said: "[It's important to] know for sure what is allowed and not allowed and how it's worded and how well it's enforced, and what the other docs in the department are doing . . . contraceptive management is really broad. You cannot prescribe [all] classes of medication, even if you're prescribing them for non-contraceptive benefits. So if they're really strict about that, I would say just walk away. *You can't really do your job.* If they really have a long history of the 'don't ask, don't tell' kind of mentality, then it's probably okay."

To be sure, a few respondents referenced having one physician on staff who stood out as ideologically aligned with the ERDs, even going so far as to report transgressions in provider behavior to the local bishop. For the most part, however, Catholic doctors I spoke with share Catholic women's skepticism about the Catholic Church's official position on contraception, sterilization, and, to a lesser extent, abortion. Catholic physicians are no more likely to work in Catholic hospitals than physicians with other religious identities. Still, certainly, many Catholic doctors end up doing so.[5] Dr. William Murphy is Catholic, and he strongly opposes the religious restrictions on reproductive care. Like other Catholic doctors I interviewed, he was drawn to work in a Catholic institution because of his belief in its original mission of serving the poor, and despite the national statistics to the contrary, his hospital does serve the low-income community of his county. But he sees the Church's preoccupation with controlling reproduction as derived directly from the patriarchal authority structure. He explained:

> The more positive side of the Catholic Church to me is the social-justice and the sticking-up-for-the-disenfranchised part of it. And that part of it has a lot to do with providing healthcare. So, in that sense, there's a lot of things I like about [my hospital] . . . [We] have an interest in providing healthcare to the underserved and providing education for people to provide excellent healthcare . . .
>
> I think the whole thing [around reproduction] is misguided and detached from experience with real women with real problems . . . you can't lock [women] out of power. It doesn't make sense. And I think that the Church's teachings on

these issues of reproduction have been arrived at without being informed by women. And if they had been informed by women, they'd be different.

And then you can certainly get into the question well, "Why am I Catholic," and all that kind of stuff, and it has to do with . . . it's a culture to a significant degree as well as a religion, and that I really do believe the tenets of it that are, what I believe to be, the core of it. *But these reproductive issues are not the core of it.*

Dr. Murphy and other physicians I spoke with generally characterized most of their colleagues as unsupportive of religious restrictions, regardless of their individual religious affiliation. Responding to my question about whether her radiology colleagues would balk at cooperating in a sterilization workaround (by reviewing a scan months later to confirm successful tubal occlusion), Dr. Bari responded: "That hasn't been an issue yet. And I don't think it would be . . . I've yet to meet a clinical person who wants to shove the Catholic directives down a patient's throat. I've really never heard of it." Ultimately, while some doctors, including Dr. Bari, had mixed feelings about abortion depending on the pregnant person's reason for it, they did not waiver in their disrespect for the directives restricting contraception, sterilization, and miscarriage management.

The hospitals, too, seem to have different expectations about physicians' level of adherence to the ERDs. Dr. Murphy had noted variability on his own, asking me: "I'd be interested in what you're hearing from people, but my impression from talking to people in a lot of different places across the country is there's really just a wide range of practices at Catholic hospitals. Some are very strict in terms of their contraception and sterilization approaches and some are really not."

What became exceedingly clear through interviews is that most doctors wanted to, and even expected to, work around many Catholic policies on reproductive care. The question was not *if* they would do so but, rather, *how* and in which circumstances.

Taking Patients Elsewhere

Dr. Thomas Jay, who describes himself as a non-practicing Catholic, held privileges to work in three different hospitals in the Midwest, two of which were Catholic. He told me that he warned his colleagues against working solely in a Catholic hospital, as it meant too many restrictions on a physician's autonomy over medical practice: "If that's the only hospital they're going to go to, then they're going to have to refer their patients out that want, you know, a tubal ligation or contraception. Because if you're owned by the hospital, you're going to have to practice under their restrictions."

For Dr. Jay, maintaining hospital privileges at multiple hospitals offered the most reliable workaround for religious restrictions on care. If a patient wanted or needed something he could not provide at one of the Catholic hospitals, he simply scheduled their appointment at the third. He repeated the phrase "you've got to take care of your patient" a few times during the interview, even offering up a story of going

to unusual lengths to help a highly religious Catholic patient hide her tubal ligation from her own parents:

> I actually had a patient whose parents were both physicians and she was sup-
> posed to deliver at the Catholic hospital. She had six children and it was her
> seventh baby and she had them all at [Holy Cross] Hospital and her mom and
> dad were big staff members there ... And we had to make up a big story about
> her going into labor in my office to go to the hospital on my campus, where I
> could tie her tubes during her C-section. And she wanted—'cause she had
> seven kids. I mean, she wanted her tubes tied. The rhythm method doesn't
> always work ...
>
> I still kid her about that when I see her. Like, "They never found out, did
> they?"'Cause some people are still very strict about that, which I respect if that's
> what they believe. There's ways you do things to get around stuff. I mean, you've
> got to take care of your patient.

Dr. Jay's strategy was one of the most common mentioned by my interviewees.
In practice, however, this approach requires that doctors and patients navigate disclosure, access, and even employment contracts. For example, a family medicine
physician, Dr. Tracy Lange, who does not do C-section and tubal ligation procedures herself and, thus, must be sure an ob-gyn or other surgeon is available to do
so if necessary, said of her patients: "If they were absolutely dead-set on a tubal, I
would probably refer for a single visit during their prenatal care over to one of the
surgeons [at the non-Catholic hospital] ... And I have privileges and can do their
delivery over there." As such, navigating this process includes explaining the
restrictions to the patient, and assessing her willingness to involve another physician in her care and to deliver at a different facility.

Like Drs. Jay and Lange, Dr. Sophia Chan, an atheist who practices in a Southern city, learned early on that she needed access to a non-Catholic hospital if she
wanted to provide sterilizations for her patients. Upon being hired by a Catholic
hospital, she was told that a new bishop had recently cracked down on some of the
ways her colleagues were working around the directives.

This fit with what I found to be true historically. Before being installed as pope
in 2005, Pope Benedict was known as Cardinal Ratzinger, Dean of the College of
the Cardinals in the United States. Cardinal Ratzinger was very disconcerted by
an analysis of hospital data reporting that, between 2000 and 2003, sterilizations
were happening in U.S. Catholic hospitals with regularity.[6] The reports were conducted by faithful Catholics, some within the Church, some within private academic settings, and both with the interest of purifying Catholic institutions. They
aspired to make Catholic hospitals conform to the bishops' policies and stay true
to the Catholic mission. In 2008, WikiLeaks posted a vigorous back-and-forth
between Catholic researchers accusing Catholic hospitals of widespread sterilization practice and the Catholic hospitals defending that each was somehow medically indicated. In turn, the researchers rebutted that the medical indications were
not justified. That this dirty laundry was aired publicly on the internet is considered

a Church scandal, but since it was not about abortion, it did not seem to garner comparable public interest.[7]

While these internal conflicts over sterilization may not have interested the non-Catholic world much at the time, Catholic bishops took note and began to scrutinize hospital practices. In some locations, new bishops replaced old ones. Whereas the previous local bishop governing Dr. Chan's hospital had looked the other way, the new one allowed zero exceptions for tubal ligations. Dr. Chan was warned that she should not even ask to perform them. She recounted her memory of getting oriented to the job: "The department was kind of like, 'Yes, you can do this, no, you can't' and . . . 'And no, there are no exceptions to the tubals.' Yeah, they did sit you down [to] kind of know that you're not—there's no way you can work around it. 'Cause you're like, 'What if we say this?' 'No, no, no, not going to work, no, no.' . . . there's different hoops at different places and that's, *the Catholic hoop is you have to tie the tubes someplace else.*"

Having maintained privileges at another, non-Catholic hospital, Dr. Chan was confident she could provide her patients with the care they needed. But things didn't always work out as planned. Dr. Chan told me about a patient who wanted a tubal ligation after delivering her fourth child by C-section. Dr. Chan scheduled the procedure in a non-Catholic hospital where she had limited privileges, but when the patient went into labor in the middle of the night, she presented to the Catholic hospital emergency room instead, because it was the default and primary hospital of Dr. Chan's medical group: "It felt really stupid that there was this woman having a fourth C-section and that she really wanted her tubes tied . . . We had her scheduled to be at the other hospital so we could do her C-section and tie her tubes. But when she came in in labor before that time, then she came into the Catholic hospital, which was our primary facility, and she couldn't get her tubes tied."

While Dr. Chan clearly lamented the outcome, it was by no means unpredictable. Many women go into labor ahead of schedule. Dr. Chan's privileges in the non-Catholic hospital were limited to procedures that were scheduled in advance. She justified her acquiescence to this policy in terms of patient safety. If her medical group wanted full privileges at the non-Catholic hospital, its physicians would have to start taking regular call shifts, and she and her colleagues felt the practice could not handle that: "Our patient safety issue was that we didn't want to cover two hospitals simultaneously so that we didn't have to have patients in two places at once . . . in the middle of the night. And so, when she came in, in the middle of the night, she had to just get her C-section [at the Catholic hospital]. But yeah, it was her fourth C-section and you know, there's definitely more risk each time you go in there. And when someone's having a C-section, their tubes are sitting right there."

Her patient's body, operating on a timing of its own, went into labor before the scheduled date for the C-section at the non-Catholic hospital. Thus, she did not get the tubal ligation. Dr. Chan's workaround failed.

Maintaining privileges elsewhere was the most common workaround physicians mentioned in our conversations, but, as Dr. Chan's experience illustrates, this practice has become increasingly difficult. The combination of health system consolidation and exclusivity requirements have left doctors with less flexibility.[8] Twenty-first-century health systems operate in a competitive marketplace in which success often depends on controlling the largest sector of the regional market as is possible; physician groups often are bound to specific hospitals through contracts. And, in fact, physicians frequently used the past tense when telling me about this strategy, telling me, for instance: "'So, in order to do [interval] tubals, we went across the street and did them' or 'If you wanted your tubes tied you went to the hospital across the street and the doctors all knew that.'" Even in 2011, when I conducted my earliest interviews, this model was vanishing.

The success of this particular workaround also depends on patient insurance, creating obvious inequities related to patients' employment and socioeconomic status. Dr. Terry Horn, who is a member of the Church of Jesus Christ of Latter-day Saints, works in a Catholic hospital in the South, explained how inequity is built into his local healthcare system. The city in which he works has a poverty rate almost twice the national average, with half the population being people of color. Until a few years prior to our interview, Dr. Horn had been able to offer tubal ligations at his Catholic hospital, which was the only Medicaid provider in the region and took care of 80 percent of the region's obstetric patients. At that point, a highly religious patient became upset when a physician asked if she would want a postpartum sterilization, and she reported it to the diocese, which then cracked down on the practice:

> I thought it was terrible [to lose the ability to offer tubals] because our hospital is the main maternity hospital and our patients, because we run this big maternity clinic, tend to be the lower socioeconomic patients. They're the ones who need access to contraception and need access to permanent sterilization and yet the private doctors in town are the ones going to the hospital across the street. So, you had a situation where if you had insurance, had a job or had money, you could go over across the street and get your tubal done. But if you were, you know, getting Medicaid or if you had CHIP, then you didn't have access to that, and I thought it was a *terrible double standard*.

Coming from a white male doctor in the South speaking about women of color's "need" for sterilization, Dr. Horn's comment may strike some as having eugenic undertones. And yet, research is mounting that women of color, especially those on Medicaid, who *do* want to be sterilized face increasing barriers.[9] Sterilization access was unequal and unjust in Dr. Horn's town. Privately insured patients could just go across the street to give birth if they wanted a postpartum sterilization, but Medicaid patients could not.

Although Catholic hospitals in the twenty-first century provide no more Medicaid and charity care nationally than other types of healthcare systems on average,[10] when looking individually, they are diverse. Some Catholic hospitals serve mostly private patients and others serve as a local safety net. That means, regionally, Catholic directives can have severely racist impacts if most low income patients have only the option of religiously restricted care, as with Dr. Horn's hospital and many others throughout the United States.[11] Of course, not everyone can go to any hospital they want; *many people* have private insurance plans that specify that certain services must be provided at in-network hospitals.[12] Whether publicly or privately insured, patients are additionally constrained if their only option for care comes with religious restrictions.

Some physicians explain this situation clearly to their patients. Others do not. When Dr. Bari and her partners decided "it just wasn't worth their time to maintain privileges in two hospitals for only that surgery [tubal ligations]," they recognized that they might lose some patients. She said: "I tell them exactly what's going on. I offer them what we have, you know, and I understand if they don't want to wait. I mean, it's fine. And I have had somebody leave because they wanted a tubal. I can't tell you exactly who, but I do know that's happened." As we have ·seen, however, many patients remain loyal to their doctors, even when it limits their options for care.

Catholic hospitals, like any hospitals, can have good local reputations for specific features, such as a well-regarded postpartum nursing service, access to specialists, or newer facilities. This alone can make it unlikely for patients to agree to receive care elsewhere, even when doctors explain their concerns. Dr. Tim Ward (introduced in chapter 3), who is Jewish and practiced in the West, maintained privileges at two hospitals, neither of which was Catholic at the time he started his practice. About three years prior to our first interview, his primary hospital, the one located across the street from his practice, was bought by a Catholic system. Dr. Ward maintained privileges at another hospital specifically to accommodate his patients who wanted postpartum sterilization, but he struggled to convince them to go to the other location. As he explained to me, the non-Catholic hospital is much smaller, seeing only about a quarter the volume of deliveries as the Catholic hospital, suggesting that it may have fewer resources and less specialty expertise. It is also twenty-five minutes away on a high-traffic corridor.

Childbirth is an exceptionally vulnerable physical and emotional experience. Patients who have choices in where to deliver often prioritize familiarity, quality of care, and safety in their hospital selection.[13] It should not be terribly surprising to hear, then, of women who defer a tubal sterilization rather than deliver somewhere that necessitates a change of doctors, a lengthier drive, or some other type of sacrifice in safety or quality of care. Ultimately, the workaround of taking a patient to a different facility for childbirth and then a postpartum tubal ligation works only when patients have knowledge of the religious constraints early in prenatal care, as well as the willingness and ability to seek care elsewhere. Even then, it is not always up to them.

THE OUTPATIENT "SOLUTION"

Physicians who did not or could not maintain privileges at non-Catholic hospitals but nevertheless wanted to retain their patients had to seek alternative workarounds. Depending on the nature of the procedure, one option is to provide patient care in an outpatient setting not owned by the Catholic healthcare system, whether the physician's own office or an ambulatory surgical center. This solution, of course, is limited to the kinds of low-risk procedures that can be performed safely in an outpatient setting. The physicians I spoke with mentioned this option most frequently in regard to inserting contraceptive devices and performing vasectomies and laparoscopic interval tubal ligation (meaning six weeks or more post-delivery), but new types of sterilization could be done outpatient as well.

Although the physicians did not know it at the time we spoke, one popular innovation for outpatient tubal sterilization, Essure, would shortly become unavailable. Sterilization with Essure worked by inserting a tiny metal coil into the fallopian tube transvaginally and transcervically with a hysteroscope. Over three months, scar tissue develops around the coil, permanently blocking the passage of eggs from the ovary to the uterus. In 2018, it was removed from the market in the United States due to a slew of bad outcomes, including "persistent pain, perforation of the uterus and fallopian tubes, and migration of the coils into the pelvis or abdomen." The FDA had amassed "a significant collection of recent reports" in which the device had to be surgically removed from patients.[14]

At the time of my interviews, the FDA had not yet issued its statement. A few doctors spoke with confidence and enthusiasm about having gotten training to offer Essure, unaware of its impending legacy as one more medical technology that was adopted and promoted too early at patients' expense. One physician, Dr. Frances Morgan, confidently stated: "I actually don't do tubals anymore. I do Essures." Dr. Horn echoed his optimism: "You know, what's going to be great in the long run, are these new office sterilization procedures, such as Essure and [Adiana, which] uses radio frequency to ablate the tubes. Those can be done in people's office and therefore it wouldn't involve the hospital."

For physicians working in Catholic health systems, "not involving the hospital" would mean physicians could continue to offer an alternative that was, at least theoretically, not subpar care and was less invasive than an interval tubal ligation. Dr. Horn was the only physician who mentioned radio frequency ablation, but this technology has similarly been taken off the market due to adverse patient outcomes.[15]

Except for its safety issues, it makes sense that Essure appealed to ob-gyns, even those not working in a hospital with religious restrictions. Dr. Bari explained how Essure fit the needs of older doctors; namely, the ob-gyns who no longer did obstetrics due to the intense schedule and night hours:

> And then Essure became available and kind of brought up the discussions again about the availability of those services and it took the need for a hospital out of the equation and so, since we didn't have to go to a hospital and maintain privileges somewhere else, all we needed was to find space. That became very easy because there were a lot of physicians in the community who had gotten older and dropped the OB part of their practice and needed to supplement their

income, and so they did that by leasing out the space and the equipment to us, to do those procedures.

Essure gave doctors a way to offer women a sterilization option that did not take place during delivery and, in fact, did not require a surgical facility at all. And, as Dr. Bari mentioned, Essure also was a good source of business. Essure's makers sold doctors on its safety because of the technique's minimally invasive nature. Because the device could be inserted via the opening in the cervix, it theoretically presented less anesthesia risk than surgically entering the abdomen. Dr. Bari enthused: "It's wonderful. It's definitely more safe. There's no general anesthesia, there's no hospitals involved so the errors that can happen in a hospital system are gone."

While convenient for doctors, Essure nevertheless created extra steps for patients. For this reason, some physicians saw both Essure and interval tubals as ethically suspect solutions, given the difficulties they created for patients. Dr. Ward criticized physicians who seemed to be trying to retain business for themselves by telling patients about only outpatient options instead of attempting to schedule delivery with a postpartum tubal in a non-Catholic hospital or referring to a physician with privileges elsewhere. Reflecting on the period of time after his previously nonsectarian hospital was bought by a Catholic system, Dr. Ward described how his colleagues did or did not attempt to meet patients' reproductive needs in the face of the new restrictions:

> During the time this was all transpiring none of my colleagues have gone elsewhere to practice, so they're all essentially staying near the campus here, but not offering their patients sterilization procedures here or termination of pregnancy procedures because it's not permitted . . . they just tell the patients it's not available . . .
>
> [In regard to sterilization], they don't want to relinquish the fee, you know, the possibility of earning a fee for it. They'll take them to a surgi-center sometime afterwards, post-partum, six weeks, three months, and put in a laparoscope and tie their tubes. So now the person's relegated to a second procedure, a second anesthesia and in addition, the risk of a scope going into an abdomen that's had previous surgeries because of repeat Cesarean sections. And that's all because of the medical bylaws at [the Catholic health system that now owns his hospital] and also the doctors', you know, sense of "I'm not going to lose this patient and a fee for tying their tubes."

Highly critical of colleagues who were looking out for their bottom line, Dr. Ward feels the prohibition on sterilization leads to both poor care and bad incentives in medical practice.

Dr. Ward's comments allude to another procedure historically performed in outpatient settings: termination of pregnancy. Doctors typically refer out patients to specialized abortion clinics for a host of reasons, including doubts about their own skills, desire to avoid abortion stigma, anti-abortion policies (governmental or institutional), fear of violence and harassment from protesters, or because reimbursement for it is just too low to merit combatting all the above.[16] However, as abortion has been restricted and banned in more conservative states, specialized abortion clinics are disappearing. With the growth of Catholic systems, women must travel farther for both hospital-based and clinic-based abortion care.

Squeezed on all fronts, occasionally doctors still provided abortions for their own patients in out-patient ambulatory surgical centers. For example, a Hindu physician, Dr. Neysa Vijay, whose group practice was not owned by, but saw patients exclusively in, the Catholic hospital recounted the case of one of her patients who had a liver transplant and became pregnant afterward. Unfortunately, the immunosuppressant drugs she needed to take were known to cause birth defects. Furthermore, the pregnancy was physically dangerous for her. But she was stable enough for an outpatient procedure: "We could not wait until she's like 20 weeks pregnant and look at the baby and you know, look at all the organs and make sure baby's okay. Just the pregnancy itself was going to be life-threatening to her because she had liver transplant, and so she needed an elective abortion at about 6 to 8 weeks. So, my colleague took her to the Surgery Center which is at short drive from the hospital . . . to do the abortion . . . which is not affiliated with the hospital."

It was rare to hear about doctors doing abortions for patients' outside of the Catholic facilities, like this instance described by Dr. Vijay, especially if the Catholic healthcare system was their employer. Occasionally, physicians who were not employed by a Catholic system and wanted to perform restricted procedures made use of outpatient options to serve and retain patients for other procedures. However, this approach caused unanticipated problems for some, such as Essure patients with bad outcomes. And, by definition, there were limits to the outpatient "solution;" the hospital is the only safe and appropriate venue for certain procedures and certain patients.

CARVE-OUTS AND COLLABORATIVE AGREEMENTS

A carve-out, in this context, is a legalistic approach that designates some portion of the healthcare facility as non-Catholic specifically to allow certain restricted reproductive services there. In some cases, religious authorities allow the administration to agree to sell some part of their building to a separate, non-Catholic fiscal entity of some sort. Within that non-Catholic space, the tubal ligations or other prohibited services are then permitted (though rarely abortion). A prime example is the "tubal room" of Drs. Altera and Sherman, discussed in the introduction. In their case, one of the hospital's operating rooms was sold to their non-Catholic clinic so they could perform C-sections with tubal ligations there. To ensure the Catholic hospital would not be complicit in any way with the sterilization, the non-Catholic owners were required to provide all medical staff and supplies needed for the operating room, from the beginning of the C-section through the tubal ligation and all other aspects, such as pathology and janitorial services.

Many kinds of carve-outs exist throughout the United States. As mentioned in chapter 2, the 2018 revision of the ERDs added several directives that the bishops explicitly included to put an end to such carve-outs and creative collaborations. The revision pits the business side of Catholic health care against the religious side in stark ways. John Haas, president of the National Catholic Bioethics Center told Modern Healthcare reporter Harris Meyer just after the 2018 revision was released publicly that he expected the bishops would ask his organization to review many of the collaborative agreements. Philip Boyle, an administrator in Catholic health-care system Trinity Health, told the same reporter about his concern that an arrangement in Troy, New York, may not survive such scrutiny, even though the local bishop approved it a decade earlier. Meyer wrote:

> One carve-out that could be called into question is the Burdett Birth Center in Troy, N.Y., a separately incorporated women's health and birthing center that's located within Samaritan Hospital, which is now part of the Catholic systems St. Peter's Health Partners and Trinity Health. Burdett offers post-partum tubal ligations and contraceptive services. It also provides treatment for women in cases of miscarriages or ectopic pregnancies, which can become an issue under Catholic care rules . . .
>
> Philip Boyle, Trinity's senior vice president for mission and ethics, said the Burdett arrangement to offer services that violate Catholic religious directives inside a hospital that must follow the directives might look like "smoke and mirrors." But it won the approval of the local bishop and is based on permissible moral theory, he added.
>
> Still, he acknowledged it's possible under the revised Ethical and Religious Directives—though unlikely—that the church could go back and rescind the arrangement . . . As he and other Catholic healthcare ethicists note, much depends on the views and interpretation of the local bishop. That's cold comfort to hospital administrators, who can't be confident that their facility's services will survive church scrutiny. "Some bishops might interpret it one way, some another," Boyle said.[17]

A unique compromise—which seems unlikely to survive bishop review—was struck when the community of one of my respondents fought a Catholic health system's plan to take over their sole hospital in the region. The doctor I spoke with told me that a separate, non-Catholic fiscal entity was created to pay other entities to supply transportation and provide prohibited healthcare services, including abortion, about an hour away.[18] This doctor thought that few knew about the entity, and that it was rarely used. Additional creative solutions that a few doctors mentioned were designed to aid Catholic hospital resident physicians who want to get training in prohibited services. Residents would be placed on leave or "let go," then re-hired by a separate entity to employ them while they learned and performed vasectomy and other contraceptive procedures elsewhere, after which they were re-hired by the residency program.

Other arrangements I heard about during interviews that also could be on the list to be revisited involve fertility services. Recall that the ERDs prohibit in vitro fertilization and related procedures, both because they separate procreation from sex and because it can lead to the destruction of extra embryos. The physicians I spoke with nevertheless found their Catholic employers eager to find ways to provide the highly lucrative and popular service. Dr. Bari explained: "Because it's a Catholic facility, we don't do in vitro fertilization or embryo storage, embryo transfers, artificial insemination—none of that." That said, she noted: "They're getting a little crafty with how they get around it and they go off-campus . . . in fact, the chairman of the entire OB/GYN department of all [our] hospitals *is* an infertility specialist, who is starting up an in vitro fertilization clinic off-campus . . . We had somewhere to send them anyway before—it was just out of the system— but now the system wants the business."

Dr. Patel (introduced in chapter 2), in the Midwest, found a similar eagerness from Catholic hospital leadership to make it work. Describing a bit of a geography puzzle, he said: "Well, I cannot mix egg and sperm here [in the Catholic-owned office], so that's the religious part of the problem . . . it's a timeshare office basically. I use this to see patients and do my initial workup, consultations, and most of the blood work . . . checking the uterine cavity can be done in the office." Then he goes to an off-site building, not owned by the Catholic healthcare system, to do the other parts. He learned from colleagues that meetings were held between Catholic hospital administrators, religious authorities, and physicians to come up with an agreement that would allow them to base their practice within the Catholic system despite the many ways IVF services conflict with Catholic doctrine. Like Dr. Bari, he postulated that the money was a large incentive for them to strike a deal. "It was an amicable solution between the two [groups], I guess. It was the closest that they could come to people [i.e., fertility doctors and patients] not leaving their hospital . . . I can't get rid of you because if I get rid of you, how am I going to build a bigger hospital or how am I going to build another hospital building that I plan to build?"

Leadership managed to keep fertility care within their healthcare systems despite the fact that procedures that are firmly prohibited by the ERDs make up the vast majority of fertility medicine. Hospital administrators worked with physicians to come up with creative solutions to separate the diagnostic, clinical, and procedural activities into parts that could and could not be performed within Catholic spaces.[19] The Catholic building could be used to attract the patients, do all the background, testing, diagnosis, and post-implantation assessment and follow-up, while the parts that technically violated the directives would be performed off-site with or without informing the patient as to exactly why, allowing patients to stay entirely in the dark about the religious policies.

REFERRAL IS THE UNOFFICIAL OFFICIAL PLAN

Even physicians who are inclined to abide by Catholic hospitals' directives some-times find themselves in situations that force them to pick sides between patient autonomy and religious policies. Language in the directives focuses on avoiding becoming complicit in "immoral" procedures through "material cooperation," which basically means intentionally facilitating the goal of a "wrongdoer."[20] Until 2018 (and throughout the course of these interviews), the directives had ample lan-guage directing Catholic hospital employees to avoid "any immediate material cooperation in actions that are intrinsically immoral, such as abortion, euthana-sia, assisted suicide and direct sterilization," but did not use the word "referral" at any point. The 2018 revision of the ERDs explicitly prohibited "referrals" for "immoral procedures" in the context of affiliation agreements in Directive 73: "Before affiliating with a healthcare entity that permits immoral procedures, a Catholic institution must ensure that neither its administrators nor its employees will manage, carry out, assist in carrying out, make its facilities available for, make referrals for, or benefit from the revenue generated by immoral procedures."

CHA theologians have muddied the waters by stating: "The prohibition on refer-rals needs to be carefully explained so that we do not abandon patients."[21] Despite all this, in reality, when doctors cannot take care of patients' reproductive needs in the Catholic hospital or elsewhere, many of them refer them to someone who can.

Doctors' referral practices vary.[22] Some doctors put considerable effort into making direct referrals, even going so far as to make a "warm hand off" by com-municating with the abortion provider over the phone, sending paperwork to the clinic in advance, and following up with the patient afterward. Others make indi-rect or minimal referrals and simply tell the patient to call an abortion clinic her-self if she is interested in abortion care and have little involvement otherwise. And many, like Dr. Bari, offer different levels of the support depending on the stage and indication for the abortion.

> We make those referrals all the time . . . When it's a purely elective early termi-nation of pregnancy, like an eight-or-nine-week pregnancy, we give the patient the paperwork that they need to take to whatever clinic they're going to go to and we have a typed-out, pre-printed list of places within the area that take cer-tain insurances for that procedure and we just tell them to make the appoint-ment when they want to go and this is the paperwork they need to show . . .
>
> If it's a later thing like what you talked about, a genetic anomaly, and those are usually second trimester or later terminations, those we fax usually directly to the office and the other end has their own protocol. You know, you can't just, as a patient, call up and say, "I have a baby with Down syndrome and I want to terminate my pregnancy." They have their own protocols. They want the paper-work ahead of time, they only do them on certain days of the week, they have to have the patient come in, usually on consecutive days, for cervical dilators to be placed. So, the whole thing is this big, coordinated effort . . . they're emotion-

ally distraught as it is. So, I told my staff, I don't want to add to it by making them have to navigate through the bureaucracy of healthcare on their own, you know, and try to explain to five different people on the phone what the deal is.

As well-intentioned as Dr. Bari is, her extra efforts to help patients with fetal anomalies navigate abortion care remind us that doctors tend to see patients who are terminating a wanted pregnancy due to a health problem as more deserving of support than other abortion patients, despite the reality that those who terminate pregnancies due to poverty or interpersonal violence or for any other reason deemed "elective" also can be struggling emotionally and logistically.[23]

It is questionable whether referrals should be conceptualized as a workaround, in that the physician making the referral does not actually provide the restricted service; however, doctors themselves frequently spoke of referrals in this way, and on a systemic level, one can see them as such. Catholic hospital doctors funnel patients steadily to family planning clinics to get what Catholic facilities prohibit, developing alternate pathways to reproductive care just as coronary collaterals develop to work around a blockage in an artery. Collaterals develop to relieve the pressure that comes from the need for abortion that never dissipates, despite the bishops' most sincere wishes. With the vanishing of abortion rights post-*Roe*, these collaterals have been rerouted and blocked with yet unknown consequences for patients.

Dr. Horn did his residency at a Catholic hospital in a large Southern city. He went on to work in a mid-size city for another Catholic hospital that served a large rural and suburban population. As a member of the Church of Jesus Christ of Latter-day Saints, he explicitly chose to work in a Catholic hospital to avoid being in a position where he could be asked to perform an abortion, yet he still wanted to meet his patients' contraceptive needs and makes sure to refer them to people who can perform contraceptive services he cannot. He explained:

> I personally am not a big advocate of abortion and I prefer not to perform them, which is one of the reasons I've always worked for a Catholic system. However, I am a big proponent of contraception and so that's where it's kind of a hard situation. I'm okay with tubals, I'm okay with all kinds of contraception and in fact I think that's probably a better solution, is to prevent unwanted pregnancy. And so that's a little frustrating at times, but I feel okay in that we can refer our patients to places where they can get access to contraception in the community.

I asked him if he had heard about Sister Margaret McBride, in Phoenix, Arizona, who was excommunicated for approving an abortion for a patient with life-threatening pulmonary hypertension in 2010 (for more about this see chapter 7). I wanted to know what his hospital's approach to problem pregnancies like that would be. My question opened up a discussion about the larger pattern of referral-making in Catholic facilities.

> DR. HORN: What we typically do is refer them to the high-risk Maternal Fetal Medicine doctors, who are in [a large Southern city a hundred miles away]. And so then they can, they have a broader, you know, they have more options.

LORI: They have more options? They're not managed under a Catholic system?

DR. HORN: Correct. Which is interesting. Because we had a Catholic [clergy member who] . . . came in and spoke to us about the Catholic ethic about a couple of years ago. And one of the things he recommended was that if we have a situation where a patient needs something that can't be provided by the Catholic institution, that *we should refer them to, you know, refer them away to the place where they could get things taken care of, you know, as quickly as possible.* I thought that was interesting. I think he was from [a large Midwestern city]. I'm not sure all of the more conservative nuns in the hospital where I was a resident would've agreed with that, but he was very open about it.

ME: This was in your new hospital?

DR. HORN: This was in my new hospital, yeah. I think he was a consultant of the Catholic Church who came from [that Midwestern city] to talk to us . . . I was really surprised. He was like, you know, "If you know if somebody wants a tubal, you know, refer them to a doctor that can do a tubal at another hospital." I thought that was interesting 'cause usually you would think they would say, "Well we don't want them to have a tubal. That's not the right thing to do."

LORI: Right, and they do seem to have some language around not making referrals.

DR. HORN: Right. Now that was just in reference to tubals. I don't know what his thoughts would've been like for an abortion or something.

LORI: Okay. Yeah. How about abortion? Does it come up in your medical setting at all, maybe for fatal fetal anomalies or anything like that?

DR. HORN: Yeah. And that again, same situation. That [Arizona case] was pulmonary hypertension. If we have a patient who has a known encephalic baby, a baby with, you know—and they want to terminate, then we refer them to [large Southern city] and they usually can get them referred to somebody who can take care of that.

Several things stood out to me about this conversation. First, although Dr. Horn stated that he purposely sought residency and employment in Catholic hospitals to protect him from participating in or having to opt out of doing abortions, he also seems relatively concerned that women retain the ability to get abortion care (at least in certain situations). He reassures me that his hospital can refer women to the big city where, should a woman have a medical condition or the fetus have a major fatal anomaly, they could get her to someone who "can take care of that." I also found it striking that Dr. Horn considered a hundred-mile one-way drive a "reasonable" workaround. It is also worth noting his state and neighboring ones have since banned abortion, so patients now will need to go much further.

One of the most common types of referrals involved requests for contraception. Indeed, a thick irony emerges from the number of times physicians specifically cite Planned Parenthood as the most logical place to refer patients in need of services, whether contraception or abortion, that they themselves cannot provide. That is, around the same time as the United States Conference of Catholic Bishops was petitioning the Senate to "withhold federal funds from the Planned Parenthood Federation of America and its affiliates," and instead "to reallocate federal funding, so that women can obtain their health care from providers that do not promote abortion" through targeted defunding legislation,[24] Catholic hospital physicians clearly and repeatedly asserted their reliance on the organization in all corners of the country.

Knowing that the name "Planned Parenthood" itself would raise a red flag within some Catholic health settings, physicians can be reluctant to put this particular referral in writing. Dr. Horn, for instance, explained that his practice accompanies a generic list of clinics for postpartum care that can likely provide contraception with a verbal suggestion that patients go to Planned Parenthood: "We've tried to comply and so mainly the workaround is that we do provide a list of doctors that they can go to [for] their post-partum visits, or clinics, and without directly including like Planned Parenthood, we know that those doctors in the community can provide them contraception. So, there's a little bit of a workaround . . . And I can verbally tell them. I can say: "You go to Planned Parenthood."

When I asked Dr. Horn how he and the people he works with regard Planned Parenthood, he grounded his positive association with them in the fact that his local Planned Parenthood focuses on other needed services besides abortion. "My office is just five physicians and five midwives, and we are supportive of what Planned Parenthood does here 'cause they mainly provide contraception, do PAP smears and that kind of thing." This Planned Parenthood provides only referrals for abortion, but at the time we spoke, it is possible they did offer medication abortion services.

While it remained unclear whether Dr. Horn would offer a direct referral for an abortion with no specific health indication, other physicians, like Dr. Miriam Teel, who is a Protestant Christian and describes her religion as very important to her, had no trouble writing a referral to a family planning provider. Recalling her experience working in a Catholic hospital in the past, Dr. Teel said:

> I don't think we were really allowed to prescribe contraception under the hospital auspices, but generally what we would do is just recommend that they go to the local family planning clinic for their birth control pills or whatever, and I think I would just write them out a referral to go there. And nobody seemed to care about that. I could tell people whatever I wanted to. It was just you couldn't write a prescription for birth control pills on a [St. Peter's] prescription pad . . . I don't recall anybody telling me that I couldn't counsel patients in any way that I thought fit.

Thus, while Dr. Teel described a similar reliance on family planning providers to fill the gap in care, she felt no need to hide it from staff or superiors. Dr. Franklin Quarles, an ob-gyn who works in a Planned Parenthood in a region of the

Midwest dominated by Catholic hospitals, describes a similarly unobstructed referral process on the receiving end, noting that he was especially familiar with the Catholic hospital ob-gyns because of their prevalence and the fact that their referral pattern is so consistent and thorough: "Whether or not they're allowed to, I don't know. We do get lots of paperwork from them because we—I guess—'require,' is the right word, copies of ultrasounds that are done and genetic amniocentesis and that kind of testing and copies of prenatal records when it's available so that we can make sure that we know exactly what we're getting into. And we have had virtually no problem obtaining that kind of stuff from them."

Although the directives technically prohibit such referrals, they also prohibit care that women regularly need. Physicians I spoke with know quite well that family planning clinics and non-Catholic hospitals will fill this gap, sometimes with federal funds, sometimes with philanthropic funds. I would even argue that the relationship is symbiotic because demand for Planned Parenthood increases as Catholic hospitals deny care. The more Catholic health systems grow, the more family planning clinics also must expand to serve their patients' contraception and abortion needs; their mandate is even stronger. That said, the overturning of *Roe* has disrupted the symbiosis between Catholic hospitals and brick-and-mortar abortion providers within conservative states.

One patient's experience of getting a referral to Planned Parenthood sheds light on why so many doctors have leaned on them. Sara needed an abortion and was referred to Planned Parenthood by her physician. The physician was not working in a Catholic hospital, but his own religious views prevented him from performing abortions himself. Nevertheless, he wanted to help her find care. She explained: "It was an unexpected [pregnancy], and we did decide to terminate, and he—his religious views would not allow him to do anything about it. But he was respectful of me . . . He actually gave me a couple different referrals for OBs who might be willing to help but said that the best place would be Planned Parenthood."

I asked her why he particularly recommended Planned Parenthood. Somewhat to my surprise, she conveyed her impression that her physician wanted to protect her from the possibility of delays, denials, or disrespect by the obstetricians on his list: "Just the ease of getting in and getting out and not a million questions. Because he thought that the other OBs that he had mentioned would help, but he did not know 100 percent that they would be reliable or how that experience would go."

This physician, like so many of those working within Catholic healthcare systems, walked a thin line in trying to make sure his patient could get adequate care without actually providing it himself. Sara found this acceptable, as did countless other patients when they were treated compassionately and skillfully by the referring physician and the abortion provider.

Perhaps the thinnest line I heard of physicians walking is when they referred patients with fetal anomalies out to a high-risk ob-gyn outside of the health system to initiate the abortion by administering medication to stop the fetal heart. After that, the patient returns to the Catholic hospital's obstetric unit for an induction of labor for fetal demise. Dr. Chan described this infrequently mentioned practice:

It's not unheard of for people to drive to [large city], see this specialist, get an injection of potassium intra-cardiac, you know, into the fetal heart, and then come back with an intrauterine fetal demise. And then you have no problem with it whatsoever . . . The baby's already demised . . . an induction at 24, 27 weeks can take a day or two and some of the people would just rather be at home. So they don't necessarily want to stay in—their family and their support system live here in [mid-sized city] and they don't want to stay in [large city] . . .

LORI: And can I ask about this [large city] physician? . . . Did anyone at the Catholic hospital care?

DR. CHAN: I mean, I think if you had made a big deal to the admin-, you know—I mean, there's nuns on the board. If we'd all advertised it, probably would have. But on a local Labor & Delivery basis, no, not really.

However, not all physicians make meaningful abortion referrals. A national survey of physicians in the United States showed that 29 percent do not feel it is their duty to refer a patient to get care they will not provide, and 14 percent do not feel obligated to even give information about that care.[25] Conscience laws protect both individual clinicians and major institutions from being penalized for withholding both information and care. Fortunately for their patients needing abortions, many of the doctors I interviewed feel professionally and ethically obligated to at least make some effort to refer their patients to where they can get the services they need.

PUNTING AND DUMPING

It is reasonable to conclude that if Catholic hospitals' physicians *actually* followed the letter of the law when it comes to the directives, some of their patients might die, some others could have reasonable grounds for successful malpractice suits, and many more would experience greater numbers of unintended pregnancies and abortions than they do already; all various forms of doctrinal iatrogenesis. In relation to obstetric emergencies, it is illegal for a hospital to turn away a patient who arrives medically unstable or in labor due to Emergency Medical Treatment & Active Labor Act (EMTALA) laws instituted to ensure public access to emergency services. But EMTALA is the bare minimum; many are not content to stabilize an obstetric patient in distress and watch her while withholding or delaying treatment due to religious policies.

Thus far, this chapter has focused on how physicians attempt to deliver care without completely violating hospital policies when they or, in some cases, their own personal beliefs restrict their ability to provide the services a patient needs. Over the course of my interviews, however, I became aware of a curious and disturbing phenomenon of physicians being advised *by their own Catholic hospital ethics committees* to "send patients out." This happened on notable occasions when it was clear to both the physicians and religious authorities that obstetric patients needed a termination of pregnancy but the patient did not yet meet ERD criteria (infection or other life-threatening pathology). Fundamentally, this means the ethics committee knows the hospital cannot provide the standard of care. By recommending it, religious authorities acknowledge that termination is preferable for her wellbeing and that watching and waiting in the hospital would simply be less safe.

Two doctors from the same urban and previously non-Catholic hospital in the West told similar stories about how their hospital actively diverts patients it considers at high risk of bad outcomes under the medical directives. When it was bought by the Catholic health system three years prior to the interview, administrators repeatedly assured physicians that their medical judgment would be paramount. Dr. Noa Fine recalled:

> We were told that there really wouldn't be much of a change in terms of how we practice medicine, except for the fact that they did not want us—they would not allow us to perform abortions at the hospital, nor would they allow for tubal ligations, either at the time of Cesarean section or just elective in general.
>
> We were told there would be exceptions made if it was—you know, if the mother had health issues, then we would approach an Ethics Committee, which would then review our appeal or request, and then they would make a decision. And we were also told that it would be a medical decision, meaning, you know, if we determined as physicians that the mother's health was at risk or if future fertility would harm her health, that, you know, of course that wouldn't even be a question

Dr. Fine's colleague, Dr. Ward, in contrast, was never so optimistic that medical exceptions would be made. He was opposed to the loss of reproductive services on principle and implored his colleagues fruitlessly to fight the deal: "Everyone sort of poo-poo'd it like it wasn't important . . . I remember one of the oncologists saying to me, 'Well they're going to put $300 million into the hospital and they're going to have a new CAT scan machine and they're going to have new equipment and they're going to aesthetically make the place look beautiful . . .'"

Furthermore, many simply did not believe they would end up having to deny their affluent patients what they needed. As a highly religious Jewish ob-gyn, Dr. Fine additionally thought the hospital's opposition to abortion would align well with her own desire to avoid performing abortions. She was surprised, then, when the hospital's ethics committee told her and her colleagues to "send out" two complex cases where she thought abortion was not only justifiable but medically critical. Dr. Fine recalled:

> The first case [that upset me] was a woman who, during her pregnancy, was diagnosed with a brain cancer, a brain tumor, a malignant brain tumor. And it was in the beginning, in her first trimester of her pregnancy, and she needed aggressive treatment. And it was chemotherapy, and she could not have that done while she was pregnant. The chemotherapy would be harmful to the pregnancy. And so, the OB who was taking care of her approached the hospital and said, "Hi, I've got one of those cases where you said there wouldn't be an issue. I've

got a woman whose life is threatened by a brain cancer. She's pregnant and I need to do a termination." And they refused. They said, "Go take her to another hospital, take her to another place. Those places are available to you. We don't have to do it here." And so that, in my mind, is not adhering to their original commitment to, you know, putting the woman's health first. And they said, "If we were the only hospital, maybe we would do it, but we're not. There are other hospitals." They punted, and that's not the way I think medicine should be practiced, and so I think that was egregious. That just was not okay.

In this case, the hospital leadership made no pretense that this woman would not have an abortion before starting cancer treatment. Chemotherapy can harm or kill a fetus, especially in the first trimester, as the goal is to attack cells that reproduce quickly. The ethics committee clearly understood that the medical standard was to perform an abortion so that, among other possible bad outcomes, the patient would not suffer a uterine infection after fetal demise, taxing her body further during cancer treatment. In their response, they indicated it might even be possible to terminate the pregnancy in a Catholic hospital if the woman had no other place to get care, essentially acknowledging that even they would not suggest she continue the pregnancy and watch it be harmed or destroyed by the treatment. But the abortion of a live fetus was simply not permitted. At that point in time, both the woman and the fetus were stable, so according to the ethics committee, there was no theological justification to intervene. Dr. Fine went on to tell me another story about a twin molar pregnancy, for which the standard of care is abortion because the nonviable fetal cells can be cancerous. The ethics committee once again insisted she be sent elsewhere for an abortion, even though she had presented to the ER bleeding, with the additional complication that the pregnancy might be cancerous.

Neither of these patients were Dr. Fine's, but hearing their stories from colleagues left her incensed. Both episodes made her reassess the extent to which Catholic hospital management actually aligned with her own views about abortion:

> [The ethics committee] made such, I mean, such illogical decisions, in my opinion. . . . I feel like if it was my patient, personally, I would advocate so much that I would make their lives so bad they would have to agree. You know, maybe it's just like hubris. I'm just thinking well if it were me, I would not stop knocking on their door until they agreed to do it, just out of principle. I don't know if these two physicians did it or if they just kind of threw up their hands and said, "Okay, we'll just move them to another hospital."

Dr. Fine was particularly alarmed because she no longer maintained privileges elsewhere. Had either of these patients been hers, she, too, would have had to transfer their care to someone else. She considered this sort of "patient dumping" professionally irresponsible: "These two physicians have privileges at another hospital. I don't have privileges at another hospital, right? So if it was my patient, then

I'd have to dump the patient on another hospital. That's dumping, you know? I don't know if there's a neglect aspect to it or, you know, any kind of a malpractice, but I would have to punt the patient off to another hospital with another doctor. It's not like I could even do it at another hospital. So that would really tick me off. I mean, I only work at this hospital." As more and more hospital systems require exclusive contracts, more and more doctors find themselves in this position.

Some physicians who spent years proactively observing this pattern of ethics committee decision making talked about trying to stay ahead of the problem. Instead of "dumping," they were preventatively diverting. For example, Dr. Patel maintained privileges in five hospitals when we spoke, three of them Catholic. During call shifts at Catholic hospitals, he had been on the receiving end of women with pregnancy complications who were sent by ambulance in labor—with sterilization papers ready—just to be denied. He said: "*Well, we just have to funnel patients in a different way*. And you know, now that you've been working for a long enough time, you know what is going to be done and what is the answer anyhow." He advises his patients to call his clinic before proceeding to the ER during an obstetric complication, if possible. When he can, he directs them to the non-Catholic hospital to avoid restricted care.

Another physician, Dr. Hakeem Roy, in the West, expressed bitterness about his hospital being purchased by a Catholic network. He started by describing a possible path for obstetrics complications that will, by now, be familiar: "The patient ruptured membranes sixteen weeks, seventeen weeks. They're lying in the hospital. You say, okay, there is no—the chance that she's going to be fine is extremely minute and the chance of a healthy birth is ridiculously minute, and the patient doesn't wish to take those odds. They will not permit you to end the pregnancy . . . you have to take the patient out of their center elsewhere . . ."

He explained how he and his medical group adjusted practice to stay ahead of likely obstetric complications by sending the miscarrying patient to a non-Catholic hospital early and transferring her out of his care, ideally before anything goes wrong. He said: "We send the patient to [local private] or [local university] hospital and just, you know, we relinquish the care of the patient to somebody else . . . we figured out a pattern, right? So, if a patient now has a problem, we discuss with her before she goes to the hospital—the rules of the hospital—so we don't have to deal with that as much as we did earlier on, when it was our habit to just say 'go to the emergency room' or 'I'll see you at the hospital.'"

Of course, this solution assumes the patient's insurance network includes a non-Catholic hospital that is relatively nearby. As such, that patient arrives as an emergency patient without a preexisting relationship with an ob-gyn, and possibly no medical records, in the new facility, which can cause delays and confusion, and, typically, worse care.

Another physician, Dr. Nancy Unni, works in both hospitals of an academic medical center. The original university facility is non-Catholic, and it had partnered with the Catholic hospital just across the street. According to Dr. Unni, the

Catholic hospital operated on an explicit agreement that it would send all patients seeking tubal ligations and all miscarrying or ectopic patients across the street, even if they were unstable. Dr. Unni recalled: "Even if the mom was septic and going to die, they would transfer" to the non-Catholic university hospital. When I asked if this was seen as an EMTALA violation for the system to move patients from its Catholic to non-Catholic facility while unstable, she simply said no, that all parties involved know "we accept them into inpatient service [at the university hospital] because we understand [St. Mary's] doesn't do this," which doesn't exactly answer the question. But it does indicate widespread acceptance of the agreement. When I asked her if she was aware of any instances in which the Catholic hospital's ethics committee approved life-saving treatment instead of sending patients across the street to the university hospital, she said no. She then proceeded to offer a terrifying example involving an ectopic pregnancy emergency:

> So, three, it was like three years ago that a provider who was a couple years above me in training and he actually had [a patient with] a ruptured ectopic with a heartbeat at [St. Mary's]. They got the Ethics Committee involved. Ethics deemed that she was stable enough to get transferred to [University] and she was bleeding into her abdomen. I mean, if [I was her doctor] I would have shat my pants and never come back. Literally shat my pants. I don't know. And that provider, when I talked to him later, he was very calm about it. He was like, you know, "There are things that are good at [St. Mary's] and there are things that are very, very frustrating" and that's the example that he gave me . . .

Generally speaking, Dr. Unni thinks the proximity and coordination between St. Mary's and University hospitals allows them to take greater risks with patients' lives and more strictly follow the ERDs: "I think the Ethics Committee has definitely been involved in those cases and said no. And I think it's because they have the luxury of saying, 'Just have them go to [University]. It's so close and we don't have to violate our beliefs.' So there's that luxury with that [St. Mary's/University] relationship."

Dr. Unni's example reiterates how the continued success of Catholic hospital systems relies, sometimes quite heavily, on non-Catholic hospitals. It remains unclear what will happen to these patients in communities where non-Catholic options disappear and/or abortion ban proliferate.

CONCLUSION

In the past, Catholic hospital doctors had a variety of ways to ensure their patients still received some of the prohibited but standard ob-gyn care. But recent changes within the Catholic Church have presented challenges and eroded some such workarounds as the bishops have cracked down on exceptions for postpartum tubal ligations and creative collaborations with non-Catholic partners. The different techniques doctors mentioned to work around the barriers presented by the ERDs included taking patients to a non-Catholic hospital to deliver; changing a care plan to one that can be executed in an outpatient facility; referring the patient to another doctor or a family planning clinic that is unrestricted; creating a carve-out agreement to designate some facilities not-Catholic and, therefore, less restricted; and, finally, punting and dumping, which involves sending a patient mid-crisis, despite the risk to her health, to be treated by a different doctor not necessarily in the same system.

These approaches have allowed physicians working in Catholic hospitals to minimize doctrinal iatrogenesis and ensure their patients access reasonable levels of care. Most of these techniques involve the physician's discretion and their desire to "help" a patient stymied by the system. This opens the question: Who are they likely to stick their neck out for? Whose pleas are they likely to ignore? The informality and inconsistency of workarounds physicians mentioned raise serious questions about potential bias and racism.

Nearly *all these approaches* involve obtaining care outside of Catholic hospital systems, whether it involves taking patients to another hospital or getting them treatment in an outpatient setting. All these approaches assume patients have access to non-Catholic care, but this is a classist and urbanist assumption. What of the rural patients who have to drive 120 miles to get to another hospital? What of the patients with bad insurance? Or on Medicaid? What of the patients in states where abortion is banned? In other words, what do doctors do when they *have* to treat patients in the system?

CHAPTER 6

Under-the-Radar Workarounds

We would lie—not lie—but we would present something in a certain way so that we could get what needed to be done.   *—Dr. Acker*

When a patient needs care that is not allowed under Catholic doctrine, physicians who want to keep the patient within their Catholic facility have three options: deny the prohibited care, seek an exception from hospital religious authorities, or somehow fly beneath their radar. Physicians who concede the denial simply tell patients they cannot have the service they seek, whether a tubal ligation, contraception, or miscarriage treatment in the presence of a fetal heartbeat. Hospital rules forbid it. Doctors who follow the second path can petition the Catholic hospital's ethics committee to approve the prohibited procedure, usually on the so-called principle of double effect.[1] Given that physicians who request exceptions are working within the hospital's system, it might be considered yet another workaround, a way of bending but not quite breaking the rules. In practice, however, doctors know they are more likely to obtain that exception if they stretch the boundaries of the truth in their description of the situation. And, sometimes, the ethics board turns them down anyway. What happens next?

This chapter explores the practices physicians have developed to serve their patients *within* the Catholic hospital or clinic, either by circumventing or ignoring the official policies. For the most part, these strategies to overcoming religious barriers to care are nonsystematic. They can be loosely grouped into four physician approaches: justify; conceal; rename; and rebel. As will become clear over the course of the chapter, this informal, highly idiosyncratic approach to delivering care almost guarantees unequal access. Some patients are more comfortable or skilled than others at lobbying doctors to bend or break the rules on their behalf, and some doctors are more willing to do so for some people than for others. The strategy varies by a physician's tolerance for risk and reproduces countless forms of patient privilege and provider bias, the ethical implications of which are even more concerning post-*Roe* in places where there may be no alternatives for patients who are turned away.

Ultimately, delivering reproductive care within Catholic hospitals requires doctors, patients, and even hospital administrators to stretch the truth. This informal, unsettling system of providing care allows the Catholic hospital system to have

111

it both ways: restricting care to most patients but providing it to those patients who would be most likely to cause trouble for the hospital.

JUSTIFY

The Catholic directives make clear that neither contraception treatments nor sterilization can be offered for the purpose of contraception. Similarly, a woman's uterus may not be emptied during miscarriage simply because she no longer can tolerate the symptoms of cramping, bleeding, pain, and uncertainty. A fetus with a known, fatal anomaly cannot be terminated so long as it is alive. In all cases, there must be some other medical reason—most compellingly, that the life of the pregnant patient is threatened—to proceed.

Physicians I spoke with regularly and unselfconsciously mentioned the need to make up some different reason for why a patient might need contraception, tubal ligation, miscarriage management, or pregnancy termination. Having seized upon a workable diagnosis, the doctor would record the condition in the patient's chart. This approach was so common, and so widely viewed as necessary, that most did not characterize it as lying per se. Dr. Elena Albu, an Eastern Orthodox ob-gyn who did her medical training in a Catholic hospital in the Midwest, put it simply: "Oral contraceptives were used for any use except oral contraceptives. So, patients had heavier bleeding, patients had painful periods, but it was never really used for the intent of contraception, even though that may have been the prime reason that the patient came in."

Dr. Pete Gold, a Jewish ob-gyn, had worked in two Northeastern Catholic hospitals in his career. He explained how he routinely recorded some other justification for contraception in the chart, even if the patient never mentioned it: "Well, they were called pills for menstrual irregularities. And so everything was coded in the chart that the patient had complained of menstrual irregularities, even though they didn't, they 'complained' that they didn't want to have another child. And so we gave them birth control pills to regulate their menstrual cycle."

For some physicians, it was important that the discussion in the chart match the patient's reality, if for no other reason than to reduce their own professional liability. But getting a patient to verbalize something that was not necessarily true required elaborate playacting in some instances, particularly if the physician was unable or unwilling to explain the hospital's policies. Dr. Chan (introduced in chapter 5) shared her feelings of resentment about the ritual: "So not everybody's aware of it . . . that's when it starts to be, 'Well what are your periods like? You know, are they kind of heavy?' So yeah, it just sort of comes, you know—They don't always know it ahead of time but we can usually ask the right questions . . . Yeah. Like I said, that part I just find awful."

This guessing game was unpleasant for some physicians; they were not always successful in getting patients to play along. Dr. Albu recalled observing as a medical student that some patients failed to catch the hints and, thus, left their appointments without their prescription: "You know, [some] patients who didn't get the hint that they had to have a medical problem for contraception being just for contraception . . . they didn't actually get the hint when you would say, 'Well you're having heavy periods, aren't you? You're having painful periods, aren't you?' And they'd say, 'No.' 'Well you know the treatment for heavy periods are birth control pills. Well you know the treatment for this is birth control pills?' And they just wouldn't get it."

While some patients did not "get it," the physicians, arguably, had other options than offering opaque hints, like: (a) explaining the policy; (b) making a referral; and (c) not participating in the system. Technically, there was nothing prohibiting them from being transparent about the policies, but the culture of the hospitals varied in regard to how openly they felt they could speak about prohibited care, and a few mentioned being concerned about upsetting religious staff who might overhear the discussion.[2] Doctors gave various reasons for participating in the guessing game with patients rather than routinely explaining the policies or making referrals, such as not wanting to shame the patient by articulating the Catholic Church's views on sexuality and reproduction; being too squeezed for time to meaningfully discuss why and how the health system can constrain physician behavior; and not wanting patients to lose respect for them or their medical group by explaining that they must bend the rules. For Dr. Albu, all this was too much: She chose option "c." After medical school, she made what she referred to as "a conscious choice not to practice at Catholic institutions."

The patients I spoke with who had experienced similar coaching found the exchanges perplexing. Katie, who is not currently religious but was raised Catholic, sought contraception from a Catholic clinic. She was working temporarily for a Catholic university system, and this was the clinic covered by her insurance at the time. She recalled being confused by the hints her "helpful physician" tried to throw her way:

I worked with [a Catholic] University Health System . . . and attempted to receive a renewal of my birth control—at the time I was on the pill still—through that system, and received some pushback from the nurse when I initially told her that was the purpose of my visit, and then ultimately had a helpful, understanding provider who went, "So your cramps are really bad, right?" Wink, wink, wink at me, and I went, "No, I've actually never had a cramp in my life," and he was like, "Are you sure you've never had a cramp, because I'm hearing your cramps are really bad," and was able to ultimately provide me with a prescription for the pills despite their health system routinely not providing reproductive prevention methods along those lines . . .

It did not occur to me what was being implied by that statement until he more or less literally had to wink at me. Like he was staring at me with an "are you dumb; you need to play along with this" face while we were having this conversation. And I was oblivious because I had never had trouble getting birth control before. I had also never gone through a Catholic health system before, and I was literally working [for them], so I'm kind of shocked that it hadn't come up in my day-to-day job that this, of course, is something they routinely don't do. But as soon as I sort of made a confused face at him and went, "Yeah, I guess my cramps kind of suck," he was like, "Okay, great. I'm going to prescribe you birth control for your cramping to minimize those symptoms," and I was like, "Oh okay, whatever you—yeah, mm-hmm."

Later, Katie's mother, an ob-gyn nurse, explained what had happened. Although Katie remembered the experience as odd, she also was relieved to have found a provider willing to bend the rules, by fabricating a diagnosis, on her behalf: "Coming out of it I felt like I was almost colluding in a happy way with someone who had my best interest at heart but seemed to be hamstrung by a system that he may or may not have believed in himself. My guess is not, given that he was so willing to work around the confines of his system. So I felt like I was helped by having someone in my corner willing to bend the rules a little bit to get to the result that was medically appropriate for me."

As Katie demonstrates well, such exchanges can have the effect of building patient loyalty to a provider in a healthcare system that betrays them—here was a physician who went to bat for her; this was how he showed he cared. It is a likely outcome of discretionary rule-breaking and sheds light onto one way the system is sustained.

Few patients I interviewed understood and articulated the workarounds as clearly as Katie. Perhaps this is inevitable, given the wide range of transparency or disclosure among the physicians I spoke to. While Dr. Albu and Katie's physician were indirect with varying success in getting patients to play along, others, like Dr. Jay (introduced in chapter 5), let the patient in on the ruse. Dr. Jay, an older physician who worked in two Catholic hospitals in the Midwest, would tell the patient about the non-contraceptive benefit of reducing period cramps and heaviness, hand her a prescription directly "and tell them, you know, 'If anybody asks, that's what it's for.'"

Miscarriage management was another area where physicians sometimes had to fudge the charts to justify treatment. While the principle of double effect allowed physicians to evacuate the uterus to save a patient's life once infection or some equivalent threat had presented itself, some physicians learned to lower the bar to speed up the justification process. Dr. Gold explained how he massaged the numbers to reduce his patients' exposure to suffering and risk:

And in the Catholic hospital you had to wait till they get sick, which was kind of foolish when you knew the prognosis was so poor. So you have to wait till they got an infection. So, if the temperature, normal temperature was 98.6, true infection's probably not till 100.6, but we would cut corners, and so if they got to 99, we would call it a fever. And we would induce them. Because we were protecting their life and trying to salvage their uterus, so they didn't get a serious infection, that they needed a hysterectomy. So we cut corners there when the prognosis was poor, and we would just say, "Well, there's an overwhelming internal infection" when their temperature was 99 rather than 100. And then we would induce them so they don't get into trouble.

Similarly, Dr. Deborah Zander, who is Jewish, mentioned some of the diagnoses she used to get approval to do a tubal ligation during C-section. To my surprise, some of these even were suggested by the ethics committee.

> Hospital leadership, including clergy, did their best to look the other way. . . . We had this list of criteria. And it's generally known if you can't figure out what your criteria falls under for her C-section to have the tubal—I mean, anybody on the committee would have told you, "Oh, it's a reproductive hazard," or it's like "a serious pathology related to the reproductive tract, scarred uterus." If you have a serious medical condition, there's some sort of verbiage about that. If you have a genetic risk—so if you're over thirty-five, you clearly have a genetic risk. So we kind of, I mean, we were kind of massaging things.

Some physicians framed this strategy as "massaging" language to generate a diagnosis that would justify the treatment per the principle of double effect. Others, like Dr. Chan, named it for what it was: lying to overcome a barrier to care. "If anything, it's that the Catholic Church makes you lie, you know? That's what I think. It's always like, 'Oh, gee' and you just kind of roll your eyes."

In our conversation, Dr. Chan stressed that doctors have, by now, become accustomed to stretching the truth to work around bureaucratic hurdles, whether or not they work in Catholic hospitals. She continued: "In a lot of ways, that's insurance in general though. You know what I mean? There's a lot of workarounds for, 'Okay, we're going to call it this because that'll get paid for and this won't.'" Her comments help us understand why physicians who work in Catholic hospitals so readily rationalize lying, false charting, and misdiagnosing: they are already doing it anyway—to a certain extent—to make a rigid reimbursement system work for their patients and themselves.[3] What is different, and particularly troubling, about the Catholic context is that doctors were perpetuating untruths to adhere to rules supposedly based on faith-based morality that neither the patients nor the doctors necessarily subscribe to.

Conceal

For physicians, who tend to be rule-abiding and risk averse as a group, the threat of losing privileges looms large. Losing privileges can gravely disrupt a physician's medical practice, and it leaves a professional stain on their record and reputation. It also can interfere with a physician's ability to get privileges in another hospital, to get hired into a practice, or to get patients at all. Physicians can lose privileges in a hospital due to poor bedside manner, failure to meet the medical standards of their specialty, and, most relevant here, failure to follow hospital policies or procedures. Physicians may lower the risk of being accused of not following hospital policy if they get patients to play along. But for most physicians working in Catholic hospitals, the best way to avoid the consequences of breaking the rules is to avoid getting caught. For that reason, multiple physicians mentioned that they or their colleagues simply hid some treatments and practices they perceived to be both critical to patient wellbeing and of low risk to their professional standing.

Who were they hiding their activities from? Often, nurses. A consistent thread throughout physician narratives was the need to keep nurses out of the loop, as nurses are tasked with rule enforcement and protocols. In Catholic hospitals, some nurses also track physicians' compliance with hospital religious rules. Given that nurses have less autonomy and power in medicine than physicians, in some cases making them more vulnerable to retribution by a hospital employer, some nurses may prefer not witnessing workarounds. Physicians ensured this by building in private spaces—a desk drawer, a locked closet, time alone with patients—less accessible to the nurses. Physicians shared stories of covertly delivering a private stash of oral contraceptives or an illicit prescription and counseling for contraception behind closed doors. They also described practices that seem difficult to pull off without nurses' knowledge; for instance, not checking for heart tones when miscarriage was inevitable or performing a tubal ligation after a C-section. Because I interviewed only two ob-gyn nurses, I cannot speak to their awareness of such practices. It may be that this form of "concealment" involves some nurses' willingness to ignore things they are not intended to see.

Many Catholic hospitals do not stock oral contraceptives in their pharmacies. When a patient is on oral contraceptives and becomes admitted to the hospital for an unrelated reason, physicians sometimes have to navigate the awkwardness of asking family to covertly bring the pills in so she can continue to take them herself, unlike other medications that a hospital would routinely supply and nurses would formally administer to the patient in the course of care.

The lack of contraceptives in Catholic hospital pharmacies can present more urgent problems managing patients who come to the ER with abnormal menstrual bleeding. When such a patient arrives, physicians first assess the patient's stability. If a patient is unstable for having lost too much blood, what physicians often call "dysfunctional bleeding," they may be admitted for additional assessment and management to stop the bleeding. Management ranges from medication (usually oral contraceptives) or a procedure such as transfusion, D&C, removal of bleeding fibroids, and, in extreme cases, a hysterectomy. But if a patient is stable, the American College of Obstetrics and Gynecology recommends prescribing birth control pills. While such a prescription would be easily justified as medically necessary, there are reasons the doctor would want certain patients to start taking the medication while still in the hospital, including simply verifying that the oral contraceptives are enough to stop the bleeding or wanting to ensure the patient has access to the pills if they are uninsured or underinsured. For example, one patient I interviewed, Sheila, had gone through several episodes of dysfunctional bleeding with pain from cysts, and she had the bad fortune of having an episode when she had a gap in her insurance coverage due to a change in employment; she could not see an ob-gyn without paying out-of-pocket. Eventually, because of the pain from the cyst, she went to the emergency room of the only hospital in her area, which was Catholic, but they sent her home with a follow-up appointment at a doctor's office after determining that no immediate action was needed for the cyst.

SHEILA: I was also bleeding so heavily I was worried. And they were like, "Well, we really can't do anything for you because" the medicine that I needed to stop everything was just Provera, again, but there at the hospital, they were not allowed to write that prescription . . . because it is in the same class as birth control and they're Catholic.

LORI: So what happened?

SHEILA: I had to wait until I could go to an ob-gyn because their offices were separate. That's how they get around it, which I've always thought crazy.

LORI: Okay. So you're in the ER, you're bleeding, and they figured out that you need birth control related medication to stop the bleeding. What did they say to you about it? Do you remember?

SHEILA: I was being seen by the physician's assistant and she told me flat out, "What you need we can't write you a prescription for. You're going to have to go to your ob-gyn and . . . tell them what happened and they will write you the prescription you need." And I told her, "I'm in between right now. I can't go to my doctor." And she said that they weren't allowed to write it. [So] I went home. I just dealt . . .

Sheila did not leave with pills in hand, which is what she needed, nor was she able to get into the ob-gyn office because of her insurance lag and not having enough money to pay out-of-pocket, so she continued to bleed heavily. "It went on for two or three weeks pretty heavy. Yeah, it was really, really unpleasant."

Some physicians who have experience working in Catholic hospitals that do not allow any stocking of oral contraceptives know that if they want to ensure the patient gets the contraceptives they need in the ER they must keep their own stash on hand. Others have to learn this the hard way. Dr. Ward told me about a time his practice partner "was called in to see somebody with dysfunctional bleeding, significant bleeding from the emergency room and—an indigent person," shortly after their Western hospital had been purchased by a Catholic system. "She left the hospital and got a call about an hour later, 'We don't have any birth control pills here on formulary,' and so they didn't even have the medication for a non-contraceptive use." Dr. Ward and his colleagues were still coming to terms with the impact of the religious affiliation on their ability to help patients. Ultimately, his colleague "went to her office, got packages and went in there [to the ER] and gave them to the patient without the hospital's awareness of it."

Dr. Bari (introduced in chapter 5), a physician who works at an East Coast Catholic hospital, corroborated the existence of this practice among physicians savvy about Catholic hospital policies, especially if their offices are nearby: "They don't keep birth control pills in stock for [dysfunctional bleeding in the ER], so most of us have offices on campus, so we would go get them from our office. . . . Literally walk over—yeah. And that's a whole other—you have to do that kind of on the sly. The nurses can't really document that because you're just getting it out of your own closet."

Not charting prescriptions or handing patients medicine without the nurses' knowledge might be considered a deeply suspect practice in other settings. In a Catholic ER, however, consulting ob-gyns view these same practices as the most ethical and straightforward way to help their patients.

Instead of following approved Ethical and Religious Directives for Catholic Healthcare Services-sanctioned medical protocols, physicians are moved to bend the rules, get creative, and conceal workarounds from monitoring eyes. But are they moved equally by all patients to take such risks? The layers of discretion and judgment involved in working around the ERDs brings up questions of bias. Which patients appear most sympathetic and deserving of physicians' efforts to retrieve a personal stash of sample packages of birth control from the office? This is where unconscious racial bias can become highly problematic, which plagues medicine as surely as it does other facets of society.[4] The expansion of Catholic healthcare systems not only limits women's access to care; it also can magnify existing racial disparities by relying on physician discretion about when and whether to take professional risks or go the extra mile to meet patients' needs.

Contraceptive counseling is another activity physicians sought to hide from nurses and other hospital staff. The ERDs prohibit the "promotion of contraceptive practices." When not justifying contraception through an acceptable diagnosis, some doctors simply hid their counseling. Dr. Roy (introduced in chapter 5), a maternal-fetal medicine specialist who holds privileges in three Catholic hospitals and two non-Catholic hospitals, said that while in the Catholic facilities: "I continue to counsel about contraception and all that. I don't know if somebody hears it or not . . . I do it behind closed doors . . . but I mean, if a nurse walks in I continue my conversation." Dr. Jacob Halpern, a Jewish perinatologist who had experience working in Northeastern Catholic hospitals, although his primary hospital was not Catholic, felt that hiding contraceptive counseling and failing to document his prescriptions was a way to be considerate of the nurses charged with enforcing hospital rules. "I think the nurses knew that this was going on. I mean, it wasn't that they were policing us. We just didn't put them in the position of . . . they wouldn't get us in trouble for talking about it but sort of the documentation that went in the chart would be sparse around the contraceptive counseling."

None of the individuals in the study disclosed having performed tubal ligations covertly. I nevertheless wondered if it had happened. Many mentioned the exceeding simplicity of tying the fallopian tubes during a C-section, as did Dr. Gold, who told me: "If you're in the delivery room and you have a C-section and tubes are right there . . . they're very easy to tie."

Dr. Jay told me a story about how one of his teachers in a Catholic hospital used to do covert tubal ligations long ago: "We had an old professor. Gosh, he's got to be dead now anyway. That was 25 years ago [in the late 1980s]. But he would do a C-section and if the patient wanted to have a tubal ligation, do the C-section, take the uterus out to sew it up and at the same time put clamps on the tubes, you know, and just destroy them, 'cause the patient wanted that. And he'd always—he knew who would assist him that wasn't going to say anything about it."

This story of covertly sterilizing patients is alarming, to say the least. It is notable that it involves a teacher, which means that multiple new physicians observed the procedure and went into practice knowing this was at least a possibility. While one interpretation puts the physician on the patient's side, covertly doing what she asked him to do, risking his own professional standing on her behalf, it is just as easy to imagine a situation in which the patient did not thoroughly consent, given the lack of any formal documentation. Worse yet, any biases the doctor might have about who should or should not reproduce would be additionally concealed by the practice. Dr. Jay's telling says that the patient "wanted" it, but we also know that involuntary sterilizations went on systemically into the 1970s. It is entirely possible, or perhaps even probable, that the original physician "learned" to do this as a way to tie the tubes of indigent women without their consent. Given the stark history of involuntary sterilizations along with the power dynamics, the nurses' "increased policing" could have several different explanations, including protecting patients from racist/classist doctors. Ultimately, "concealment" as a workaround privileges physician authority over true accountability.

Rename

Some Catholic hospitals occasionally allowed prohibited procedures to take place after someone—usually someone with authority in the Catholic hospital context—renamed or reimagined the prohibited medical procedure. For example, several physicians mentioned that tubal ligations were performed under a slightly different name in the era before the sterilization crackdown. It is very difficult to ascertain the scale to which this happened, but given that multiple interviewees from different corners of the country reported the practice, it is reasonable to suspect they were not exceptional.

Dr. Theresa Drake told me about witnessing a procedure the physicians called "uterine separation" during her training at a Catholic medical school on the East Coast. She found the experience both memorable and peculiar: "When I was doing my third-year rotation there was a woman having her eighth baby who wanted a tubal and they wouldn't do it. And so somebody renamed it 'uterine separation.' I just remember that, that like you give it a new name and it's okay now. I just thought it was kind of funny . . . They separated the uterus from its surrounding structures." Similarly, Dr. Albu recalled that in Midwestern Catholic hospital where she trained "instead of doing a tubal ligation after a woman had a baby, they called them 'uterine isolations.'"

Dr. Gold's hospital even had a special committee devoted to rubber-stamping requests for tubal ligations by another name:

> We had very, very sick patients and many of them probably would die if they had another pregnancy. So, in a public hospital, you just call it a simple tubal ligation. But as it is a Jesuit University, you can't do a tubal ligation, so we had a committee, it was called the "*Uterine Isolation Committee.*" You had to write

them a letter explaining why this patient, [why] it would be against her best health to have any more children, and then you automatically, it was a rubber stamp, you got a letter back saying go ahead and you can do a uterine isolation procedure, which was really just a tubal ligation. So they got around the whole Jesuit thing, with just calling it something different.

Catholic theologians were not fooled by this. Ultimately, the term "uterine isolation" circulated widely enough that the Vatican prohibited it. The guidance was clear and exactly as it had been for tubal ligations—which makes sense because it is exactly the same procedure. The Vatican's guidance reiterated that Catholic hospitals may not ever perform direct sterilization for the purpose of contraception, even if a subsequent pregnancy would put the woman's life at risk.

That said, per the principle of double effect, physicians can perform hysterectomies if there is something wrong with the uterus. Enter the concept of the "tired uterus," a somewhat unscientific term used when a uterus does not effectively contract and shrink back down after birth, possibly due to exhaustion during labor, and sometimes due to having given birth many times. Dr. Acker described encountering use of this term in the 1980s to justify surgery: "I'll tell you one thing they used to do . . . instead of doing tubal ligations, they would do Cesarean hysterectomies, believe it or not. And I remember this one guy, he would say, 'It's a *tired uterus.*' And a Cesarean hysterectomy is a pretty dangerous operation."

He added that, in the past, Catholic hospitals frequently performed hysterectomies for non-pregnant women who wanted to be sterilized, even though tubal ligations were safer. The term "tired uterus" fit with the Catholic doctrine of "remove the pathology" and opened the door for doctrinal iatrogenesis. Generally, the uterus can effectively contract again with the help of medications, but calling something a tired uterus to get around sterilization restrictions exposes the patient to a higher level of risk; hysterectomy is a more dangerous operation than a tubal ligation. The removal of the uterus also has the potential of long-term side effects such as pelvic prolapse. Thus, this renaming practice is ethically dubious to the point of malpractice; one can only hope it is, by now, obsolete.

The most extreme story of reimagining prohibited care as something else was recounted by Dr. Zander, from the period when she served as chief of the ob-gyn department. One day, the hospital's clergyman, who we will call Father Tom, asked her to arrange an abortion that he insisted was not actually an abortion.

Dr. Zander began her story by saying: "I did have a very bizarre experience once." She explained that a patient's fetus had been diagnosed with anencephaly, which means that a major portion of the brain, skull, and or scalp has not developed. The condition is fatal; such a fetus cannot survive long outside the womb. By now, it was quite late in the second trimester, leaving little time to get a termination of pregnancy done in most states. The physicians arranged for a termination at an abortion clinic they trusted would provide her safe and compassionate care in a large city a couple of hours away. It was then that things started to get strange: "So apparently, she was one of Father Tom's parishioners and she went to Father Tom and she said she really didn't want to carry this pregnancy, but she really didn't want to go to an abortion clinic and why does she have to go to an abortion clinic? Why can't she stay at [St. Vincent's]? And this baby's not gonna make it anyway. And she did this whole thing with Father Tom."

The patient was clearly distressed about carrying the pregnancy to term, which is a sentiment expressed by many women when they learn their fetus has a severe or life-threatening condition, but she also was deeply disturbed by the idea that she would be an abortion patient seeking an abortion in an abortion clinic. Committing such an act would pose a deep threat to her identity as a devout Catholic; the stigma of the abortion clinic permeated the entire conflict.

Even though Dr. Zander was now working as the chief of ob-gyn services at a hospital that resolutely refused to perform abortions, she herself was definitively pro-choice. She supported Planned Parenthood and even had provided abortions herself before taking the job at St. Vincent's. Given the irony that Father Tom was a representative of the Catholic Church that promulgated the doctrine he now wanted her to ignore, she took umbrage at his request:

> So then Father Tom calls me and he said, "Well, you know, it's really okay for you to do this procedure at [St. Vincent's] Hospital. And this is why." And he starts giving me this convoluted story about why it's okay . . . It seemed so completely random to me that I absolutely couldn't recreate it. And I was in a position of saying, "You know, we don't have a protocol for doing this. We don't have a nursing staff that's prepared, we don't have a protocol for when it's okay. This is very confusing to people. We've never done this. We don't have protocol that says when it's okay and when it's not. She has like two days to get to [large city]. If we can't make this happen, she will miss her opportunity all together." And I frankly had no intention of putting in—I mean, I just really didn't feel like putting in the energy, in two days, to figure out *how we were gonna make this okay.*
>
> So I called the president of the hospital, and I explained the situation to him and I could practically hear him getting down on his knees [to pray]—I mean, the one thing he hates is bad publicity and he is like . . . "Well, you know, you don't have to do anything you don't want to do." He said, "Just remember, you don't have to do anything you don't want to do. You don't have to do this. It's your choice." And I could hear this like pleading quality in his voice—like, please. . . .

The president of the hospital, reluctant to tell Dr. Zander not to do it, seemed to hope (or pray) she would refuse so their Catholic hospital could avoid the kind of public scandal that might erupt if word got out that they had performed an abortion (more scandalous yet, at the urging of a priest).

Ultimately, it was the fiction itself that Dr. Zander objected to most fervently. She continued:

> I mean, the whole thing was crazy, and it was crazy for *me* . . . The fact of the matter is, it's an abortion . . . They do this in abortion clinics . . . I didn't really

feel a great need to bolster her fantasy that this is not an abortion. So, the whole thing was so confusing on so many levels . . .

I like really didn't know what to do and I'm kind of sleeping on it. And I wake up the next morning and I run into one of my colleagues . . . [and] I'm telling him this story and he said, "This feels bad to you because this is just not in your current medical practice. It's like somebody asked you to do something that's not in your current medical practice and you don't want to do it, so don't do it." I mean, he was just like very straight. And I said, "I'm not doing it," and that was the end of the little episode.

Dr. Zander ultimately determined that, despite Father Tom's sincere wish that this was somehow not an abortion, the chances of her persuading all the hospital staff to share in his delusion were slim. Perhaps more to the point, she had no interest in contributing to abortion stigma by distinguishing between "worthy" and "unworthy" abortions. While on the one hand Father Tom was simply endeavoring to work around the religious restrictions on behalf of his parishioner, as doctors did daily for their patients, because he was a clergy member of the very church that authors and promulgates those restrictions, it chaffed. She did not want to assist the patient and Father Tom in their game of pretend, a dangerous game designed to limit care to those with access to the power to rename.

REBEL

While stories of physician rebellion to defy or subvert Catholic hospital policies were rare, I did hear a few. Some acts were brazen, whereas others were quite subtle. One standout was Dr. Acker's story of providing cab fare for extremely poor patients in the 1980s to shuttle to and from a non-Catholic hospital for a sterilization procedure immediately after delivery; a medically risky way to meet their needs:

It turns out some of the women had signed consent forms to have their tubes tied. So the first one came in, she had her baby, and the next morning I said to the nurse on the post-partum floor, "Well, let's get her ready because she's going to have her tubes tied." And she just went white. She said, "Are you nuts? Absolutely not. We don't do that in Catholic hospitals, blah, blah, blah." I said, "Okay." So I called [City] Hospital, which was our other—our secular hospital that was also part of the system and I talked to the chief there. He said, "Ah, bring her over. We'll do it here." So, in those days, before they had any of these security things, the women just walked around the halls, you know, post-partum, and everything like that, and would carry their babies and stuff. So I said to the woman, "If you want this to be done, I'll give you cab fare. You go down, you go out in the front of the hospital and get in a cab, go to [the non-Catholic hospital], I'll meet you there, we'll tie your tubes, we'll bring you back here, nobody will know any different." . . . It's like a twenty-minute drive. So we did and it worked out really great and I probably did about two or three of those before they caught me . . . God, were they mad.

It is very hard to imagine such a practice succeeding in the current era marked by security, managed care, and electronic medical records. The fact these women were traveling postpartum, and then post-surgery, in taxis by themselves is quite medically precarious. Dr. Acker presented himself as a bit of a medical cowboy on a social justice mission; such subterfuge perhaps appeals most to risk-takers but by no means guarantees the best outcome for patients.

Rebels·such as the physicians in Dr. Bari's hospital who regularly provide oral contraceptives to patients in the ER lacked Dr. Acker's level of action and drama. She explained: "The ER doctors routinely prescribe whatever they need to prescribe . . . they have electronic medical records and electronic prescribing and it's all very traceable and they do it anyway." Based on our conversation, I wondered if Dr. Bari's hospital is particularly permissive; she went on to explain that she typically does not check for heart tones before treating a woman whose miscarriage is inevitable: "If you write the diagnosis as 'inevitable abortion at five weeks,' at five weeks you may not see a heartbeat anyway. And if that's what your diagnosis is, most people won't really question you about, 'Are you sure this isn't a viable pregnancy?' You know, when they're bleeding and it's obvious that that there's blood all over their perineum, they don't usually question it."

Dr. Bari explains that, in her hospital, the use of the term "inevitable" is important; without it, the nurses will require proof that there is no cardiac activity before allowing treatment to proceed: "[The nurses] have got check lists for everything . . . if you're coming in for a D&C or failed pregnancy, they need proof that the pregnancy really has failed, that you're not trying to sneak in an elective termination."

Dr. Bari frames the confirmation of no cardiac activity during miscarriage treatment within a normal domain of nursing practice: the checklist. Medical care requires such an extensive number of safety protocols that the integration of checklists is increasingly common, and studies show they improve health outcomes.[5] But, in Catholic hospitals, the nurse's checklist may include compliance with the hospital's religious policies as well as more routine safety checks.

Dr. Fine, whose Western hospital had been recently made Catholic, had already found (in chapter 5) that it was compromising medical practice there. She did not accept the presence of ERD-driven tasks on the checklist. When I asked her whether she had been in a situation where she was unsure if she could offer treatment during an inevitable miscarriage because of the presence of fetal heart tones, she replied: "I wouldn't even ask. If they want to come get me later, let them." Dr. Fine spoke with bravado; she asserted that confirming a lack of cardiac activity was medically irrelevant in such cases, as she clung to her medical authority and autonomy. That the nurses assisting her felt the same way is certainly plausible, because it is highly unlikely physicians would successfully evaluate patients, make a decision, and proceed without any assistance from any nursing staff whatsoever.

Dr. Unni (introduced in chapter 5) works in an especially strict Northeastern Catholic hospital. Even if the nurses wanted to help her skirt the rules, the hospital has implemented procedures that make it hard to avoid the restrictions on miscarriage management. Her hospital requires the ER physicians do an ultrasound to check for cardiac activity in every patient who presents with vaginal bleeding. She, therefore, cannot claim ignorance if she deems a termination is in the best interest of the patient before ERD criteria are met.

The day of our interview, Dr. Unni had operated on a woman with an ectopic pregnancy. During the surgery, staff members repeatedly asked whether there was a heartbeat, even though ectopic pregnancies are not only nonviable but potentially lethal. When I asked who is generally the most concerned about this issue, she stated: "Nursing staff and OR staff . . . I don't know if it's because they believe in the rules that are set by the Catholic Church or if they just want to make sure they're not getting in trouble. It could be both." Whatever their objections, they ultimately assisted her in the operation; no one walked out of the room despite the fact that nurses have less power and could be at more risk than the physician when breaking hospital rules. The consequences of this action, however, were not clear at the time of our conversation.

In another emergent case, she did not check heart tones because she felt it was irrelevant. Although she relied on her authority as the attending physician and the urgency of the clinical situation to compel staff to disregard the requirement to check heart tones, staff nonetheless peppered her with questions about fetal cardiac activity. She deflected: "'Oh, no, it's definitely not a pregnancy that's going to survive,' is what I tell people to get around that. . . . That's only happened to me once and this lady was really hemorrhaging, and I was transfusing her in the OR and she really was not doing well and so no one really questioned that at that point."

Rebellion entails various levels of risk depending on the clinical scenario, the culture of the hospital, the autonomy of the health professional, and the degree of surveillance by clergy. Getting caught could have serious professional consequences for doctors and nurses. A family nurse practitioner (FNP) I spoke with who took a job in a Catholic health system's outpatient clinic that strictly adhered to the ERDs refused to omit contraceptive counseling and prescriptions from her practice, and then charted openly about it. Her honesty was met by a firm reprimand from her supervisor, who then refused to recommend her as permanent hire, extending her probationary period in the clinic because she "required additional chart review." Yet, her supervisor was soon replaced and the new one found the FNP's practices acceptable and allowed her to advance. While doctors discussed quietly providing contraception under the radar regularly, this nurse practitioner's experience suggests that the response to a clinician's rebellion against the ERDs can vary greatly by work environments, staff, and the power of the rebel.

For patients who might find themselves on the operating table or in the exam room with a clinician willing to do what is not technically allowed, rebellion can be welcoming or confusing, or both. Yet, only certain patients gain access to restricted care. Who are doctors willing to collude with? Presumably, they do not take such chances every day, or with every patient who might need/desire prohibited services. What kind of patient inspires a doctor to act like Father Tom, to proclaim that the religious rules just do not apply to them?

Conclusion

Compared to either their patients or nurses, doctors working in Catholic hospitals are relatively powerful actors. They are, nevertheless, practicing medicine in a sea of religious and administrative constraints. Watchful staff and increasingly stringent reporting procedures make it hard for doctors to reliably work around the bishops' policies. Nonetheless, the physicians I interviewed named numerous strategies for working around the religious rules to avoid doctrinal iatrogenesis when all above-board options were off the table. Whether through justifying a treatment as medically necessary, concealing a prescription from prying eyes, renaming a procedure as something other than it is, or outright rebellion, some physicians working in Catholic hospitals have learned to be creative so as not to deprive their patients of standard reproductive treatments, and sometimes hospital systems themselves bend the rules when doing so suits them. Fundamentally, however, physician discretion over when to stretch the truth or bend the rules for a patient is not an equitable replacement for access to care. As such, the expansion of the Catholic healthcare system reproduces inequality by encouraging idiosyncratic and unpredictable adaptations that are not sustainable at scale.

CHAPTER 7

Separation of Church
and Hospital

In 2009, Catholic Healthcare West's St. Joseph's Hospital in Phoenix, Arizona, admitted an extremely ill twenty-seven-year-old mother of four with pulmonary hypertension to its intensive care unit. Importantly, she was also eleven weeks pregnant. Doctors determined she would likely die if the pregnancy continued, yet she was too ill to be moved to another facility. She consented to a termination of pregnancy.[1] A fiery conflict ensued that ultimately resulted in St. Joseph's being stripped of its affiliation with the Catholic Church. Various news sources reported that: (1) a St. Joseph's doctor performed a life-saving abortion; (2) in response, Bishop Thomas J. Olmsted excommunicated St. Joseph's administrator Sister Margaret McBride, who had authorized the procedure; (3) a public feud ensued between hospital leadership who supported the decision and religious authorities who did not; and (4) Bishop Olmsted subsequently stripped the hospital of its Catholic affiliation.

Throughout my decade-plus of researching how Catholic doctrine affects health care, it always has mystified me that some hospitals continued to be affiliated with the Church after the affiliation no longer seems to serve them. How and why do hospitals remain bound to the Ethical and Religious Directives for Catholic Health Care Services in an era of mega hospitals and health systems that do not derive financial support from the Church and have few clergy members left within them? What would the consequences be if a hospital simply severed ties?

I had heard anecdotal reports of a few hospitals that ceased to be Catholic, but no clear patterns emerged. Nor did the doctors I spoke with know much about what had transpired behind the scenes. This makes the St. Joseph's case exceptional. The break was widely reported, and in the process of conducting interviews, I met an ob-gyn, by complete coincidence, who worked there. That ob-gyn then referred me to a second, and both were willing to share their experiences. The story of St. Joseph's separation from the Church shows how a bishop can wield power, how healthcare administrators can push back, and how, ultimately, the institutional imperative to grow can bring Catholic healthcare systems and clergy back together.

It also points to the problematic imbalance of power in the relationship between physicians and institutions. In Catholic hospitals, physicians are workers whose clinical autonomy is limited by the ERDs. The example of St. Joseph's shows that change from within Catholic health care is possible, but also improbable without countervailing external forces.

A Troubled Relationship

I use the hospital's real name here because it was such a public case that anonymization would be pointless—there are simply no others like it. However, to protect their confidentiality, I refer to the two doctors I interviewed by the pseudonyms Dr. William Murphy and Dr. Adele Lee.[2] A white, Catholic man, Dr. Murphy had worked in the hospital in Phoenix quite a long time when I first interviewed him in 2011. I began by asking him the same question I asked all physicians to get the conversation going: "Can you tell me a little bit about what you like and dislike about working at your hospital?" He launched right in.

> I like my colleagues. I like the institutional interest in the underserved and the commitment to taking care of the underserved. I don't like that, at times, that commitment is not as thoroughly lived out as one might wish it would be, and I don't like that the bishop has interfered in our care of women—although he seems to be out of the picture now—and that we needlessly have to work harder than necessary to provide our patients with all the appropriate, you know, the appropriate range of care, like contraceptive services and tubal ligation at the time of C-sections, particularly. Are you familiar with the St. Joe's in Phoenix and the recent controversy we've had with the local bishop?

Starstruck, I gasped: "This is *your* hospital?" He assured me it was, and I asked him to explain what he meant by the bishop being out of the picture now. He said simply: "I mean, he divorced us." His use of the term divorce was ironic, of course; divorce is notoriously frowned upon within Catholicism. Dr. Murphy's language was peppered with the kind of humor-bordering-on-irreverence that only a member of the club can pull off.

When Dr. Murphy first began working at St. Joseph's, he did not think much about the religious policies. St. Joseph's doctors were permitted to do tubal ligations at the time of C-section, Dr. Murphy said: "with minimal justification and relative impunity," because the patient was already having a surgery. He explained that the physicians simply needed to document "an important medical or anatomic reason to do a tubal to prevent future potential morbidity or mortality for the mom or future fetuses." He continued: "And so that was the environment when I was a resident, and it was the environment for the first several years of me being an attending. And a lot of this is bishop dependent. I didn't really realize it at the time."

He added: "Nothing about St. Joe's struck me as unusual when I was a resident or a young attending." He was able to offer contraception in his own clinic, which was located in the office building next door. The office building was not owned by the hospital or the healthcare system. While Directive 52 states: "Catholic health institutions may not promote or condone contraceptive practices," Dr. Murphy explained that "our functional interpretation of that in the late nineties and to this day is 'Okay, we don't give it in the hospital. We give it in the clinic next door.'" Over there, he said, "there never has been a contraception prohibition."

For Dr. Murphy, these two flexibilities—contraception in his office and some wiggle room around sterilization for C-section in the hospital—meant he could live with the religious constraints on his practice. But things began to change in 2003 when a new bishop was installed: "They'll say 'we've never changed our policy' but they have. But it's fair to say that some bishops [take], they like to call it, a more pastoral approach, which means they're kind of supportive and they keep their nose out of the reproductive issues. Some bishops take a more, sometimes they'll say, a more magisterial approach, and they'll say 'we're more interested in making sure we follow the teachings of the magisterium.' And so, you know, Bishop O'Brien, that we had [previously] was more pastoral."

Dr. Murphy was the only doctor to distinguish between a pastoral approach and a magisterial approach. In fact, he is unusual among the rank-and-file physicians I spoke with throughout this project, displaying far more knowledge about the dynamics of the Catholic Church and its hierarchy's influence on his hospital. His pastoral versus magisterial distinction helped me understand why I heard tales of bishops' cracking down on tubal ligation practice in some places and not others. The pastoral approach refers to the style of clergy member that doctors think of as supportive, empathetic, and nonintrusive. One Catholic critic of the pastoral approach likened it to having "a truncated set of values,"[3] and another asserted that it signified a willingness to "turn a blind eye to breaking church law."[4] In contrast, those clergy who adopt the magisterial approach are more likely to follow the letter of the law. The Catholic Church regards the magisterium as the authentic, legitimate, and even infallible teaching authority passed from Christ through the Apostles to their successors: the bishops in union with the pope.[5] A magisterial approach includes a strict enforcement of Church law, and in the U.S. healthcare context, this includes the ERDs written by those very bishops themselves.

Compared to other physicians I interviewed, Dr. Murphy was more cognizant of individual directives and their variable implementation. Having done some informal research of his own, he explained: "My impression from talking to people in a lot of different places across the country is there's really just a wide range of practices at Catholic hospitals. Some are very strict in terms of their contraception and sterilization approaches, and some are really not." His curiosity might have been fueled by his personal background, but he also took a special interest in what was happening at other Catholic hospitals as conflict started brewing at his own.

Dr. Murphy returned to the saga at St. Joseph's:

> What changed was we got a new bishop. We had a bishop named O'Brien, who
> had his own little scandal that led to his downfall, that involved drinking and

running somebody over with his car and apparently not noticing and driving his car home and all that kind of stuff.[6] So that led to him going away and that led to the appointment of Thomas Olmsted, a bishop named Thomas Olmsted, who's the current bishop of the Dioceses of Phoenix. And he came, I want to say 2003. Although things didn't start to change in 2003.

Around 2005, Bishop Olmsted "started pressing the hospital about these issues a little bit more." The bishop's pressure did not emerge in a vacuum; it reflected the international concern of devout Catholics about sterilization practices in Catholic hospitals far and wide, visible in their public writings, with some pressure traceable to Pope Benedict XVi in Rome.[7]

In 2005, Dr. Lee, a white ob-gyn with no particular religious identification, was in practice with Dr. Murphy at St. Joseph's hospital. She similarly recalled a relatively permissive environment related to contraceptive services, at least at first: "I felt in terms of birth control I could provide my patients what they needed . . . I was not uncomfortable with how we were practicing." Although she recalled restrictions on performing tubal ligations for women who had not had C-sections, she accepted the workaround of taking these patients to a nearby surgical center about six weeks postpartum. She and her colleagues understood themselves to be in compliance with the ERDs because they were not performing the procedure within the Catholic hospital. But soon enough, the fact that they were employees of the hospital became an issue.

Around 2007, the hospital administration told the ob-gyns to stop taking patients to the nearby surgery center. The parent system, Catholic Healthcare West (CHW), wanted to keep such business within the system, so they instructed the doctors to take patients to a CHW affiliate thirty miles away, which was not required to follow the ERDs fully, to do the tubal ligations. Not long after that, however, they were told to stop doing interval tubal ligations altogether. Dr. Lee recalled: "Initially we were going to a surgicenter that was right by our hospital to do the tubal ligations, but then they decided they wanted us to at least stay in their health-care system . . . Then eventually, they decided we just couldn't do them anymore, that we would have to refer those patients somewhere else altogether. And you know, you have a relationship with patients."

For Dr. Lee, the rupture of the patient-physician relationship that resulted from sending them to another doctor was unwelcome. She found the system limitations on where she could go and what she could offer her patients increasingly suffocating. She said: "We kept getting squeezed a little bit more, a little bit more. Family planning was important to me, so I wasn't happy with that." She continued:

When I first joined it was fairly new in the history of St. Joe's employing [their own] physicians . . . they didn't pay that much attention to us, we were fairly autonomous . . . as long as our numbers were OK, everybody left us alone. But over the time that I was there, they brought in a new chair, and they said you guys are going to do this, and this, and this . . . It's hard to remember exactly what we were being told when but there was definitely this sense that the bishop in the community—and the Catholic Church a little bit—were poking around and paying a lot of attention to exactly what we were doing."

Dr. Lee did not know much about Catholicism or Catholic health care before she started residency at St. Joseph's. The gymnastics involved in working around the directives bothered her, as did the surveillance. As a self-described rule follower, Dr. Lee was not used to stretching the truth in her charts, as others were accustomed to doing to get around the ERDs. She wrote down exactly what she did for the patients, and why:

> I didn't want to put in the chart, "oh, the patient has heavy periods," or "the patient has a problem with their periods," when that wasn't really true. If they were getting an IUD [intrauterine device] for birth control I wanted to write that they were there for birth control, and I was putting in an IUD for birth control. And so, it was a little bit gray: How we were supposed to document that and what people thought we were telling the patients. Our stance, as a small group of us physicians, was that what happens between the patient and the physician in the exam room is just between the patient and the physician and the administration and the Church can't come in and look at our charts. It's none of their business.
>
> But it wasn't totally clear—what if something bad happened and it became known that I put this IUD in . . . I wasn't sure, if there was a complication, if that chart went to be reviewed by another committee in the hospital, [what would happen?]

She could not shake the lingering fear that she would face some sort of punishment, or worse, that she would not be legally protected by the hospital's malpractice coverage. It bothered her. "Everything was sort of nebulous: What we really should be doing and what was expected of us. I didn't like that it was sort of gray." Dr. Lee eventually left.

Dr. Murphy, in contrast to Dr. Lee, was unphased by the culture of working around what he considered to be unrealistic and unjust health doctrine. He was, after all, a seasoned left-leaning Catholic. He became less comfortable as enforcement increased.

> It really wasn't until probably the eighteen months that preceded December of 2010 that the bishop really started putting pressure on the hospital and saying, "we don't want you to do any tubal ligations at the time of Cesarean delivery."
>
> And this is a big deal for us because we're a big hospital and we're a tertiary care center and we run a high-risk obstetric service and we get maternal transports and we get people transported with bad medical problems and complicated pregnancies and people who pregnancy really does jeopardize their health.
>
> And so when he [Bishop Olmsted] really started putting pressure on the administration and the administration consequently started putting pressure on the clinicians not to do tubals at the time of C-section, it was really making us uncomfortable and unhappy and causing some conflict.

This was a turning point for Dr. Murphy. For the first time, the Church's authority was directly affecting the quality of hospital care. He felt "inappropriate care patterns were being recommended."

I asked Dr. Murphy if he could remember how that conflict manifested at work and between colleagues. He recounted the interactions from approximately two to three years prior: "It manifested by the Chief Medical Officer coming to Ob-Gyn Department meetings and saying, you know, 'Guys, we're really getting some pressure from the bishop and we would really like to not be doing these tubals at the time of C-section,' which resulted in me saying, 'You know, at times that's going to result in inappropriate care,' which resulted in him saying, 'No, I don't believe that,' which resulted in me saying, 'Yes, you do,' and—which is the conflict that I'm referring to—it's at a department meeting."

Compared to my own experience of department meetings, this struck me as quite tense, but Dr. Murphy experienced it as not uncollegial: "It wasn't *that* tense. I mean, I've known the guy for a long time . . . administrators can have a tendency, when some pressure is exerted on them, they can have some tendency to want to make that problem go away and to want to comply." Nonetheless, Dr. Murphy openly expressed resentment about being required by his administration to withhold this care. "They're not on the front line," he said. "They don't get that sick feeling of feeling like you're not doing the right thing for somebody."

As he continued, his comments revealed an increasing sense of moral distress regarding in his position vis-à-vis patients:

> But if you're on the front line, you have a terrible feeling when a patient is transported, who had a plan for a tubal ligation, who went into pre-term labor at twenty-eight weeks, who needs to be delivered, who maybe has, you know, one disabled kid at home and now is going to deliver this preemie who might have a lot of challenges and require a lot of resources and you're told that you shouldn't do her tubal. When you're the person on the front line in that situation, it makes you want to go have an argument with someone.

RUPTURE

The ob-gyns at St. Joseph's did not comply with the orders. Such bold and transparent disobedience was extraordinarily rare among the physicians I spoke with. Dr. Murphy said: "Sometimes we did them [tubal ligations] and sometimes we didn't do them, but mostly we did them anyway and, you know, got a letter saying you shouldn't have done that." He specifically noted that they never performed sterilizations covertly: "We never did any tubals and like didn't document it or didn't write it in the chart or just clamped somebody's tubes and then—we never did that." However, the fact that the physicians chose not to obscure their practices meant that Bishop Olmsted took note. Dr. Murphy said: "As we continued to do that, and then the bishop continued to put pressure on hospital administrators . . . it was coming to a head." The sterilization dispute was fuel for an explosive situation, he continued, "but the termination of pregnancy, that one case really blew it up."

The patient at the center of this disputed abortion was in no way seeking to end her eleven-week pregnancy when she was admitted to St. Joseph's. She arrived at the tertiary care heart and lung care center with severe pulmonary hypertension in November 2009. Dr. Murphy explained: "She was actually admitted to the Intensive Care Unit on the pulmonologist service. She was not admitted to the obstetrical service." He went on: "I'm not sure how terribly sick she was when she got admitted, but then she continued to deteriorate. I mean, the classic textbook thing with pulmonary hypertension and pregnancy is, some of them do okay and get to carry to viability or even term and deliver, and some of them go *really bad*. Most of them do okay. You don't usually get to a situation as bad as this one. This is an unusual case. There's no question it's unusual."

I asked if it was a difficult decision for his ethics committee to approve the abortion procedure, but Dr. Murphy was disinclined to think of what the ethics committee did as "granting permission." He replied: "I wouldn't have even said 'a decision for the Ethics Committee.' It was a decision for the clinicians that they ran by the Ethics Committee, and it was a, you know, it was a sad and difficult case, but it was not a difficult decision to recommend that she end that pregnancy 'cause she was dying."

While that may have been true, Bishop Olmsted did not agree, and Sister McBride, an administrator and member of the Ethics Committee, received a rapid rebuke when the bishop learned of the abortion months later. In his May 2010 statement, Bishop Olmsted asserted: "I am further concerned by the hospital's statement that the termination of a human life was necessary to treat the mother's underlying medical condition. An unborn child is not a disease. While medical professionals should certainly try to save a pregnant mother's life, the means by which they do it can never be by directly killing her unborn child."[8]

He immediately excommunicated Sister McBride from the Church and she was demoted from her position of vice president of mission integration.[9] Journalists noted the contrast between the bishop's swift decision to punish Sister McBride and the Church's notoriously slow reaction to clergy sexual abuse.[10] The medical ethics director for the Diocese of Phoenix, Rev. John Ehrich, as well as the National Catholic Bioethics Center, backed up Bishop Olmsted.[11] Fr. Ehrich said: "She [McBride] consented in the murder of an unborn child . . . There are some situations where the mother may in fact die along with her child. But—and this is the Catholic perspective—you can't do evil to bring about good. The end does not justify the means."[12]

The hospital administration stood by Sister McBride and the other staff involved. In an October 27, 2010, statement defending Sister McBride, CHW included a lengthy moral analysis by a Marquette University professor and Catholic ethicist, arguing that it was theologically correct to approve the abortion because of the imminent risk to the mother's life.[13] The bishop, however, was undeterred: "I appreciate the diligence with which it [the statement] was drafted," Bishop Olmsted wrote. "At the same time . . . it disregards my authority and responsibility to interpret the moral law and to teach the Catholic faith as a successor of the apostles." He stated: "The Catholic Church will continue to defend life and proclaim the evil of abortion without compromise, and must act to correct even her own members if they fail in this duty . . . We always must remember that when a difficult medical situation involves a pregnant woman, there are two patients in need of treatment and care; not merely one. The unborn child's life is just as sacred as the mother's life, and neither life can be preferred over the other."[14]

From this perspective, the eleven-week fetus was no less valuable than the mother, regardless of the fact that it certainly would not survive if she died.

This back-and-forth appears to have caught many analysts by surprise. Mainstream and progressive news outlets exploded with interest in the drama, with titles such as that of ABC News, "Nun Excommunicated after Saving a Mother's Life with Abortion."[15] In contrast, some Catholics took note of the fact that abortions were happening in Catholic hospitals at all.[16] Within this latter group, significant disagreement existed around whether an abortion was ever justified, let alone justified by these particular medical circumstances.

Dr. Murphy told me that, in his experience, some portion of faithful Catholics will never accept "that the need for emergency abortion ever really happens." He expanded:

> If you get on the blogosphere and among conservative Catholics, you'll certainly see two themes of ideas that are incorrect. One is that medically these cases never really happen, these cases where somebody's pregnancy is going to kill them, and they have to end the pregnancy or else they're going to die . . .
>
> So one idea that I see floating out there is that the idea—usually from some doctor who's not a high-risk obstetrician—that [1,] these cases don't really happen, [and 2,] that they must have been exaggerating how sick mom was or they must have wanted to do an abortion. . . . And both of those things are not true. These cases are legitimately uncommon cases, even rare cases, but sometimes they do happen and, you know, this was one of the times when this woman was dying, and she would've died without a termination. This was not a choice between mom or baby. It was a choice—the fetus had no chance—this was a choice between letting two people die or saving the one that you can.

Recall that Directive 47 allows for the possibility of emergency abortion through the doctrine of double-effect, meaning that an abortion is permissible it if happens "unintentionally" (albeit predictably) while treating a patient to save her life. But in this case, Catholic authorities dismissed this justification, saying that the point of the intervention was to remove the pregnancy. Termination itself was the treatment rather than an unintended side effect of some other procedure. For these purists, the only theologically correct treatment would have been to continue pulmonary hypertension treatments, even knowing that, by so doing, they would save neither the pregnant woman nor her fetus's life. This disagreement over emergency abortion provides a window into the theological, gendered, and practical divisions between the Catholic right (the U.S. Conference of Catholic Bishops and the NCBC; mostly men) and the Catholic left (some nuns and the Catholic Health Association; more women) in the leadership of American Catholic healthcare institutions.

Dr. Murphy considers the bishops' stance unacceptable, as it prevents doctors from reliably saving the life that can be saved. Because of this, he questions if a rigid interpretation of the ERDs can coexist with a hospital that serves women properly:

> You might say, "Well maybe [if] Catholic hospitals are going to take this incred-
> ibly conservative view of the ethical and religious directives, maybe they just
> shouldn't run obstetrical services." Well this woman—it wouldn't have saved you
> from this case because this woman—was not admitted as a woman with a preg-
> nancy complication. This woman was admitted as a long-term pulmonary hyper-
> tension patient whose pulmonary hypertension was getting worse. She was
> admitted, and then they found out she was pregnant. So, what this says is you
> can't even take care of women. If you're going to run a hospital with a hyper-
> strict interpretation of the ERDs, you can't just run it and not have an obstetri-
> cal service. You have to never admit a woman to your hospital.

DISAFFILIATION

On November 22, 2010, Bishop Olmsted wrote Lloyd Dean, the CEO of CHW, a letter demanding that the hospital fulfill three requirements to retain its affiliation
with the Catholic Church. It was not money on the line, as neither the Church nor
the bishops fund the hospital. But to be able to continue to be known as a sanctioned institution of The Catholic Church, an identity meaningful to the founding
sisters and board members of the hospital, St. Joseph's would need to comply. Someone released the letter to a local news website, which posted it publicly.[17] Specifically, Bishop Olmsted first required that CHW publicly acknowledge its violation
of Directive 47, apologize for performing the abortion, and promise never to do so
again. Second, the Diocese of Phoenix must be allowed to conduct a thorough review
and ongoing oversight of the hospital's broader compliance with the Catholic directives. Finally, Bishop Olmsted demanded that St. Joseph's commit its clinicians to
ongoing training by either the diocese or the NCBC about the ERDs and their implementation. The hospital president, Linda Hunt, stood firm, issuing a public statement that the hospital was not only *not sorry* that it permitted its doctor to perform a
lifesaving procedure but that it would do nothing differently if presented with the
same clinical scenario.[18] Among the hospitals ob-gyns, the rumor was that the
decision not to comply came directly from CHW's corporate headquarters in San
Francisco.

Dr. Murphy recapped the situation: "That's the thing that we would identify as
the reason that we could really not comply with the bishop's demands . . . one of
the demands was that you had to say that you did the wrong thing and accept my

interpretation of the morality of the situation . . . we felt like we did the right thing, and we would do it again."

The entire situation was unprecedented; in my research sample, this is the only time in which a bishop initiated what Dr. Murphy referred to as "divorce."

Technically speaking, St. Joseph's being formally stripped by the bishop of its affiliation with the Catholic Church had little organizational or financial significance. A 2011 article in a Catholic news source reported that St. Joseph's remained a member of the Catholic Health Association: "The Catholic Health Association said it 'does not enter into' questions of how 'individual Catholic facilities and systems work with their local ordinary [bishop],' and it recognizes the local bishop's 'complete authority regarding the interpretation of' the bishops' ethical and religious directives."[19]

The hospital also remained religiously sponsored by its founders, the Sisters of Mercy, which continued to regard Sister McBride as one of their own in good standing.[20] The hospital's president, Linda Hunt, publicly stated that the Catholic identity and mission remained in place. Bishop Olmsted was able to make, however, one important change. The bishop's declaration effectively deconsecrated the space, meaning the hospital's chapel could no longer function as a de facto outpost of the Church. Mass could no longer be performed on site, a loss for religious patients and their families who were comforted by it. Nevertheless, in President Hunt's statement, she ensured that priests would still be allowed to see patients as they could at any other hospital.

Dr. Murphy agreed that Catholic patients were the most affected:

> The people who have been hurt by this are our patients who are Catholic and would like to go to Mass in the chapel at the church. But when the bishop says that he's taking away your Catholic identity, then you cannot have Mass . . . you cannot keep the Eucharist, the consecrated bread that to Catholics is the body of Christ . . .
>
> People have responded by saying, "But you can have Mass in an airport. You can have Mass, you know, in your back yard." And the answer to that has been that it's a matter of perception, and nobody's going to accidentally perceive an airport as a Catholic institution.

Indeed, Bishop Olmsted was quoted to this effect in a *National Catholic Reporter* article about the disaffiliation of St. Joseph's in 2011. He stated: "The Catholic faithful are free to seek care or to offer care at St. Joseph's Hospital but I cannot guarantee that the care provided will be in full accord with the teachings of the Church. In addition, other measures will be taken to avoid the impression that the hospital is authentically Catholic, such as the prohibition of celebrating Mass at the hospital and the prohibition of reserving the Blessed Sacrament in the Chapel."[21]

Bishop Olmsted's concern that the public might misperceive St. Joseph's as officially Catholic if Mass were continued there is poignant, if not paradoxical. Patients regularly mistake Catholic hospitals for facilities that are not restricted by the Church, but the Diocese of Phoenix is, of course, less concerned with clarifying limits on health care than limits on religion.

President Hunt was keen to reassure patients immediately after the split that this change in status did not have to impair their spiritual experience at the hospital. An Arizona business news source that interviewed her asked how the average patient would be affected by the fact that the "Roman Catholic Diocese of Phoenix has stripped St. Joseph's of its Catholic standing," and President Hunt replied:

> If you came into our hospital in early December and you came in today, we would look no different. The one thing we cannot do is Mass in the chapel. We still have worship services, they're just not Catholic worship services. But we do have rosaries, we have spiritual hours, we have people who are there to allow you to pray and to provide that spiritual comfort, just as we did in the past. . . . We acknowledge that (Bishop Thomas J. Olmsted) has the authority to no longer designate us a Catholic hospital. We're all very sad about that. . . . But we will always take care of people who are here and do what we can do to make sure they are safe, and that they receive the care that they deserve. . . . it came down to we had to save the life we could and we did."[22]

St. Joseph's stayed within the parent system of CHW. It was renamed Dignity Health in 2012, at which time Dignity Health as a system became nondenominational. Publicly, they stated they did so to accommodate the several non-Catholic (SCV) hospitals they acquired, which are allowed to offer contraception and sterilization, while the vast majority of Dignity's holdings remain officially Catholic and bound to the complete ERDs.

Regarding material losses besides the Eucharist, I asked Dr. Murphy if St. Joseph's lost any funding. Dr. Murphy did not think St. Joseph's suffered financial losses. He heard from colleagues that all the major hospital donors were going to continue giving and had no "qualms about the situation." Dr. Murphy summed up how he answers the very common query about Church money. People ask him: "'Is the Church giving you—you know, did you lose that financial support?' And I mean, the hospital runs a business. The Church doesn't financially support the hospital. The Church doesn't have any money, so the Church was never a source of income or anything for the hospital . . . So the concern was, you know, you're going to lose your charitable donations and things like that. And the answer I have heard—I mean, I don't see the books—but the answer that I've heard from multiple sources is no."

In fact, soon after the news broke, he heard from colleagues that some donations had increased from donors pleased with St. Joseph's handling of the situation.

According to Dr. Murphy, his colleagues were overwhelmingly pleased with the decision: "Oh, everyone was happy." Without Bishop Olmsted's surveillance haunting them, the doctors continued offering tubal ligations during C-section, although a justificatory medical-not-contraceptive reason was still required by the Sisters of Mercy involved with hospital administration. Even the sole conservative

Catholic physician on staff seemed happy, albeit possibly for a different reason. Dr. Murphy recalled: "He didn't think the hospital administration was really Catholic" so they may as well just "quit pretending." He stayed on staff.

The one exception to the rule, Dr. Murphy observed, was President Hunt: "I think it's always tough when you're the leader of the—the captain of the ship and your ship gets un-Catholic'd and your ship's been Catholic for 115 years, and it means something to you personally and professionally and in the community and all that kind of stuff. And so that is, you know, I think it's very hard on her. I think she still wonders if she did the right thing, even with a lot of reassurance from a lot of people that she did."

The patient at the center of the story also was upset, feeling guilty about the fall-out from her case. When Sister McBride was receiving a leadership award in 2011 at a conference of nuns titled "Call to Action," she recounted a touching reunion she had with the distressed patient that provided emotional healing for both of them.[23] As for Sister McBride herself, she was back on her feet shortly thereafter, and she reported the excommunication had been lifted because she complied with Bishop Olmsted's two conditions: that she go to confession and step down from her position.[24] President Hunt also reappointed her to a comparable position in the hospital.

The whole episode was quite fresh at the time of our first interview, in 2011. In 2019, I reached out to Dr. Murphy again to ask if there had been any changes in ob-gyn practice or the Catholic affiliation in the wake of the widely publicized merger of Catholic Health Initiatives and Dignity Health that year under CommonSpirit, based out of Chicago, which became the largest Catholic health system in the United States and fourth largest health system period.[25]

He reported that St. Joseph's remained officially unaffiliated with the Catholic Church at the time of the merger, and that staff and administration seemed anxious about what changes the new organization might bring. Dr. Murphy specifically mentioned uncertainty about whether clinicians' C-section tubal ligation practices—specifically the justifications written on the required form—would once again come under scrutiny. At the time of our interview, the hospital administrators had instructed Dr. Murphy and his colleagues to just keep filling out the form to cover their bases, come what may. Fundamentally, for Dr. Murphy and his colleagues, the lack of the affiliation, thus the lack of the bishop's scrutiny of their medical practices, had meant they had enough clinical autonomy to work around most conflicts between Catholic doctrine and standard ob-gyn care.

Around this time, one administrator told Dr. Murphy that Bishop Olmsted had sent her a letter with a long list of things St. Joseph's could do to get its Catholic affiliation back. According to Dr. Murphy, however, this same administrator doubted whether it would ever be possible for St. Joseph's to please the bishop. She did not think they should try. He recalled telling her, by way of response, how happy he was with the way the Sisters of Mercy were running the hospital without the formal affiliation. He told her he felt they were providing good moral leadership.

REAFFILIATION

However, the wheels of reaffiliation were in motion already. On March 24, 2020, early in the COVID-19 pandemic period, the Phoenix Diocese website posted a statement announcing that Bishop Olmsted had allowed the chapel to reopen and resume Mass at St. Joseph's again. It said: "On the Feast of Saint Joseph, March 19, 2020, Bishop Thomas J. Olmsted, in a spirit of reconciliation, mercy, and healing has extended permission for St. Joseph's Hospital and Medical Center to begin reserving the Most Blessed Sacrament in the tabernacle in their chapel. He also extends the permission for Mass to be celebrated in the chapel, according to the current liturgical restrictions, in order that it may be live-streamed to patient rooms and be watched by staff, nurses and doctors."[26]

A day later, on March 25, 2020, Dignity Health St. Joseph's Hospital and Medical Center posted a statement on its website announcing not only that Mass had resumed but that allowing Mass was but a first step in a larger initiative. Dignity Health St. Joseph's Hospital, CommonSpirit Health, Creighton University (which is Jesuit/Catholic), and the Diocese of Phoenix planned to "deepen our shared missions and ministries."[27]

Even as the statement seemed to reaffirm the hospital's good stead with the Catholic Church, it attempted to reassure patients (and potential patients) that the initiative would not change day-to-day medical operations or treatment: "As the world deals with the COVID-19 pandemic, our collaborative efforts will help us better serve our community. The committee and its initiatives will not impact day-to-day hospital operations or the medical treatment provided to our patients. Instead, it will look for ways to share opportunities and partner on projects that fulfill our missions, and enrich our culture." Both statements seemed to indicate that St. Joseph's Catholic affiliation might have been formally reinstated. The next day, *The Catholic Sun*, a Catholic news source, reported that the collaboration was in fact a step toward that goal:

> "We've been looking for the right time to do this," said Fr. Ignatius Mazanowski, FHS, director of medical ethics for the Diocese of Phoenix. "This was a very important time," he added, noting the increase in patients expected to go through the hospital in the midst of the coronavirus pandemic. "We wanted to offer spiritual strength to patients, nurses, doctors and medical professionals of St. Joseph."
>
> A collaborative mission committee made up of representatives of the diocese, St. Joseph's and Creighton Medical School—a Catholic university whose students receive hands-on training at the hospital—has been working to reconcile and restore the hospital's Catholic status.[28]

I reached out to Dr. Murphy again. He said the reunification had happened quietly. He gave me a long back story he had since learned that preceded the pandemic and involved the powerful imperative of institutional expansion. He explained that it started with the fact that Creighton University, a Jesuit medical school based in

Omaha, wanted to expand an already-existing program in Phoenix. For a decade, St. Joseph's had hosted and taught Creighton's medical students, who rotated through the hospital in their final two years of medical school. Now, Creighton aspired to create a second four-year medical school site in Phoenix. The Creighton University Arizona Health Education Alliance (the Creighton Alliance) had been established in 2017 to begin working toward this goal. The Creighton Alliance's members included St. Joseph's Hospital, Valleywise Health (Arizona's only public safety net hospital), and District Medical Group, which employs all the doctors of Valleywise Health Medical Center.[29] The hospitals' residency programs would come under the umbrella of the Creighton Alliance, lending them greater academic prestige than they had as community residency programs. Creighton University is Catholic, but Dr. Murphy and his colleagues were told that the non-Catholic partners in the Creighton Alliance, such as the county hospital, would not be subject to the ERDs. Dr. Lee, who had since relocated to work in the county hospital, concurred that she had been assured her site would not experience any new restrictions on reproductive health care beyond those already in place due to the state's strict prohibition on using public funds for abortion.

The process of establishing the Creighton Alliance had catalyzed conversations between Creighton, St. Joseph's hospital, and the diocese because, as a Catholic institution, Creighton wanted to be in good standing with the religious powers in the area. Dr. Murphy, a leader in his department, occasionally was brought into such conversations. He recalled: "One of the Creighton administrators, who is Jesuit, a sweet guy, came to me. He said, 'We can't be here without the blessing of the bishop. And you know, we want to have Mass here. Don't you think that it would make sense to get back in his good graces.' And I told him, 'No, I don't!' Later on, I realized it may have been one of those conversations where a decision had already been made. He might have been trying to see—if I had agreed—it would have looked like I had a voice in decision making."

But of course, Dr. Murphy had not given the Creighton administrator the answer he was looking for, and he soon realized the plans were quite far along by the time he was "consulted."

Dr. Murphy didn't agree with the decision, but he saw its logic. Through conversations with the hospital president and other administrators within St. Joseph's and Creighton, Dr. Murphy began to understand that establishing this medical school in Phoenix was enormously important to all parties involved, to their professional legacies, and to the prestige of their institutions. No one wanted any hiccups in the process. He continued:

> This is Creighton really putting a footprint in Phoenix. And apparently to do that the understanding is, the written or unwritten rules of the Catholic Church are: Listen, to operate in a bishop's diocese, that local bishop has to give you his blessing. You can't be a Catholic entity functioning in the diocese without the local bishop saying "ok you're on my turf, you are good with me . . ." You gotta get the local bishop's blessing to move in as a Catholic school . . .

They realized they could not accomplish their goals without having a reasonable relationship with the bishop. . . . The goals being, "We want to start a medical school, not a community medical school, but we are an academic medical center, and we want all that goes along with that," and that is what Joe's and Valleywise and Creighton all want to do. I think this is the Westernmost Catholic medical school.

The institutional excitement about establishing a new medical school made sense to me, but I still did not understand why they needed the bishop's blessing. Jesuits are known for leaning left within the Church, and Bishop Olmsted is as far right-leaning as a bishop can get. Why, at the end of the day, would Creighton *need* his blessing? More specifically, I asked Dr. Murphy, what would the consequence be of not getting the bishop's blessing? Dr. Murphy wondered the same thing; he could not say for sure. He gathered they were motivated by respect for Church hierarchy, fear of public conflict with the bishop, the influence of religiously conservative donors, or possibly just a deep abiding commitment to playing by the rules, be they written or unwritten. Whatever the motivation, the result was that St. Joseph's relationship with the bishop was rekindled in the process of establishing the Creighton Alliance.

In contrast to the drama in 2010 when Bishop Olmsted excommunicated Sister McBride and then disavowed the hospital, the process of reconnecting was much subtler. Dr. Murphy noticed a very gradual change in the language the St. Joseph's administration used about their Catholic status, while he was presumably left out of some of the behind-the-scenes discussions: "What I noticed was a gradual creep in St. Joe's administrator talk . . . For several years they would *not say we are* a Catholic hospital, and then they would begin to say we *want* to be a Catholic hospital, and then they would begin to say we *are* a Catholic hospital. And there was never an announcement."

As feared, with the reaffiliation, Dr. Murphy began to note a slight change in how obstetrics and gynecology was practiced at St. Joseph's. Contraception was still easy to prescribe in the medical offices—because the building was not owned by St. Joseph's—and somehow the C-section tubal ligations remained available with the required form that documented a non-contraceptive purpose for the procedure. (He added: "I have never failed to be able to find a reason.") However, he did notice an increase in reminders about filling out the form at department meetings: "I will say in the last six to twelve months . . . there is scrutiny about if the form is filled out, and if some medical reason is given."

He also noticed a difference in practices for obstetric complications and miscarriage management. In his 2011 interview, he told me he never had encountered resistance to initiating treatment for an inevitable miscarriage when the patient was ready, so long as he could in good conscience note such signs as "a little uterine tenderness, a little elevated white count, certainly a fever and not too much." But things were tightening:

I would say that in the last couple years it has gotten a touch stricter in the particular cases I'm thinking of: [when the patient's water breaks] . . . Are they infected or not and can you move things along? It seems to me like people are more hesitant if the patient wants to be induced and deliver that pregnancy and be done. It seems to me, like in the past we would say "is there any evidence of chorioamnionitis [infection in the lining of the uterus]? Just give me a little evidence, gimme a little evidence, and we'll move that along if that is the patient's desire." And now people are like "no, there has to be some stronger evidence that this person is infected."

Tenderness is not enough anymore.

I asked Dr. Murphy how he observed these changes on a daily level. The changes were subtle but noticeable. During morning rounds, for instance, he noticed that supervising attending physicians had begun advising residents to wait a little longer to offer treatment for patients experiencing obstetric complications. When his group of residents discussed the details of such cases, he would ask questions about why they did not offer medications or intervene to empty the uterus. "They'll say, 'The attending was worried about that,'" by which Dr. Murphy understood they meant that attendings worried that giving labor medications would cause leadership to perceive treatment as an abortion.

Dr. Lee also reported that the implications of the Creighton Alliance were starting to concern physician residents. Now that the joint residency program between St. Joseph's and the county (Valleywise) was subsumed under Creighton University, residents had to pay a separate premium to get birth control while on Creighton's insurance, which they had not had to do previously.

A Creighton administrator came to speak to the residents about what becoming part of Creighton meant for their medical training. His talk only exacerbated residents' and attending physicians' fears. Some reached out to Dr. Lee: "I was working on Labor and Delivery and people were blowing up my phone . . . The main thing that people were upset about, at some point he kind of implied that those who are pro-choice are sort of unethical . . . that was hurtful."

The residents actually were far more supportive of abortion rights and training than the Creighton speaker understood, and many took offense. Furthermore, they told Dr. Lee the administrator hoped to recruit the kind of residents who would not want to do abortion training at all. Dr. Murphy, who was at that meeting, reported a similar account of the meeting. He even recalled one of his residents standing up to challenge, "Why did you come here?! We're a public hospital!" (referring, of course, to the county, not St. Joseph's).

Around this time, someone apparently emailed the bishop a picture of an individual walking into a clinic where abortion services occur wearing a Creighton white coat. Dr. Murphy got an earful from a very anxious St. Joseph's administrator about it, who told him, in Dr. Murphy's account: "I can't have the bishop coming up to me and telling me he's getting email from one of his spies with a picture of somebody walking in with a Creighton white coat on a Saturday morning."

He concluded: "Health care administrators want the legacy of building something big, and they're getting harassed by the bishop. And properly training women's health providers can get sacrificed in pursuit of this bigger goal of 'let's build a medical school in Phoenix.'" Dr. Murphy's interactions with the various leaders of the Creighton Alliance drove home to him how important the success of the medical school was to them. It will likely come with additional strings attached.

CONCLUSION

What is the point of highlighting this story when, in the end, St. Joseph's is back where it started? Is it a nothingburger of a story? I think not. St. Joseph's disaffiliation from and re-affiliation with the Church is important because it sheds a rare bright light onto commonly obscured spaces in the relationship between Catholic hospitals, the religious hierarchy, and the evolving structure of U.S. health care. It is necessary to look closely when we get a glimpse to understand how religious power operates in American medicine and, in turn, affects providers' work and patients' lives. In doing so, we can see that Bishop Olmsted's magisterial style of surveilling and policing reproductive care at St. Joseph's crossed a clinical and moral line for the doctors, the Sisters of Mercy, and CHW, causing the split with the Church. We also can see that the organizational and financial consequences of the split were not particularly disruptive to the hospital or health system—at least from Dr. Murphy's vantage point—which simply begs the question: "Why don't more hospitals split with the Church?" Given clinicians and patients seemingly widespread discomfort with the religious policies among physicians and patients, what keeps Catholic hospitals and the Church together?

The story offers some clues in answer to this question. The attraction of establishing a new medical school, the Westernmost Catholic one, was strong for people somewhat high in the power structure of Catholic health care. Without being able to interview them personally, I can only guess what that meant to them, what the attraction was. In the case of the hospital president, Linda Hunt, Dr. Murphy reported she had agonized over the split with the Church at the time. She retired during the writing of this book after over fifty years in working in health care, half of those years in the same Catholic hospital and health system. A public announcement noted that she retired from being a division head within CommonSpirit and founder of the Creighton Alliance.[30] It is unclear, and perhaps unimportant, whether she is a devout Catholic; Catholic healthcare administrators often are specialists in running health systems first. What is clear is that most of her career was built in the system and that the split with the Church repeatedly made national news. Coming together again to build the medical school repaired that rift, and doing so required deference to Church hierarchy and making good with the local authority, Bishop Olmsted. Catholic healthcare institutions (both Creighton and CommonSpirit) grew in size, strength, and prestige through the Creighton Alliance. And, even if the ERDs would not apply to non-Catholic Alliance partners in full, in small ways, St. Joseph's physicians immediately felt Church scrutiny increase over clinical matters such as obstetric complications, C-section tubal ligations, and abortion provision as a result.

Catholic hospitals are diverse in their geography, history, leadership, and how strictly they interpret and implement the religious directives for medical practice. But in proclaiming the ERDs as their hospital policies, they fundamentally restrict comprehensive reproductive health care and clinicians' ability to carry out best practices within obstetrics and gynecology. Even though St. Joseph's administrators remained loyal to the premise of the ERDs during the period of estrangement from the Church, they continued to reserve the right to interpret those ERDs in a way that would diminish doctrinal iatrogenesis. They drew a life-saving line in 2009 in supporting the physician's judgment to intervene, and again in 2010 by pushing back on the bishop's demands and standing by the decision.

Dr. Murphy's observations of recent shifts in practice suggest that being back in relationship with Bishop Olmsted may bring chilling effects on clinician practice. But it is, nevertheless, unclear at this point what would happen if a pregnant woman with a similar life-threatening medical condition were to be admitted to St. Joseph's today. Indeed, Bishop Olmsted's retirement was announced in January of 2022,[31] and whether the successor has a more magisterial or pastoral style remains to be seen. What is clear, however, is that there are now several more institutions, both Catholic and non-Catholic, with skin in the game. They do not want abortion-related conflict to enshroud their new medical education enterprise in an increasingly conservative state.

Conclusion

Savita Halappanavar died in 2012 in an Irish hospital where she had gone to get help when she began experiencing severe back pain while losing her pregnancy of seventeen weeks.[1] She was an Indian immigrant to Ireland and a dentist with the kind of education one might hope for when navigating health care. The doctors there managed her miscarriage expectantly, giving her no other options. After spending a day in severe pain, she begged them to terminate the pregnancy but was told it was not allowed—Ireland is a Catholic country.[2] Her husband later told reporters she endured another two-and-a-half days "in agony" until the fetal heartbeat ceased and the fetus was removed; shortly thereafter, she died of sepsis in the intensive care unit.[3] While Savita's case did not take place in an American Catholic hospital, the doctors there were similarly hamstrung by the Catholic prohibition on all abortions. This took place a year after I started conducting interviews for this book.

Savita died in the same scenario that commonly killed women a century ago, when the maternal mortality rate was about 608 maternal deaths per 100,000 live births.[4] She died even though it was entirely avoidable. In 2020, the mortality rate in the United States was about twenty-four maternal deaths per 100,000 live births. The rate in the United States is the worst in the developed world, but it is much improved from a century ago because the field of medicine now knows how to manage obstetric complications without putting women's lives at such risk.[5] Savita's medical outcome—sepsis resulting in death—is one that ob-gyns fear. It is an outcome that Black women in the United States suffer at twice the rate of white women.[6] And it is the outcome that doctors who work in American Catholic hospitals sometimes stretch the clinical truth to avoid. Although Irish pro-choice activists had been advocating to reform abortion laws for years, it took the protests following Savita's death for the Irish government to finally act. Abortion was legalized in Ireland in late 2018.

The United States is not a Catholic country. The United States was founded on the notion that Church is separate from State. Yet, with a blind eye toward their intermingling in health care, American medical regulation and law does little to prevent completely foreseeable obstetric tragedies induced by religious restrictions. Catholic authorities in Ireland argued that medical treatments that may risk the fetus's life are "ethically permissible" so long as "every effort has been made to save the life of both the mother and her baby."[7] This statement reflects Directive 47, which allows that "operations, treatments and medications that have as their direct purpose a cure of proportionately serious pathological condition of a pregnant woman are permitted when they cannot be safely postponed until the unborn child is viable." But waiting until she has a "serious pathological condition" is unsafe and unethical obstetric policy. If the woman does not wish to continue to risk her life for a pregnancy that is already doomed, the safest thing is to empty her uterus before she becomes so ill, not after.

In an interview on the Diane Rehm show, the president of the National Catholic Bioethics Center, John Haas, acknowledged a greater problem of religious medical policy implementation while discussing emergency abortion. "You know, a lot of people overlook Directive 47," he said, to explain why doctors failed to provide miscarriage management to a patient when she needed it.[8] Such an observation does not help patients. A massive sector of publicly funded health care in the United States promulgates Catholic policies that contradict best ob-gyn practices, with the caveat that, if physicians know how to ask and, then, if the Catholic ethics committees agree that the patient has developed a "serious pathological condition," they may grant permission to bypass the policy. Not only does awareness of the life-saving loophole of Directive 47 vary among doctors, gatekeepers' interpretations of when to use it vary, too. Religious authorities, like Bishop Olmsted and some of the ethics committee members in this book, think abortion or tubal ligation is never warranted within Catholic hospitals, not even if a woman might die without them. Because this process is incredibly opaque, with no public record of how exemptions are made or who is involved in the process, religious institutional power over patients' bodies remains deeply problematic.

Just before Savita died, a U.S. public health worker named Faith Groesbeck, who was trying to reduce fetal and infant mortality in Muskegon, Michigan, began to notice disturbing trends.[9] Her job was to confidentially investigate the medical care provided during cases of fetal and infant death to help hospitals improve care. The nearest hospital without a religious affiliation is located twenty miles from Muskegon. While interviewing patients about their experiences of hospital care, she noted that several women had similar experiences of medical neglect, showing emotional trauma after losing a previable pregnancy. The theme in these cases was denied or delayed care during pregnancy loss and stalled induction of labor. One woman she spoke with, Tamesha Means, went on to tell her story publicly: how she was sent away twice from Mercy Health Partners while miscarrying at eighteen weeks pregnant, being told there was nothing they could do. Attorneys for the American Civil Liberties Union (ACLU) took her case and sued the United States Council of Catholic Bishops for issuing the directives that restricted miscarriage management. Notably, the ACLU sued the bishops, not the doctor or the hospital. The Sixth Circuit ruled that Tamesha Means needed to show present injury and also argued that the case was outside its jurisdiction.[10] Although the ACLU did not win the case, it did draw more attention to the issue.

Soon after Tamesha's lawsuit, the ACLU unearthed more problematic cases, including that of Jennafer Norris, who was denied a tubal ligation during an emergency C-section. Norris could not travel to a non-Catholic hospital thirty minutes away, so the physician closed Jennafer back up without the sterilization despite the presence of multiple medical problems that would make a future pregnancy unsafe for her. Mindy Swank was refused an emergency abortion five times by her Catholic hospital after her water broke at twenty weeks of pregnancy. Doctors finally intervened when she hemorrhaged at twenty-seven weeks; the fetus, which had a genetic anomaly, then died.

While Jennafer and Mindy did not sue, others did. Rebecca Chamorro preemptively sued to be allowed a postpartum tubal ligation in her Catholic hospital, which her physician wanted to provide, since the nearest alternative was seventy miles away, but the judge did not find seventy miles too burdensome to go for childbirth. And, of course, Evan Minton sued after his gender confirming hysterectomy was abruptly canceled. He won in California, but Dignity Health's efforts to overturn the decision are ongoing, although the Supreme Court declined to hear the case.[11]

Patients are not the only ones suing, either. Two doctors in Colorado, a state with a very high concentration of Catholic hospitals, also sued. In 2013, a cardiologist sued after being disciplined by his Catholic hospital employer for counseling his patient that if her test for a connective tissue syndrome came back positive, she might need to get an abortion to save her own life. Incidentally, the cardiologist did not even know his own hospital forbade abortion.[12] And in another case in 2019, a geriatrician sued for wrongful treatment by the health system in relation to an aid-in-dying case.[13] This is not an exhaustive list of lawsuits, but they paint a picture of recent legal efforts to draw a boundary between clinical and religious control over medical practice. So far, the courts have consistently favored religious institutional power over that of the patients or doctors.

This book has not focused on tragic deaths, like Savita's, or the publicly shared stories of harm that have animated the lawsuits just mentioned. The people I interviewed told me more about how Church policies compromise medical treatment without ever putting Catholic hospitals' abilities to thrive in American health care in jeopardy. My research indicates that the worst outcomes of doctrinal iatrogenesis, like Savita's death, are rare largely because of the many strategies physicians use to work around restrictions on care. But harm still exists for both patients and physicians who are bound to this system for one reason or another. While Tamesha Means, Evan Minton, and others were willing to speak openly about what happened to them, the patients in this book did not want to take their harm public. Not Jaelyn, who suffered several hours longer than necessary during a miscarriage, described in chapter 4; not Amy, whose tubal ligation denial led to a life-threatening unintended pregnancy, described in the introduction; nor Kayden, whose reproductive procedure was canceled, as described in chapter 3, when he told the pre-op nurse he was transgender.

In fact, among the people I got to know, those who seemed to have the most devastating denials of care were the least interested in having their experiences scrutinized by the public. They were simply too vulnerable. They shared their stories on the condition of anonymity. These stories were personal and often involved stigmatized matters: sex, reproduction, pregnancy loss, religion, gender identity, and abortion. They did not go public because they did not want their lives exposed and criticized. But, also, some quite reasonably questioned whether sacrificing their privacy would make any difference. Lawsuits have been filed and nothing has changed, yet.

Regardless of the outcomes of these lawsuits, this book has demonstrated that the institutional arrangement in which Catholic hospitals use public funds to limit reproductive care to patients who may or may not subscribe to Catholic beliefs is unethical and unjust in at least four key ways. First, the Ethical and Religious Directives for Catholic Health Care Services deny patients the standard ob-gyn treatments allowed in other hospitals, thereby systematically providing inferior reproductive care as it is, in some instances, less safe and, in many instances, less patient-centered. Second, Catholic healthcare systems deliberately lack transparency about religious restrictions, which violates patients' reproductive autonomy. The ERDs limit treatment without patients' advance knowledge and without their choosing; ample research shows that if patients understood the policies and had the resources to go elsewhere for reproductive care, they would. Third, the restrictions simulate clinical conditions of resource scarcity, creating moral distress for physicians caught in the middle, who must stretch the truth or creatively work around restrictions in other ways to avoid patient harm. Fourth, and finally, the ERDs may exacerbate reproductive injustice when Catholic hospitals are the only source of care. Moreover, providers' extra efforts to work around restrictions for some patients likely reproduce the racial discrimination and disparities already rampant throughout health care. While certainly not the early Catholic hospital founders' intent, these systemically entrenched injustices perpetuated on a massive scale in modern healthcare are simply unacceptable.

The Evolving Role of the Catholic Hospital

Catholic hospitals, originally established to care for the "deserving poor" in their time of greatest need, have become corporate mega systems in American health care.[14] They prospered, consolidated, and proliferated over the past century through strategic compromises and political leverage, and they built economic strength from the national coordination of hospitals bound together by the Church. In the early twentieth century, Catholic hospitals made pragmatic choices to become part of the burgeoning American healthcare system; most significantly by developing a Catholic code that appeased religious authorities while providing a theological justification for abortion if done to save a woman's life, which was required to gain public trust, accreditation, and legitimacy.[15] As American medicine grew, Catholic hospital leadership strategically and successfully lobbied for healthcare bills that would fund their hospitals without controlling how they ran them. They lobbied against early attempts to establish universal health care, instead lobbying for a patchwork approach to supporting the autonomy of disparate nongovernmental hospitals across the country.

After *Roe v. Wade* legalized abortion, Catholic hospitals and systems continued to expand, both legally and economically. The legal fiction of conscience rights emerged in application to institutions, not just individuals, enabling the bishops to keep standard reproductive services out of their buildings. Economically, Catholic healthcare systems grew strong by merging with or acquiring other facilities; the new non-Catholic acquisitions generally were made to comply with the ERDs as well. Internally, Catholic organizations wrestled to balance margin and mission as they grew. Politicians and healthcare leaders leveraged Catholic hospitals' reputation for charitable works as an excuse for infringements on patients' reproductive rights. The halo effect from their charitable image persists even as their actual charitable contributions and proportion of Medicaid patients have declined below average.

As a result of successful growth nationally, millions of hospital patients are now treated in facilities that follow the ERDs, precluding some of the safest treatments in obstetrics and limiting patient autonomy. The services that are restricted reach far beyond abortion—the most well-known of Catholic prohibitions. The ERDs also compel less safe and/or less autonomous patient care in the areas of contraception, tubal ligation, management of obstetric complications, transgender surgery, rape treatment (emergency contraception), dysfunctional bleeding, and infertility treatment.

The structure of the American medical system, if it can truly be called a system, has enabled the Church and the U.S. bishops to develop an outsized influence over reproductive bodies, also known as *reproductive governance*.[16] That the bishops and religious healthcare institutions hold such power cannot be separated from the fact that the state has avoided responsibility for health care by repeatedly failing to develop universal health care, instead getting out of the healthcare business, often selling county hospitals to religious systems or subsidizing Catholic systems to provide care in underserved areas. At times of healthcare growth, change, and regulation, conditions for religious systems have remained favorable—with both ample funding and freedom—all while reproductive autonomy and wellbeing has been continually regarded by regulators as relatively unimportant and expendable.

The existence of Catholic hospitals is a testament to the importance of religious freedom in the United States. The doctrine of religious freedom animated the establishment of the country. In certain eras, it has made this nation a haven for immigrants who could not have religious freedom in their home countries. It has allowed people from diverse backgrounds to come together to work, get an education, and raise families in ways that feel authentic and safe.

Today, however, religious freedom means something else politically and legally. In the early twenty-first century, we have seen it twisted to restrict people rather than liberate them.[17] Hobby Lobby and similar corporate employers will not cover contraception in their employee insurance plans because of the owner's deeply held beliefs against it; janitors, bus drivers, and pharmacists threaten to refuse to do their job if they feel it aids someone getting an abortion; the Trump administration *almost* broadly legalized discrimination by expanding conscience rights protections to workers who refuse not just services but to serve particular people *to whom* they morally object. (More than twenty democratic states sued the administration and won).[18] To put it more succinctly, *conscience rights* have been leveraged by the *religious right* to push back on expanding sexual and reproductive *human rights*.[19]

The story of Catholic health care is an institutional one of great consequence that resides within this social, political, and legal space. Founded in the name of the Catholic Church and its people at a time when they were treated poorly for being Catholic, Catholic hospitals historically cared for the underserved, especially immigrants. Today, they care for religiously and economically diverse patients within enormous, prosperous nation-wide health systems that outcompete or swallow up others, reducing reproductive health services to the entire area. The newly acquired hospitals are then governed by religious directives that restrict contraception, miscarriage management, and fertility treatment, even as these beliefs are far out of step with most Americans' beliefs and practices.

Violation of Patient Autonomy

Patients find themselves in Catholic facilities for reproductive care because it happens to be where their insurance, geography, or physician leads them. In some areas, patients also are drawn to a Catholic facility because that is where their friends and family steer them or because it is the only option. Even when patients actively choose a hospital that operates within the Catholic healthcare network, they may not know about the religious affiliation. Even fewer understood what that religious affiliation meant for their reproductive care. Patients only learned about the downsides of Church-controlled reproductive care when their treatment was delayed or denied.

Several patients in this study were remarkably supportive of the freedom of Catholic hospitals to limit care according to religion, at least in the abstract. However, after becoming informed about how bishops' policies limited their care or the care of others, they grew less so. Some suffered physically and emotionally during a doctrinally protracted miscarriage, and others suffered discrimination from being denied services based on who they were. Many blamed themselves for not researching the hospital more extensively to anticipate and avoid the religious restrictions. But how could they have known?

Many patients do not necessarily know how the religious policies affected their care or whether religious restrictions, as opposed to any other number of factors, caused a harm they are aware of. It is difficult for patients to discern what is substandard care in medical domains that are already haunted by stigma and controversy. Many feel lucky to be cared for at all, finding it hard even to imagine a world in which it could be better, where their reproductive needs are not shameful on some level. Expectations are low.[20]

The consequences of encountering specific religious restrictions can be transitory or enduring for patients, ranging from mild inconvenience to prolonged pain and suffering. The directives expose patients to greater risks, often without their knowledge. Doctors do not tell patients that the bishops have foreclosed more appropriate approaches to patients' care. Why? Perhaps it simply boils down to what Dr. Murphy so aptly pointed out: These are the policies you get when you lock women out of power for centuries. A famous feminist retort similarly challenges: If all men were born with uteruses, there would be contraceptives in the vending machines and abortion would be a "sacrament."[21] Applied here, physicians also would provide very good information about comprehensive treatment options so the patient, and not the bishop, could make the most informed decision affecting treatment and future reproductive capacity.

Only recently has there been any attention in the fields of bioethics and medicine to this injustice. In 2007, ACOG published guidelines for physicians with personal or institutional conscience-based limits on care urging them to ensure adequate referral procedures were in place for patients to get what they need quickly.[22] More law articles than can be counted have challenged the morality and legality of using religion to restrict care individually and institutionally.[23] In 2018, prominent ob-gyn ethicists Frank Chervenak and Laurence McCullough mainstreamed the topic for ob-gyns in a commentary in response to our survey showing that women largely did not know much about how their care is restricted in Catholic hospitals. In their piece, they urged physicians to be transparent about religious restrictions and implored hospitals not to impede best practices during obstetric complications.[24] Unfortunately, these expressions by leaders in the field of obstetrics and gynecology do not (and likely will not) change policies. Instead, they urge individual solutions to large structural problems. They have shed some light on these ethical conflicts. Yet, the bishops remain tremendously powerful players in American medicine, with seats at every table, and the Supreme Court has been definitively on the side of religious institutional power in health care, favoring religious freedom in one decision after the next.[25]

MORAL DISTRESS

If the directives mandate substandard care, why do we not hear about more doctrinal iatrogenesis in the news? Why don't things go wrong all the time? The answer, in short, is because doctors have developed workarounds. Doctors work around directives that are bad for patient care often and in many ways. Some of the ways are more "legitimate," so to speak, than others. The "above-board" workarounds include moving patients from the Catholic facility to a non-Catholic hospital, surgery center, or clinic to perform a sterilization procedure or embryo transfer. In some cases involving so-called carve-outs, that non-Catholic facility might be located within the walls or in the parking lot of a Catholic hospital. When all else fails, referrals are the unofficial official plan, encouraged by Catholic healthcare leaders despite the fact that Directive 73 states that employees may not "make referrals for, or benefit from the revenue generated by immoral procedures." In emergencies, though, referrals are simply punting, dumping, or abandoning the patient in place of providing care the doctor is well trained to give.

Other workarounds do not follow Church law in letter or spirit. Physicians use several strategies to provide what they technically are not allowed to provide when they want to respond to their patients' reproductive needs more quickly and effectively. They justify, conceal, rename, and rebel. More specifically, they find theological and clinical loopholes to justify treatments; they hide some of their practices from other staff; they call some prohibited procedures by new names; and in some rare cases, they unapologetically violate certain elements of the ERDs, seeking neither permission nor forgiveness.

Physician burnout is a major problem in medicine. When physicians do not have enough time or resources to address patient problems, burnout can result from moral distress. Such moral distress is especially acute when clinicians do not have the means to act in accordance with their professional values.[26] How are we to understand doctrinal iatrogenesis in this context, where clinicians are actively defending the patients against significant morbidity and mortality their policies essentially prescribe; when they must offer care that is less than they might otherwise provide? Pragmatic and compassionate doctors want to supply their patients with *something*, because between the bishops' rules, reproductive stigma, and right-wing assaults on funds for family planning, they worry she will get *nothing*. To be sure, some doctors who are motivated by their bottom line do not make extra efforts to protect their patients from the restrictions. They do not describe all the contraceptive options or medical treatments they do not provide so as to not draw attention to their practice's shortcomings and lose business. Whichever approach doctors take, expectations for patient autonomy become disturbingly low in restrictive settings.

Many of the ob-gyns I interviewed wrestled openly and conscientiously with how to do the best for their patients given the constraints. Some worked in the Catholic facility because the Catholic system merged with or took over their hospital and/or established practice or because their family was living in a town with few, if any, other choices of employer or hospital to practice in. Some worked for their Catholic hospital for the laudable reason that it served low-income patients to a greater extent than the competing facilities in their town, which continues to be (or continues to seem to be) true in many regions despite the changing national picture. Some devoted considerable time and effort into getting exceptions approved for patients or in developing more reliable workarounds. And some physicians took the job when workarounds were so well established that colleagues confidently reassured them that patients could get "everything" they needed (except abortion, of course). As time went on, the reliable pathways became less so.

That said, many physicians I spoke with passively accept the status quo of patriarchal religious governance. They found advantages to practicing in certain

Catholic hospitals (geographic, technical, logistical, financial) and did not dwell on the ethical problems. Some rationalized or normalized the imposition on patients' rights, seeing them as simply part of the very imperfect reality of American health care, folding in religious constraints on care with economic and bureaucratic ones. Ultimately, the doctors perspectives were diverse, as were their approaches to informing patients about religious restrictions and recognition of their role in maintaining patriarchal structures.

And yet, no physician I interviewed believed that the ERDs in their entirety were in patients' best interest. While some physicians opposed abortion, even they provided some form of abortion referrals, indicating respect for patients' own abilities to discern what is good for them. To be sure, I did not recruit from the Christian Medical and Dental Association's 19,000 members or the Catholic Medical Association's approximately 1,000 members, which together account for a very small portion of all doctors (less than 3 percent).[27] They might hold different views. Those I interviewed who articulated support for the abortion restrictions valued that the ERDs allowed them to avoid the discomfort that abortion requests might present for them as well as the work of finding an alternate provider, if they felt any duty to do so. Overall, however, most physicians experienced moral distress—to varying degrees—over being bound to policies that were bishop-not-patient centered.

DISCRIMINATION AND REPRODUCTIVE INJUSTICE

The various workarounds described in this book are an insufficient remedy for the bishops' overreach because workarounds are idiosyncratic and not universally applied. Some patients will receive what they need; some will not. The patterns of who does or does not get good care remain murky and deeply concerning. The religious policies very well may exacerbate reproductive injustice and further racial disparities in maternal health care in the United States. Given what we know about racial bias in medicine, working around policy idiosyncratically is not likely to benefit women of color. Working around religious policy is not an actual policy, even though physicians represented it almost as if it were.

In lawsuits, Catholic health systems defend the ERDs with the argument that they do not discriminate against women or transgender people because they apply equally to all people. Although equally limiting reproductive care for all may be the bishops' intent, impact is not intent, and equality is not the same thing as equity. Discrimination is not a surprising outcome when the impacts of a policy vary by race, sex, and gender.

The first case of discrimination according to sex can be posited simply. The ERDs discriminate against all people with uteruses by not allowing standard medications and procedures so they can avoid pregnancy just as people without uteruses are able to do. The second case of discrimination by gender is a bit more complex, but perhaps even stronger. In *Dignity Health v. Minton*, Dignity Health argued that they abruptly canceled Evan Minton's gender-affirming hysterectomy because Catholic hospitals simply do not do sterilization procedures for anyone, and, thus, Minton was no different.[28] However, Minton's lawyers won at the state level by showing that Dignity hospitals do perform hysterectomies quite regularly for medical reasons, but only the ones they find justifiable and worthy. Gender dysphoria is not one of them. And yet, are one person's bleeding fibroids less tolerable than another person's gender dysphoria, given high suicidality in people who struggle with it? Still, Catholic institutions retain the power to decide which cases are worthy of exemptions to their own religious policies.

The impact of the ERDs may differ by race, as well. Institutional racism pervades health care in the United States, meaning the systems and structures in place systematically disadvantage certain people, and especially Black people.[29] Racial disparities in health ensue across insurance and socioeconomic status. Studies have documented differences by race in both preventative care and life saving treatments, from children's respiratory infections to limb amputation to breast cancer chemotherapy regimens.[30]

Disparities in maternal mortality and morbidity have been increasingly well documented in recent years,[31] with more acknowledgment of racism as the causal mechanism.[32] We know that in nineteen states Black women are more likely to deliver in Catholic hospitals, a reality stemming from geography and health insurance.[33] Thus, Black women are structurally more likely to be impacted by the ERDs than other women, which could both cause and exacerbate existing racial disparities in both family planning and obstetric care. Increasingly, Black women are asking: Why do we have a disproportionate burden of navigating these barriers? Racism is inflicted through both individual clinician bias and institutional practices. Catholic health systems are predisposed to both because they are frequently the only choice of care and because they require physicians to use their individual discretion to work around religious constraints to avoid harm.

While laudable in terms of putting their patients' needs first, physicians' informal strategies to circumvent restrictions also raise concerns about how equitable the distribution of these extra efforts are. If a patient is not a squeaky wheel, does she get her contraceptives? If she seems uncomfortable stretching the truth to claim the justificatory symptoms she does not have, will she get what she needs? What if she does not play the expected deferential and compliant "role" of the patient in their interaction, and she triggers the physician's own insecurities and racism?[34] When clinicians do not feel their authority is respected, because "deference" is read subjectively, situationally, and culturally, will clinicians stick their necks out to bend the rules *equitably*? In cases where the patient is uncomfortable discussing reproductive care at all because of societal shame around sexuality, how likely is it that the doctor will help her initiate that possibly much needed conversation? Will the doctor interpret her discomfort as that of a highly religious person who opposes contraception and, therefore, be scared to risk bringing it up, or will they, instead, see it as the far more common sheepishness that so many patients exude when new to talking about sex? What if the patient is a sexually active teenager?

Workarounds may ultimately protect the hospital's reputation for care and serve the needs of some patients, but they do not do anything for patients whom clinicians deem unsympathetic in one way or another or who struggle to communicate their needs. Ample research shows that discretionary leeway paves the way for bias in policing, criminal justice systems, and social services.[35] Similarly, the expansion of Catholic systems in which clinicians must pursue informal strategies to meet patients' needs may magnify existing bias and reproduce inequality. ERD workarounds are informal, idiosyncratic, unpredictable, and not sustainable at scale.

The Future of Religious Restrictions

This book has focused on Catholic hospitals, the largest and most powerful segment of religiously affiliated hospitals in the United States. A handful of health services researchers have compared Catholic health care with non-Catholic health care in various ways unrelated to reproductive health care, and turned up little meaningful distinction. One 2001 study showed that Catholic ownership did not portend more compassionate care or stigmatized services, but that all not-for-profit hospitals were more generous than investor-owned hospitals.[36] Given that "empirical evidence of the uniqueness of Catholic health care remains virtually nonexistent," another research team turned to measuring patient satisfaction in Catholic and non-Catholic hospitals in 2014 and found no meaningful difference there either.[37] As stated above, research on health outcomes barely exists.[38] Studies do show differences in access to reproductive services within Catholic hospitals, which should not be surprising. Sterilization and abortion services decrease when a hospital is made Catholic, but they do not entirely disappear.[39] As we have seen, doctors and hospitals pick and choose who gets access to these procedures based upon variable medical criteria, aspects of their hospital culture around it, and, likely, their affinity for the patient.

Other religious and nonreligious hospitals also have restrictions on reproductive care, although as far as I know they focus primarily on restricting what kinds of abortions take place in their facilities. In fact, my own team's research about ob-gyn residency programs and the abortion policies of their largely nonsectarian training hospitals found that 57 percent restricted abortion more narrowly than state law; 48 percent had policies restricting nonmedically indicated abortions; and 28 percent had policies restricting medically indicated abortions.[40] Research from Lee Hasselbacher and colleagues at the University of Chicago showed that a Protestant hospital in their area prohibited abortion in more extreme ways than their own edicts indicated they would. They restricted abortion due to stigma, the influence of Catholic leadership, and, perhaps relatedly, because the Catholic Church owned the land on which the institution sat.[41] Elizabeth Reiner Platt and colleagues at Columbia Law School showed that Protestant hospitals across the U.S. South, where Catholic hospitals are not as prevalent, have outright prohibitions on abortion that are on par with the severity of those in Catholic hospitals.[42]

While these studies show that abortion restrictions actually are quite common in one form or another, the Catholic Church, a singular entity with a massively outsized influence on American health care, has paved the way for anti-abortion institutional policies by being so extreme and expansive. Their enormous model empowers other institutions pressured by anti-abortion politics and stigma to follow suit. Not only do Catholic hospitals constitute roughly three-quarters of all religious hospitals, but by promulgating the most restrictive and out-of-step reproductive doctrine, they make other milder restrictions on reproductive health care seem relatively less objectionable. *"Well, at least they permit sterilization and contraception,"* or *"At least they do terminations for fatal anomalies."* Catholic hospitals set the bar for religious control over women's bodies in health care. The enormity of the systems' scale normalizes clergy control over patient decisions in Catholic hospitals, which helps justify it elsewhere.

However, it stands to reason that if such reproductive rules can be issued from one organizational body (USCCB) and then influence countless other institutions, one incisive governmental policy change also could make an immense difference for patient care. No shortage of blood, sweat, and tears has gone into this effort by healthcare advocates around the country.

As discussed, reproductive rights advocates have brought several legal cases against Catholic hospitals. They frequently lose these cases because the courts privilege institutions' religious freedom over patients' rights. Granting conscience rights to large healthcare systems and corporation has been an enormous failing of our legal and medical system,[43] from Dignity Health to Hobby Lobby. Such institutional conscience rights are an example of legal fiction: "An assumption and acceptance of something as fact by a court, although it may not be so, so as to allow a rule to operate or be applied in a manner that differs from its original purpose while leaving the letter of the law unchanged."[44] This entire fight has little bearing on what the media and public are most concerned about when it comes to religious rights in health care. Most Americans support the right of individual people to opt out of abortion care if they can do so without harming anyone.[45] The individual physician's right not to perform abortion, in non-emergencies only, is widely valued. In contrast, the institutions' or corporations' right not to allow their employees and attending physicians the autonomy to perform abortions (or other standard reproductive procedures) inside their buildings is ethically flimsy if not corrupt.

We all know medical institutions and corporations do not have consciences. People do. In this case, the people are U.S. bishops whose doctrinal and patriarchal beliefs govern the institutions and the people inside them. Hence, the bishops' values determine how their healthcare employees are allowed to practice and what care patients in their institutions are allowed to have. This book's title intentionally centers the bishops because this is an unambiguously top-down situation. Bishops have control over people's bodies; patients depend on their health facilities for reproductive care either because they do not understand the problem or because they have nowhere else to go.

If medicine were not a limited resource and if the restrictions were transparent, this might not be a difficult problem. However, there are only a limited number of health facilities and employers. Medicine may act like a free market in some ways, but competition is not open, and medical institutions are highly regulated. A new hospital cannot be built unless there is a demonstrated community need. The invisible hand of the market will not solve this problem. Only legal, policy, and regulatory change can.

Given how the Supreme Court has favored religious institutional power since the confirmation of Amy Coney Barrett tipped the balance rightward, healthcare advocates have turned toward state legislatures in more favorable political climates to attempt to make change. Yet, a huge roadblock called the Weldon Amendment has headed off several strategies. Included alongside the Hyde Amendment since 2005, the Weldon Amendment states that U.S. Department of Health and Human Services (HHS) funds may be held back from local and state governments that are deemed to "discriminate" against entities that refuse to provide, pay for, or cover abortion services.[46] That means, if a state were to decide not to work with or support a Catholic health system in some way because of its religious restrictions, that state could stand to lose a significant amount of HHS funding. Thus, no local, state, or federal policy change can compel change without compromising a much broader funding stream. The Weldon Amendment is deeply important to the bishops, as it cements protection for institutional conscience rights specifically, ensuring that they lose no funding opportunities and no religious freedom to run the hospital as they see fit.[47]

As such, legislative efforts at the state level have been creative, though not revolutionary. Washington State was the first to institute a law in 2019 that requires all hospitals to fill out a form about which reproductive services they provide "related to abortion, contraception, pregnancy, infertility, STDS and HIV," and post it on their website.[48] This information could be helpful, if a patient foresees needing those services and knows to look for information about restrictions in advance. Unfortunately, this research shows that many patients do not understand that religious restrictions could impact their care until they run up against them. In 2021, New York and Oregon passed health equity and merger review legislation for all health facility transactions to slow the expansion of religiously restrictive facilities.[49] Together with California's preexisting law that requires the attorney general to approve mergers, these three states are poised to stave off the loss of reproductive services with some success.

Advocates in the religious healthcare space have suggested pursuing strategies along the above lines of disclosure, transparency, and merger reviews, as well as working to create protections for clinicians' positive rights of conscience. This latter approach would mean providing employment protection for clinicians who are willing to violate hospital restrictions.[50]

POST-ROE

Most of the conflicts that arose in this research were not directly about abortion, at least not the in the way most Americans think about abortion. Americans typically regard abortion as a procedure chosen by a medically stable person to intentionally end a pregnancy they do not want to continue. However, physicians and patients ran up against abortion prohibitions in Catholic institutions when pregnant patients who were medically precarious or experiencing an obstetric complication needed medical help and abortion was the safest option for them. Before *Roe* fell, doctors I spoke with had the luxury of sending stable "ordinary abortion" patients to highly skilled physicians in abortion clinics or other comprehensive health settings.[51] They did it over and over again. Catholic hospitals have intimately and consistently relied on the safety valve of skilled abortion provision. This was a lifesaving, health saving, and mental health saving act.[52] Pregnant patients no longer have this option in many states.

Two months after *Roe* was overturned, thirteen states had already banned abortion. The slim exceptions to these extreme laws include rape or incest (in some cases) and to save the pregnant patient's life (in most cases). That last part sounds simple, almost reassuring. But this book shows that it is not so simple. How to determine the exact moment when abortion must happen to save a patient's life is ambiguous, yet it now carries criminal penalties for doctors who do it "wrong." In media statements, anti-abortion pundits point to Catholic hospitals as a model for how to provide obstetric care without abortion; Alexandra DeSanctis wrote in the *National Review* that abortion supporters are making too big a deal about the danger of abortion bans, stating: "Never mind that for decades now, Catholic hospitals, which don't perform elective abortions, have somehow managed to treat pregnant women with ectopic pregnancies or miscarriages."[53] Sadly, the care has been as safe as it has been only because of the safety valve that abortion providers lent them. It is a horrific catch-22.

Will we see more cases like that of Savita Halappanavar? I simply do not see how we cannot. States that implemented abortion bans already had higher maternal mortality rates and worse outcomes before *Dobbs*.[54] Additionally, the threat of criminalization looms so large for doctors, they will be incentivized to wait as long as possible to intervene to ensure that the threat to the patient's life is evident, so that no staff member, family member, or colleague will accuse them of performing an abortion for which they might be prosecuted. It is chilling.

Many Americans in states with bans, largely those who have the resources and wherewithal to do so, already are traveling long distances for procedures in other states.[55] Some women have employed unsafe herbal methods and physical trauma to cause an abortion.[56] Increasingly, however, people are procuring medication abortion pills online or elsewhere to manage their own abortions,[57] which, though illegal, is largely safe.[58] While some portion of people will ultimately get the abortions they need after this harrowing physical and emotional journey, and all the risk of criminalization that goes with it, sick women will not be among them. Those who need to be in a hospital are not safe for travel, and they are not eligible for having an abortion at home without medical supervision. Women who urgently need hospital-based abortion care, like Savita Halappanavar and Tamesha Means, will be stuck between fearful physicians and the law, hoping against hope for a good outcome. The bishops paved the way for this reality.

Appendix

POSITIONALITY, METHODS, AND
SCHOLARLY JOURNEY

I conducted this research in my early to mid-career years. I am a white woman, a sociologist, and a professor in a medical school. Most interviews were done over the phone with physicians and patients. As such, the subjects of those interviews may not have been able to read my race and privilege completely, but it was likely assumed (or Googled), and that may have affected how participants responded to me. It also may be worth knowing that I have had many experiences of my own with reproductive care, both empowering and disempowering. As is evident throughout the book, I strongly support the right of patients to receive any standard reproductive care and treatments they deem right for themselves, unencumbered by bishops or right-wing legislators.

My interest in Catholic health care was piqued in 2006 while conducting my sociology dissertation research about ob-gyn practice related to abortion.[1] The ob-gyns I interviewed who had experience working in Catholic hospitals never expected to perform abortions there, but they were frustrated to find they also were barred from treating miscarriages in some cases due to religious rules.[2] I found this surprising and wanted to learn more. So when, in 2011, physician-researcher Debra Stulberg asked me to collaborate with her on a qualitative study to understand how ob-gyns felt their Catholic hospital's religious policies influenced their medical practice, I jumped at the opportunity. In this case, the physician subjects were drawn from respondents to a nationally representative survey fielded by her colleagues at the University of Chicago.[3] Many respondents had worked in both Catholic and non-Catholic hospitals and could compare and contrast working in the different environments. After doing thirty-one lengthy telephone interviews with doctors from fifteen states around the United States and publishing four peer-reviewed qualitative articles with collaborators,[4] I went on to interview sixteen more physicians and other Catholic hospital personnel as opportunities arose through professional networks, related research projects, and snowball sampling. Altogether, the providers explained in several ways how their hands are tied by religious restrictions, whether patients know or not, while relaying that patients often do not know or fully understand the role of these restrictions in care delivery.

From there, we decided to dig into that question: What do patients know? Furthermore, what do they want? And when I say "we," I really mean an amazing, ever-expanding team of researchers based at the University of Chicago and University of California, San Francisco.[5] We conducted a nationally representative survey that we titled "Patient Awareness of Religious Restrictions in Catholic Healthcare (PARRCH)." In 2016, we surveyed 1,430 American women of reproductive age and found that many (37 percent) who identified the name of a Catholic hospital as their main hospital did not know it was Catholic. We also learned that only 35 percent of those women think it is important to know a hospital's religious affiliation before seeking reproductive care. But after following that question with, "Sometimes hospitals restrict care according to religion. How important is it to know what is restricted?" suddenly 81 percent think it is important to know. This indicated that, for about half the population, the idea that a hospital could or would restrict their care per religion was not even on their radar as a possibility.

Within PARRCH, we also took the opportunity to replicate Maryam Guiahi's methodology from her 2014 Colorado-based survey[6] to assess women's awareness of the various religious restrictions in Catholic hospitals, this time at the national level. We learned, as Dr. Guiahi had in Colorado, that patient awareness was sorely lacking. Nationally, women expected contraceptive pills (77 percent) and sterilization (70 percent) to be available in Catholic hospitals, and many thought one could even schedule an abortion if the fetus had a fatal anomaly (42 percent),[7] but the ERDs prohibit all these things. Dr. Stulberg and I collaborated with University of Wisconsin researchers Renee Kramer and Jenny Higgins to gather more detailed state-level data, replicating a version of the PARRCH survey that ultimately showed that, in rural areas where women had fewer healthcare alternatives, they had even less awareness of religious restrictions, more denials of reproductive care, and long delays accessing it elsewhere.[8]

To learn from their own words what getting reproductive care in Catholic facilities was like for women, we returned to qualitative research supported by two grants from the Society for Family Planning and one from the Greenwall Foundation's Faculty Scholar Program. I interviewed patients in-depth in two phases. The first set of twenty-three phone interviews were done with patients recruited by Sara Magnusson, Molly Battistelli, and I through internet ads and appeals to professional networks in parts of the United States heavily saturated with Catholic health care. In these interviews, I asked patients to tell me all about their experiences with reproductive care in local hospitals to see what would emerge. For the second set, I worked again with Dr. Stulberg's team to follow up with thirty-three people who had indicated in our national PARRCH survey that they had attended a Catholic hospital or clinic for some sort of reproductive care, whether or not they perceived themselves to have been denied it.[9] Altogether, from 2015 to 2020, I interviewed fifty-six patients over the phone to gather their diverse reproductive experiences and perspectives.

During this same span of time, we conducted other related research, such as a mixed method study about insurance plans. This included key-informant interviews with human resources executives to understand the role insurance networks play in access to reproductive care and a national survey of 1,001 employees of S&P 500 companies to understand their experiences and preferences around healthcare denials.[10] The survey showed that 14 percent of women and 10 percent of men were aware that someone on their insurance plan had been denied reproductive care.[11] Additionally, most insured employees think hospitals, insurers, and employers all have a responsibility to remove barriers to postpartum tubal ligation.[12] I also advised on a qualitative study with physicians and patients in Illinois conducted by Dr. Stulberg's team to understand how to improve postpartum access to contraception for women who birthed in Catholic hospitals.[13]

Glaringly underrepresented, I will be the first to acknowledge, are the perspectives of nurses, administrators, members of Catholic ethics committees, and bishops. I do not have a great excuse for this other than the lack of resources and time and the disinterest of Catholic leadership in being involved. I had good access to physician subjects, which, in addition to the general ob-gyns, included a handful of family medicine physicians and high-risk ob-gyns (maternal-fetal medicine [MFM] physicians or perinatologists), lending breadth to the physician perspective. The perspectives of other hospital staff are represented only by a few particularly rich interviews with patients who coincidentally happened to be nurses and healthcare administrators within Catholic facilities, and one nurse practitioner who had been reprimanded for providing contraception to her patients in her Catholic clinic, so she found me because she wanted to tell her story. And, finally, I had lengthy discussions with six ethicists who have worked in Catholic hospitals when I met them at national conferences and professional meetings. But only the two ethicists who were not Catholic would allow me to record an interview; the three who were devout Catholics were at times outwardly supportive of the research and talkative but did not agree to a recorded interview; and, finally, one, who also was clergy, was so hostile toward my research I was too scared to ask. As far as the bishops, who hold titular court in this book due to their immense authority and power over reproductive bodies in the United States, well, I had reason to believe they would not speak with me.[14] Their perspectives come through the physicians' stories in the book about how bishops interacted with hospital administrators and through what they say to the media, as well as what they publish publicly.

Finally, from 2016 to 2021, I was involved with my own public institution's process of affiliating with Catholic health facilities because they wanted to broaden our healthcare network. My role within institutional meetings was to point out the ob-gyn clinical conflicts that could arise in our partnerships—based on my research experience—to leaders of both Catholic institutions and the public university system. I also pushed back on the whole endeavor where I could.[15] While that content is not integrated into the entirety of this book, it informs my perspective on how Catholic health institutions expand.

Acknowledgments

I want to start by thanking my thought partner Debra Stulberg for an amazing decade of conducting research together, which includes most of the studies that generated data for this book. I am completely in her debt for getting us started and finding us that first Greenwall Foundation seed grant to do the physician interviews. Throughout, I learned so much from her expertise as a physician, a bioethicist, a quantitative methodologist, a leader, and a genuinely good human. And we had a lot of fun.

A few folks were absolutely sine qua non in the final push. Debra Stulberg and two other personal influencers (brilliant medical anthropology friends) Liz Roberts and Mara Buchbinder read drafts and pushed me along when I was stuck. I even tried to give the project away to two of them, but both insisted I was its mother. Renee Kramer saved me from technology and my mess of endnotes, which only someone as capable and knowledgeable about the research area as she is could have done. Maryani Rasidjan helped me stop spiraling with her incisive and timely feedback on key segments. I am also enormously grateful for the deeply engaged feedback of reviewers Jessica Martucci and Miranda Waggoner; for the enduring patience and enthusiasm of Rutgers's Peter Mickulas, who checked in with me about the book project each of the ten years it took; and for the work of Audra Wolfe, who helped me say what I was trying to say better, offering concrete solutions to my overwhelm and the authoritative voice I needed to get it to the finish line.

I want to thank my book writing subgroup of Greenwall Faculty Scholars. Efthimios Parasidis, Jenny Blumenthal-Barby, and Mara Buchbinder read my half-baked chapters years before publication, when I really did not know which way was up. I am grateful for your comradery, warmth, and safety. Other generous colleagues from Greenwall were thoughtful and influential in their feedback on portions of the book, including Jen James, Brownsyne Tucker Edmonds, Danielle Wenner, Kimani Paul-Emile, Jodi Halpern, Gretchen Schwarze, Ronit Stahl, and so many more over all these years. I am especially grateful to the Greenwall Foundation and my mentors there, Alta Charo, Bernie Lo, and Keith Wailoo, for helping me grow and for bringing us all together in such a supportive way.

My research program at UCSF, Advancing New Standards in Reproductive Health (ANSIRH), together with the Bixby Center and the ob-gyn department in which ANSIRH is nested, have provided me a generative and inspiring research home all these years. I feel truly lucky for the leadership and nurturing of Dan Grossman, Molly Battistelli, Jody Steinauer, Diana Greene Foster, Rebecca Jackson, and Virali Modi-Parekh. The book project also has been blessed by helpful insights over the years from colleagues and collaborators Katrina Kimport, Bimla Schwarz, Erin Wingo, Corrine Rocca, Antonia Biggs, Sara Magnusson, Irma Hasham Dahlquist, Jocelyn Wascher, Tracy Weitz, Lee Hasselbacher, Lucy Hebert, Katie Watson, Julie Chor, Danielle Bessette, Jenny Higgins, Jen Schradie, and, of course, Carole Joffe. Thank you to the late Sharon Kaufman, a treasured mentor, for giving me confidence and a little push when needed. And a heartfelt thank you to Vanessa Jacoby, Michele Goodwin, Robert May, Lisa Ikemoto, Shane White, and John Perez for having fine-tuned moral compasses and for modeling how to speak—seemingly fearlessly—to people making institutional decisions of enormous long-range consequences for health and justice.

I am eternally grateful for those I hold close, who kept cheering me along despite having no proof that this ever would actually get done, including my dad Jonah, my sister Lisa, Bill, Candace, and, of course, my mother Judy, who has shown endless enthusiasm for all I did from day one. Thank you to my treasured birthday gals, co-paddlers, BBC, and sweetest of neighbors who all got me through. Krissy, Ana, and Ellis made my days brighter and sweeter with their hugs, shenanigans, coffee runs, and shared meals. Thank you to Gabby for the unconditional love and cuddles, to our hens for the yummy eggs, to Ici and Pickles for reducing the rat population of the coop, and to the dahlia and tomato gods for the gifts of summer.

My kids, Hannah and Ruby, have grown up through the course of this project, from elementary age to starting college. For many years, my preoccupation with religion and hospitals was curious and opaque to them. But during the pandemic, we all became clearer on how we spent our days. And as I worried about how to protect them from the perils of pandemic isolation, they questioned my writing stagnation (weirdly related and somehow motivating). They began to cheer me on. Ruby gave words of encouragement. Hannah gave feedback on chapters. Both inspired me as they grew into astonishing young adults. And I write this on the twenty-first anniversary of being married to their dad Ori, an infinitely generous and immeasurably kind person who manages to be hyper-productive while holding up more than his share of souls. I am grateful for his immense equanimity and daily model of how not to sweat the small stuff that has gotten me through these decades. Ori, Hannah, Ruby—your love is everything. Thank you.

Notes

PROLOGUE

1. Lois Uttley and Ronnie Pawelko, "No Strings Attached: Public Funding of Religiously-Sponsored Hospitals in the United States," Report, (The MergerWatch Project, 2002), http://static1.1.sqspcdn.com/static/f/816571/11352520/1300824226243/bp_no_strings.pdf?token=2YkKWWcv.

2. Lori Freedman, "Dispelling Six Myths about Catholic Hospital Care in the United States," *Rewire News Group*, n.d., http://files/2629/dispelling-six-myths-catholic-hospital-care-united-states.html.

3. Tess Solomon et al., "Bigger and Bigger: The Growth of Catholic Health Systems," Report (Boston, MA: Community Catalyst, 2020), https://www.communitycatalyst.org/resources/publications/document/2020-Cath-Hosp-Report-2020-31.pdf.

4. United States Conference of Catholic Bishops, "Ethical and Religious Directives for Catholic Health Care Services," (6th ed.), 2018, https://www.usccb.org/about/doctrine/ethical-and-religious-directives/upload/ethical-religious-directives-catholic-health-service-sixth-edition-2016-06.pdf.

5. Catholic women use sterilization and contraception at nearly identical rates as the rest of the population. For example, in 2011, the Guttmacher Institute reported that 33 percent of all women were using sterilization, and 32 percent of Catholic women were using sterilization. Rachel K. Jones and Joerg Dreweke, "Countering Conventional Wisdom: New Evidence on Religion and Contraceptive Use," Report, (Guttmacher Institute, 2011), https://www.guttmacher.org/sites/default/files/report_pdf/religion-and-contraceptive-use.pdf.

6. Catholics for Choice, "Is Your Health Care Compromised? How the Catholic Directives Make for Unhealthy Choices," Report, (Catholics for Choice, 2017), https://www.catholicsforchoice.org/wp-content/uploads/2017/01/2017_Catholic-Healthcare-Report.pdf; Belden Russonello Strategists, "Catholic Voters and Religious Exemption Policies: Report of a National Public Opinion Survey for Catholics for Choice, Call to Action, DignityUSA and Women's Alliance for Theology, Ethics, and Ritual (WATER)," Report, Catholics for Choice, October 2014, https://www.catholicsforchoice.org/wp-content/uploads/2014/11/11.17.14-National-Catholic-Voters-Survey-2014.pdf; Belden Russonello Strategists, "The Views of Catholic Millenials on the Catholic Church and Social Issues," Report, Catholics for Choice, June 2015, https://www.catholicsforchoice.org/wp-content/uploads/2016/12/2015_BRS_Catholic_Millennials-2.pdf.

7. Luciana E Hebert, Lori Freedman, and Debra B Stulberg, "Choosing a Hospital for Obstetric, Gynecologic, or Reproductive Healthcare: What Matters Most to Patients?" *American Journal of Obstetrics & Gynecology MFM* 2, no. 1 (2020), https://doi.org/10.1016/j .ajogmf.2019.100067.

8. Solomon et al., "Bigger and Bigger: The Growth of Catholic Health Systems."

9. Debra B. Stulberg et al., "Women's Expectation of Receiving Reproductive Health Care at Catholic and Non-Catholic Hospitals," *Perspectives on Sexual and Reproductive Health* 51, no. 3 (2019): 135–142, https://doi.org/10.1363/psrh.12118; Kellie E Schueler et al., "Denial of Tubal Ligation in Religious Hospitals: Consumer Attitudes When Insurance Limits Hospital Choice," *Contraception* 104, no. 2 (2021): 194–201.

10. Tom L. Beauchamp and James F. Childress, *Principles of Biomedical Ethics* (New York: Oxford University Press, 2009), http://www.loc.gov/catdir/toc/ecip088/2008000233 .html.

11. David J. Rothman, *Strangers at the Bedside: A History of How Law and Bioethics Transformed Medical Decision Making* (New York, NY: BasicBooks, 1991).

12. C. Lee Ventola, "Direct-to-Consumer Pharmaceutical Advertising: Therapeutic or Toxic?" *Pharmacy and Therapeutics* 36, no. 10 (2011): 681–684.

13. Peter Moffett and Gregory Moore, "The Standard of Care: Legal History and Definitions: The Bad and Good News," *Western Journal of Emergency Medicine* 12, no. 1 (2011): 109–112.

14. American Public Health Association, "Restricted Access to Abortion Violates Human Rights, Precludes Reproductive Justice, and Demands Public Health Intervention," Report, (American Public Health Association, November 3, 2015), https://www.apha .org/policies-and-advocacy/public-health-policy-statements/policy-database/2016/01/04 /11/24/restricted-access-to-abortion-violates-human-rights; American College of Obstetrics and Gynecologists, "Restrictions to Comprehensive Reproductive Health Care," April 2016, https://www.acog.org/en/Clinical Information/Policy and Position Statements/Position Statements/2018/Restrictions to Comprehensive Reproductive Health Care.

15. Diana Greene Foster et al., "Comparison of Health, Development, Maternal Bonding, and Poverty among Children Born after Denial of Abortion vs. after Pregnancies Subsequent an Abortion," *JAMA Pediatrics* 172, no. 11 (2018): 1053–1060; Sarah C. M. Roberts et al., "Risk of Violence from the Man Involved in the Pregnancy after Receiving or Being Denied an Abortion," *BMC Medicine* 12, no. 144 (2014), https://doi.org/10.1186/s12916-014 -0144-z; Jessica D Gipson, Michael A Koenig, and Michelle J Hindin, "The Effects of Unintended Pregnancy on Infant, Child, and Parental Health: A Review of the Literature," *Studies in Family Planning* 39, no. 1 (2008) 18–38.

16. Megan L. Kavanaugh and Ragnar M. Anderson, "Contraception and Beyond: The Health Benefits of Services Provided at Family Planning Centers" (New York: Guttmacher Institute, 2013); Ushma D. Upadhyay et al., "Women's Empowerment and Fertility: A Review of the Literature," *Social Science & Medicine* 115 (August 2014): 111–120, https://doi .org/10.1016/j.socscimed.2014.06.014.

INTRODUCTION

1. As is customary in social research, I have used pseudonyms to protect the confidentiality of study participants, with the exception of a few advocates who have public visibility and wanted to be identifiable.

2. To give a sense of how populous the environments are where study participants live and work, I classify domains in terms that are more specific than the urban versus rural

designation of the U.S. Census Bureau. In this book, rural indicates a core settlement of less than 50,000 people, small city 50,000 to 100,000, mid-size city 100,000 to 500,000, and a large city or urban area has a population of 500,000 and up. When a small or mid-size city is part of multiple contiguous cities that together hold a population of 500,000 or higher, I consider it an urban area for the purpose of understanding the extent of health-care resources and opportunities that could be available.

3. The names of all hospitals and people in this book are pseudonyms, with a few noted exceptions.

4. Catholic Health Association of the United States, "U.S. Catholic Health Care," 2021, https://www.chausa.org/docs/default-source/default-document-library/2021-the-strategic -profile-_sb_final.pdf?sfvrsn=2.

5. After delivering a baby, the temporary position of the fallopian tubes allows for a sim-pler laparoscopic tubal ligation compared to after recovery, when the tubes have returned to their natural position. Meredith J. Alston, Jennifer S. Hyer, and Morris Askenazi, "Sur-gical Sterilization," *Postgraduate Obstetrics & Gynecology* 30, no. 13 (July 2010): 1–7, https://doi.org/10.1097/01.PGO.0000383191.03059.ef.

6. Catholic Health Association of the United States, "U.S. Catholic Health Care," 2021, https://www.chausa.org/docs/default-source/default-document-library/2021-the-strategic -profile-_sb_final.pdf?sfvrsn=2.

7. Why exactly Catholic facilities and health systems prosper in some states more than others is historically contingent and widely variable. For example, South Dakota's Catho-lic hospital was the first accredited in the state and was founded by a physician in 1882 who was stranded during his westward migration, https://www.avera.org/locations/st-marys /about/history/. For more information about prevalence by state, see Tess Solomon et al., "Bigger and Bigger: The Growth of Catholic Health Systems" (Boston, MA: Community Catalyst, 2020), https://www.communitycatalyst.org/resources/publications/document/2020 -Cath-Hosp-Report-2020-31.pdf.

8. "Conscience rights" refer to legal protection for those who abstain from providing certain healthcare services for moral or religious reasons, typically abortion but often extending into contraception and end-of-life services. In the United States, religious institutions have been granted the same rights to refuse such care, including the right to prohibit those who want to offer it from doing so within their institutions. Holly Fernandez Lynch, I. Glenn Cohen, and Elizabeth Sepper, eds., *Law, Religion, and Health in the United States* (Cambridge: Cambridge University Press, 2017), https://doi.org/10.1017/9781316691274. Also see Sara Dubow, "From Conscience Clauses to Conscience Wars," in Johanna Schoen, *Abortion Care as Moral Work: Ethical Considerations of Maternal and Fetal Bodies* (Rutgers University Press, 2022).

9. D. B. Stulberg et al., "Obstetrician-Gynecologists, Religious Institutions, and Con-flicts Regarding Patient-Care Policies," *American Journal of Obstetrics and Gynecology* 207, no. 1 (July 2012): 73 e1–5, https://doi.org/10.1016/j.ajog.2012.04.023; Coleman Drake et al., "Market Share of US Catholic Hospitals and Associated Geographic Network Access to Reproductive Health Services," *JAMA Network Open* 3, no. 1 (2020), https://doi.org/10 .1001/jamanetworkopen.2019.20053.

10. Luciana E. Hebert, Lori Freedman, and Debra B. Stulberg, "Choosing a Hospital for Obstetric, Gynecologic, or Reproductive Healthcare: What Matters Most to Patients?" *American Journal of Obstetrics & Gynecology MFM* 2, no. 1 (2020); Michelle C. Menegay et al., "Delivery at Catholic Hospitals and Postpartum Contraception Use, Five US States, 2015–2018," *Perspectives on Sexual and Reproductive Health*, February 13, 2022, psrh.12186, https://doi.org/10.1363/psrh.12186.

11. By the end of their reproductive years (ages forty to forty-four), 39 percent of women and 15 percent of men had undergone sterilization. This proportion is decreasing with the uptake of IUDs and implants. William D Mosher, Jo Jones, and National Center for Health Statistics (United States), *Use of Contraception in the United States: 1982–2008* (Hyattsville, MD: U.S. Dept. of Health and Human Services, Centers for Disease Control and Prevention, National Center for Health Statistics, 2010).

12. In a national survey vignette question, 70 percent of women believed tubal ligation to be available in a fictitious hospital called Saint John's. Debra B. Stulberg et al., "Women's Expectation of Receiving Reproductive Health Care at Catholic and Non-Catholic Hospitals," *Perspectives on Sexual and Reproductive Health* 51, no. 3 (September 4, 2019): 135–142, https://doi.org/10.1363/psrh.12118. Research shows that after a hospital becomes Catholic, the number of sterilizations performed decreases by about 30 percent, but does not go to zero. Elaine L. Hill, David J. G. Slusky, and Donna K. Ginther, "Reproductive Health Care in Catholic-Owned Hospitals," *Journal of Health Economics* 65 (May 2019): 48–62, https://doi.org/10.1016/j.jhealeco.2019.02.005.

13. The 2001 revision of the Ethical and Religious Directives for Catholic Health Care Services was a two-year "collaboration among the bishops, Catholic healthcare leaders, theologians and ethicists, and the Holy See," https://www.chausa.org/docs/default-source /health-progress/a-brief-history-pdf.pdf?sfvrsn=0. In the 2018 revision, the USCCB added more healthcare professionals to the list of contributors, describing it as an "extensive process of consultation with bishops, theologians, sponsors, administrators, physicians, and other health care providers," https://www.usccb.org/about/doctrine/ethical-and-religious -directives/upload/ethical-religious-directives-catholic-health-service-sixth-edition-2016 -06.pdf.

14. The bishops speak out on a variety of political matters, especially to support immigration rights, to condemn LGBTQ equity efforts, and to oppose healthcare policy change that would improve access to abortion and contraception. The USCCB's Subcommittee on Health Care Issues is led by five bishops (including Bishop Olmsted, who features prominently in chapter 7) and a handful of consultants from major Catholic professional associations. A notable recent effort to influence healthcare policy involved the Subcommittee on Health Care Issues weighing in to condemn what they call "gender ideology" and, specifically, gender confirming healthcare, https://www.usccb.org/news/2022/bishop-chairmen -condemn-harmful-regulations-forcing-gender-ideology-and-potentially. For a close study of such efforts, see Meaghan O'Keefe, *American Catholic Bishops and the Politics of Scandal: Rhetoric of Authority* (Routledge, 2019).

15. "Remembering The Meeting 50 Years Ago That Led To 'Our Bodies, Ourselves,'" accessed March 15, 2022, https://www.wbur.org/news/2019/05/08/founding-our-bodies -ourselves-women-health.

16. D. Soyini Madison, *Critical Ethnography: Method, Ethics, and Performance* (Sage Publications, 2011).

17. B. M. Wall, "Conflict and Compromise: Catholic and Public Hospital Partnerships," *Nursing History Review* 18 (2010): 100–117.

18. More detail about the agreements from Dr. Altera's colleague: "And there was one of our young guys who is trying to keep his nose clean, even though he doesn't agree with them. He started, he had an emergent C-Section, where the patient wanted a tubal, and he started the section with hospital personnel and he called in the ambulatory surgery center on-call team . . . But they changed, the personnel changed in the middle of the case before the tubal. Well, that's strictly forbidden. Hospital staff cannot start the case, even if they're not involved in the tubal at all. So this has been a huge uproar. If it ever occurs again, it's

all over. . . . So, if you come, you know, if you want your tubes tied, you're basically playing, you know, Russian Roulette as to whether you'll get your operation done. And I as a
doctor, every time I'm on call, I'm playing Russian Roulette, because I feel that I can't look
into a patient's abdomen and as far as I'm concerned commit malpractice. I mean, to close
someone up and say, 'You need another operation,' is just malpractice. If I've left a sponge
in your abdomen, by mistake, and you need another operation to take it out, I mean, I
might as well just write you a check."

19. The quote in the previous note and other aspects of this story have been previously
printed in this 2014 article and the 2021 edited volume: D. B. Stulberg et al., "Tubal Ligation in Catholic Hospitals: A Qualitative Study of Ob-Gyns' Experiences," *Contraception*
90, no. 4 (October 2014): 422–428, https://doi.org/10.1016/j.contraception.2014.04.015,
and Julie Chor and Katie Watson, eds., *Reproductive Ethics in Clinical Practice: Preventing, Initiating, and Managing Pregnancy and Delivery*, Essays Inspired by the MacLean
Center for Clinical Medical Ethics Lecture Series (New York, NY: Oxford University
Press, 2021).

20. United States Conference of Catholic Bishops, "Ethical and Religious Directives for
Catholic Health Care Services (6th ed.)," 2018, https://www.usccb.org/about/doctrine
/ethical-and-religious-directives/upload/ethical-religious-directives-catholic-health
-service-sixth-edition-2016-06.pdf.

21. "Cardinal George: Sr. Keehan Chose Obama over Catholic Bishops," *Catholic News
Agency*, 2010, https://www.catholicnewsagency.com/news/19997/cardinal-george-sr-keehan
-chose-obama-over-catholic-bishops.

22. Catholic Health Association of the United States, "Ethical and Religious Directives,"
n.d., https://www.chausa.org/ethics/ethical-and-religious-directives.

23. Thomas Reese, "Equality Act Vote Again Pits Catholic Nuns against Bishops," *Religion
News Service*, 2019, https://religionnews.com/2019/05/20/equality-act-vote-again-pits-catholic
-nuns-against-bishops/; Barbra Mann Wall, *American Catholic Hospitals: A Century of
Changing Markets and Missions, Critical Issues in Health and Medicine* (New Brunswick, NJ:
Rutgers University Press, 2011); Barbra Mann Wall, "The Role of Catholic Nurses in Women's
Health Care Policy Disputes: A Historical Study," *Nursing Outlook* 61, no. 5 (September 2013):
367–374, https://doi.org/10.1016/j.outlook.2013.07.005.

24. CHAUSA's *Health Care Ethics USA* and the Catholic Medical Association's *Linacre
Quarterly*.

25. Four lawsuits about such denials of care for gender affirmation have been filed, the
most notable of which is *Minton v. Dignity Health*, pending at the time of this writing
before the U.S. Supreme Court.

26. Mark Joseph Stern, "When Can Dying Patients Get a Lifesaving Abortion? These
Hospital Panels Will Now Decide," *Slate*, July 29, 2022, https://slate.com/news-and-politics
/2022/07/abortion-ban-hospital-ethics-committee-mother-life-death.html; Frances Stead
Sellers and Fenit Nirappil, "Confusion Post-*Roe* Spurs Delays, Denials for Some Lifesaving
Pregnancy Care," *Washington Post*, July 16, 2022, https://www.washingtonpost.com/health
/2022/07/16/abortion-miscarriage-ectopic-pregnancy-care/; Pam Belluck, "They Had Miscarriages, and New Abortion Laws Obstructed Treatment," *New York Times*, July 17, 2022,
https://www.nytimes.com/2022/07/17/health/abortion-miscarriage-treatment.html;
Michele Goldberg, "The Anti-Abortion Movement Is in Denial," *New York Times*, July 29, 2022,
https://www.nytimes.com/2022/07/29/opinion/anti-abortion-movement.html; Ariana Eunjung
Cha, "Physicians Face Confusion and Fear in Post-*Roe* World," *Washington Post*, July 28, 2022,
https://www.washingtonpost.com/health/2022/06/28/abortion-ban-roe-doctors-confusion/;
Jessica Winter, "The Dobbs Decision Has Unleashed Legal Chaos for Doctors and Patients,"

New Yorker, July 2, 2022, https://www.newyorker.com/news/news-desk/the-dobbs-decision-has-unleashed-legal-chaos-for-doctors-and-patients; Andréa Becker and Rachel E. Gross, "The 'Abortion Pill' Is Used for So Much More than Abortions," *Slate*, July 6, 2022, https://slate.com/technology/2022/07/roe-wade-abortion-health-care-crisis-misoprostol-mifepristone-d-and-c.html; Neel Dhanesha, "A Pregnancy Turns Deadly In an Anti-Abortion State. What Happens Next?" *Vox*, July 4, 2022, https://www.vox.com/science-and-health/23191865/abortion-ban-medical-emergency-ectopic-pregnancy; Maggie Koerth and Amelia Thomson-DeVeaux, "Even Exceptions to Abortion Bans Pit A Mother's Life against Doctors' Fears," *fivethirtyeight.com*, June 30, 2022, https://fivethirtyeight.com/features/even-exceptions-to-abortion-bans-pit-a-mothers-life-against-doctors-fears/; Leah Torres, "Doctors in Alabama Already Turn Away Miscarrying Patients. This Will Be America's New Normal," *Slate*, May 17, 2022, https://slate.com/news-and-politics/2022/05/roe-dobbs-abortion-ban-reproductive-medicine-alabama.html; Whitney Arey et al., "A Preview of the Dangerous Future of Abortion Bans—Texas Senate Bill 8," *New England Journal of Medicine* 387, no. 5 (August 4, 2022): 388–390, https://doi.org/10.1056/NEJMp2207423; Rita Rubin, "How Abortion Bans Could Affect Care for Miscarriage and Infertility," *JAMA* 328, no. 4 (July 26, 2022): 318–320, https://doi.org/10.1001/jama.2022.11488.

27. *The BUMP*, a pregnancy information website, translates the complex science of Kell to lay readers: "A problem can occur when a Kell-negative mom is somehow exposed to the Kell-positive blood—say, via a blood transfusion. Once she's exposed, she develops anti-Kell antibodies, which can attack and destroy Kell-positive red blood cells. So if she becomes pregnant with a Kell-positive baby, her anti-Kell antibodies might cross the placenta and destroy the baby's red blood cells. This is called hemolytic disease, and it can be lethal," https://www.thebump.com/a/kell-factor. For a scientific explanation, see, also, https://www.ncbi.nlm.nih.gov/books/NBK2270/ and https://www.sciencedirect.com/topics/medicine-and-dentistry/blood-group-kell-system.

28. "Abortion is now Banned or Under Threat in These States," *Washington Post*, June 24, 2022.

29. Jocelyn M Wascher et al., "Do Women Know Whether Their Hospital Is Catholic? Results from a National Survey," *Contraception* 98, no. 6 (2018): 498–503; Lori R. Freedman et al., "Religious Hospital Policies on Reproductive Care: What Do Patients Want to Know?" *American Journal of Obstetrics & Gynecology* 218, no. 2 (2018): 251–e1.

30. Loretta Ross and Rickie Solinger, *Reproductive Justice: An Introduction," Reproductive Justice: A New Vision for the Twenty-First Century* (Oakland, California: University of California Press, 2017); Molly R. Altman et al., "Listening to Women: Recommendations from Women of Color to Improve Experiences in Pregnancy and Birth Care," *Journal of Midwifery & Women's Health* 65, no. 4 (July 2020): 466–473, https://doi.org/10.1111/jmwh.13102; Khiara M. Bridges, "Racial Disparities in Maternal Mortality," *New York University Law Review* 95 (n.d.): 90.

31. Kira Shepherd, Elizabeth Reiner Platt, Katherine Franke, and Elizabeth Boylen, "Bearing Faith: The Limits of Catholic Health Care for Women of Color," Public Rights/Private Conscience Project (Columbia Law School, January 19, 2018), https://lawrightsreligion.law.columbia.edu/sites/default/files/content/BearingFaith.pdf.

32. Rebecca Gieseker et al., "Family Planning Service Provision in Illinois Religious Hospitals: Racial/Ethnic Variation in Access to Non-Religious Hospitals for Publicly Insured Women," *Contraception* 100, no. 4 (2019): 296–298.

33. Elaine L. Hill, David J. G. Slusky, and Donna K. Ginther, "Reproductive Health Care in Catholic-Owned Hospitals," *Journal of Health Economics* 65 (2019): 48–62, https://doi.org/10.1016/j.jhealeco.2019.02.005.

34. By reproductive care safety net, I refer to family planning clinics and other sites providing comprehensive sexual and reproductive health care that have historically served as a safety valve for restrictive facilities like Catholic hospitals when they refuse care. Examples abound throughout the book and throughout the country.

35. See notes 5 and 6 from the prologue.

CHAPTER 1 — GROWTH

1. Katie Hafner, "As Catholic Hospitals Expand, So Do Limits on Some Procedures," *New York Times*, August 10, 2018. sec. Health, https://www.nytimes.com/2018/08/10/health/catholic-hospitals-procedures.html.

2. M. Ursula Stepsis and Dolores Ann Liptak, *Pioneer Healers: The History of Women Religious in American Health Care* (Crossroad Publishing Company, 1989); Paul Starr, *The Social Transformation of American Medicine* (New York: Basic Books, 1982).

3. Bernadette McCauley, *Who Shall Take Care of Our Sick?: Roman Catholic Sisters and the Development of Catholic Hospitals in New York City, Medicine, Science, and Religion in Historical Context* (Baltimore: Johns Hopkins University Press, 2005), http://www.loc.gov/catdir/toc/ecip056/2005000735.html.

4. Leslie J. Reagan, *When Abortion Was a Crime: Women, Medicine, and Law in the United States, 1867–1973* (Berkeley: University of California Press, 1997); Carroll Smith-Rosenberg, *Disorderly Conduct: Visions of Gender in Victorian America* (New York: Oxford University Press, 1986); James C. Mohr, *Abortion in America: The Origins and Evolution of National Policy, 1800–1900* (New York: Oxford University Press, 1978).

5. Starr, *The Social Transformation of American Medicine*.

6. Mohr, *Abortion in America: The Origins and Evolution of National Policy, 1800–1900*.

7. Kathleen M. Joyce, "The Evil of Abortion and the Greater Good of the Faith: Negotiating Catholic Survival in the Twentieth-Century American Health Care System," *Religion and American Culture* 12, no. 1 (Winter 2002): 94, 91–121.

8. In nineteenth-century America, abortion was legal before "quickening," which was considered to come with the onset of the sensation of fetal movement at about four to five months. Ads for "periodical pills" and "professional services" could be seen in newspapers and magazines posted by a variety of non-physician health practitioners, where they offered "surprising success in the treatment of diseases incident to her sex, or those suffering irregularity." See Mohr, *Abortion in America: The Origins and Evolution of National Policy, 1800–1900*, 126.

9. Joyce, "The Evil of Abortion and the Greater Good of the Faith: Negotiating Catholic Survival in the Twentieth-Century American Health Care System."

10. Joyce, "The Evil of Abortion," 93.

11. Rosemary Stevens, *In Sickness and in Wealth: American Hospitals in the Twentieth Century* (Baltimore: Johns Hopkins University Press, 1999), 160.

12. Barbra Mann Wall, *American Catholic Hospitals: A Century of Changing Markets and Missions, Critical Issues in Health and Medicine* (New Brunswick, NJ: Rutgers University Press, 2011), 12.

13. Wall, *American Catholic Hospitals*, 60; C. A. Hangartner, "Implications for Nursing Education from Vatican II," *Hospital Progress* 47, no. 10 (October 1, 1966): 63–66 passim; Stephen M. Cherry, *Importing Care, Faithful Service: Filipino and Indian American Nurses at a Veterans Hospital* (Rutgers University Press, 2022).

14. Adam D. Reich, *Selling Our Souls: The Commodification of Hospital Care in the United States* (Princeton: Princeton University Press, 2014), 113.

15. Ann Kutney-Lee et al., "Distinct Enough? A National Examination of Catholic Hospital Affiliation and Patient Perceptions of Care," *Health Care Management Review* 39,

no. 2 (2014): 134; Wall, *American Catholic Hospitals*; M. L. Palley and T. Kohler, "Hospital Mergers: The Future of Women's Reproductive Healthcare Services," *Women & Politics* 25, no. 1/2 (2003): 149–178.

16. Palley and Kohler, "Hospital Mergers: The Future of Women's Reproductive Healthcare Services," 154–155.

17. Stephen M Shortell, "The Evolution of Hospital Systems: Unfulfilled Promises and Self-Fulfilling Prophesies," *Medical Care Review* 45, no. 2 (1988): 177–214.

18. Palley and Kohler, "Hospital Mergers: The Future of Women's Reproductive Healthcare Services," 156.

19. Wall, *American Catholic Hospitals*, 141.

20. J. Gelb and C. J. Shogan, "Community Activism in the USA: Catholic Hospital Mergers and Reproductive Access," *Social Movement Studies* 4, no. 3 (2005): 209–229; D. Bellandi, "What Hospitals Won't Do for a Merger. Deals Involving Catholic Facilities Often Mean a Loss of Reproductive Services," *Modern Healthcare* 28, no. 39 (September 28, 1998): 28–30, 32; D. Bellandi, "Access Declines. Reproductive Services Fall with Hospital Consolidation," *Modern Healthcare* 28, no. 16 (April 20, 1998): 26; Deanna Bellandi, "Catholic Merger Proves Lucrative," *Modern Healthcare* 30, no. 46 (2000): 56; Leora Eisenstadt, "Separation of Church and Hospital: Strategies to Protect Pro-Choice Physicians in Religiously Affiliated Hospitals," *Yale Journal of Law and Feminism* 15 (2003): 135; M. Sloboda, "The High Cost of Merging with a Religiously-Controlled Hospital," *Berkeley Womens Law Journal* 16 (2001): 140–156; Lisa C. Ikemoto, "When a Hospital becomes Catholic," *Mercer Law Review* 47 (1995): 1087.

21. Wall, *American Catholic Hospitals*, 12.

22. Community Catalyst counts only acute care, short-term hospitals in these statistics (as opposed to rehabilitation facilities, for example), and includes previously Catholic hospitals that still follow the ERDs even if not members of CHA. See Tess Solomon et al., "Bigger and Bigger: The Growth of Catholic Health Systems" (Community Catalyst, 2020). The CHA may have different inclusion criteria, preventing precise comparison of their numbers.

23. Solomon et al.

24. Catholic Health Association of the United States, "U.S. Catholic Health Care," 2021, https://www.chausa.org/docs/default-source/default-document-library/2021-the-strategic-profile-_sb_final.pdf?sfvrsn=2.

25. Wall, *American Catholic Hospitals*, 120, 122.

26. Office for Civil Rights (OCR), "Conscience Protections for Health Care Providers," Text, HHS.gov, October 14, 2010, https://www.hhs.gov/conscience/conscience-protections/index.html; "Church Amendments," 42 U.S.C. § 300a-7 § (n.d.), https://www.hhs.gov/sites/default/files/ocr/civilrights/understanding/ConscienceProtect/42usc300a7.pdf; Mark R. Wicclair, "Negative and Positive Claims of Conscience," *Cambridge Quarterly of Healthcare Ethics* 18, no. 1 (January 2009): 14–22, https://doi.org/10.1017/S096318010809004X.

27. "Weldon Amendment, Consolidated Appropriations Act," Pub. L. No. 111–117, 123 Stat 3034 (2009), https://www.hhs.gov/sites/default/files/ocr/civilrights/understanding/ConscienceProtect/publaw111_117_123_stat_3034.pdf; "The Weldon Amendment: Interfering with Abortion Coverage and Care," (Guttmacher Institute), June 29, 2021, https://www.guttmacher.org/fact-sheet/weldon-amendment.

28. Leonard Hospital's merger case was publicly documented, and, thus, this is not a pseudonym. See P. Donovan, "Hospital Mergers and Reproductive Health Care," *Family Planning Perspectives* 28, no. 6 (December 1996): 281–284.

29. Lisa C Ikemoto, "When a Hospital becomes Catholic," *Mercer Law Review* 47 (n.d.): 49.

30. Bellandi, "What Hospitals Won't Do for a Merger."

31. Amy Pyle, "A Collision of Medicine and Faith," *Los Angeles Times*, January 3, 2000, https://www.latimes.com/archives/la-xpm-2000-jan-03-mn-50332-story.html; Gelb and Shogan, "Community Activism in the USA."

32. Gelb and Shogan, "Community Activism in the USA."

33. Pyle, "A Collision of Medicine and Faith."

34. United States Conference of Catholic Bishops, "The Ethical and Religious Directives for Catholic Healthcare Services," Report (United States Conference of Catholic Bishops, 2018): 26, http://www.usccb.org/about/doctrine/ethical-and-religious-directives/upload /ethical-religious-directives-catholic-health-service-sixth-edition-2016-06.pdf; "US Bishops Revise Part Six of the Ethical and Religious Directives," accessed March 17, 2022, https://www.chausa.org/publications/health-care-ethics-usa/archives/issues/summer -2018/from-the-field---bouchard-and-hibner---formatted-v2.

35. "New Catholic Directives Could Complicate Mergers and Partnerships," *Modern Healthcare*, July 19, 2018, https://www.modernhealthcare.com/article/20180719/NEWS /180719880/new-catholic-directives-could-complicate-mergers-and-partnerships.

36. Solomon et al., "Bigger and Bigger: The Growth of Catholic Health Systems."

37. The Lown Institute Hospitals Index. "Fair Share Spending: How Much Are Hospitals Giving Back to Their Communities?," 2022, https://lownhospitalsindex.org/2022-fair-share -spending/.

38. John Byrne, "Abortion Rights, Race at Center of City Hall Fight on Hospital Subsidy," *Chicago Tribune*, January 16, 2018, chicagotribune.com, accessed March 17, 2022, https:// www.chicagotribune.com/politics/ct-met-rahm-emanuel-presence-healthcare-vote -20180116-story.html.

39. "Emanuel Admonishes City Council Divided on Health Care Access, Abortion Views— *Chicago Tribune*," January 17, 2018, accessed March 17, 2022, https://www.chicagotribune.com /politics/ct-met-presence-health-tax-subsidy-vote-20180117-story.html.

40. The Regents of the University of California Health Services Committee, "Notice of Meeting," December 11, 2018, https://regents.universityofcalifornia.edu/regmeet/dec18 /hsx-afternoon.pdf.

41. "UCSF Walks Back Expanded Affiliation with Dignity Health," *Modern Healthcare*, May 29, 2019, https://www.modernhealthcare.com/providers/ucsf-walks-back-expanded -affiliation-dignity-health; Nanette Asimov, "Following Outcry, UCSF Ends Talks to Expand Partnership with Dignity Health," *San Francisco Chronicle*, May 29, 2019, https:// www.sfchronicle.com/bayarea/article/Following-outcry-UCSF-ends-talks-to-expand -13902018.php.

42. "Lieutenant Governor Kounalakis Statement on UCSF's Proposed Affiliation with Dignity Health | Lieutenant Governor," accessed March 17, 2022, https://ltg.ca.gov/2019/05/17 /lg-governor-kounalakis-statement-on-ucsfs-proposed-affiliation-with-dignity-health/.

43. University of California, "Community Ties: UC Health Report on Affiliation Impacts," May 2020, https://www.universityofcalifornia.edu/sites/default/files/UCH-report-on-affilia tion-impacts-may-2020-final.pdf.

44. Michael Hiltzik, "Column: UC Regents Appear Poised to Surrender to Catholic Healthcare Restrictions," *Los Angeles Times*, June 18, 2021, sec. Business, https://www.latimes.com /business/story/2021-06-18/uc-regents-catholic-healthcare-restrictions. University of California Academic Senate, May 11, 2021, https://dms.senate.ucla.edu/issues/document/?12514 .UC.Senate.Response.Regarding.UC.Healthcare.Affiliations.

45. Michael Hiltzik, "How UC Betrays its Doctors, Students, and Patients on Abortion," *Los Angeles Times*, July 21, 2022, https://www.latimes.com/business/story/2022-07-21 /university-of-california-catholic-hospitals-abortion-services.

46. D. J. Nygren, "Troubled Waters: Remaining a Beacon amid Change," *Health Progress* 94, no. 4 (July 2013).

CHAPTER 2 — INFERIOR

1. ACOG, "Prelabor Rupture of Membranes: ACOG Practice Bulletin 217," *Obstetrics & Gynecology* 135, no. 3 (2020): e80–e97, https://doi.org/10.1097/aog.0000000000003700; B Tucker Edmonds et al., "The Influence of Resuscitation Preferences on Obstetrical Management of Periviable Deliveries," *Journal of Perinatology* 35, no. 3 (2015): 161–166.

2. There is little research about Catholic ethics committees specifically, although one article reported findings from a survey in the Catholic Health Association's journal: Francis Bernt, P. A. Clark, Josita Starrs, and Patricia Talone, "Ethics Committees in Catholic Hospitals," *Health Progress* 87, no. 2 (2006): 18.

3. In the late twentieth century, hospital ethics committees were institutionalized across all types of hospitals to help clinicians, patients, and their families through difficult dilemmas in care. Whereas nonreligious ethics committees would typically apply secular principles of bioethics in ob-gyn consultation and deliberation, Catholic hospital ethics committees often are in the position of "gatekeeping" or mediating between the mandates of the ERDs and the care clinicians want to provide their patients. Two ethicists I interviewed (one formally, one informally) who worked in both Catholic and non-Catholic ethics committees noticed this distinction. The informal interviewee, a theologian, said he left his Catholic ethics committee because he was tired of gatekeeping sterilization and other obstetric services that both the physician and patient wanted and would rather participate in sincere deliberation of ethical conflicts and dilemmas faced by the different parties. The formal interviewee stated: "So the reason why the obstetrics & gynecology ones [consults] are the ones that take more of our emotion and energies, 'our' meaning the ethics people's emotions and energies, [is] because that's the one time that the healthcare providers often think that they are at odds with us, or they already presume that we will be at odds with them because of the Catholic viewpoint."

4. See United States Conference of Catholic Bishops, "The Distinction between Direct Abortion and Legitimate Medical Procedures," June 23, 2010, https://www.usccb.org/about/doctrine/publications/upload/direct-abortion-statement2010-06-23.pdf; John Seeds, "Direct Abortion or Legitimate Medical Procedure: Double Effect?" *Linacre Quarterly* 79, no. 1 (2012): 81–87; R. Hamel, "Early Pregnancy Complications and the Ethical and Religious Directives," *Health Progress* 95, no. 3 (May 2014): 48–56.

5. For a more comprehensive discussion of conflicts, see a report written by physicians and advocates cataloguing diseases and diagnoses: Susan Berke Fogel and Tracy Weitz, "Health Care Refusals: Undermining the Medical Standard of Care for Women," Standards of Care Project (National Health Law Program, 2010).

6. Stefan Timmermans and Marc Berg, *The Gold Standard: The Challenge of Evidence-Based Medicine and Standardization in Health Care* (Philadelphia: Temple University Press, 2003).

7. By medically acceptable, I mean that rigorous studies have deemed it safe, it is covered by most insurance, and it is considered a standard approach to treatment within that specialty of medicine. Boundaries around what is considered *the* standard of care are certainly debated, yet most areas of medicine have a general consensus around medically acceptable, standard trajectories of care.

8. Dorothy E. Roberts, *Killing the Black Body: Race, Reproduction, and the Meaning of Liberty* (Vintage, 1999); *Female Inmates Sterilized in California Prisons without Approval*, Center for Investigative Reporting, 2020, Revealnews, https://www.revealnews.org/article

/female-inmates-sterilized-in-california-prisons-without-approval/; Alexandra Minna Stern, "Sterilized in the Name of Public Health," *American Journal of Public Health* 95, no. 7 (2005): 1128–1138, https://doi.org/10.2105/ajph.2004.041608.

9. Alexandra Minna Stern, "Eugenics, Sterilization, and Historical Memory in the United States," *História, Ciências, Saúde-Manguinhos* 23 (December 2016): 195–212.

10. Laura Briggs, *Reproducing Empire: Race, Sex, Science, and U.S. Imperialism in Puerto Rico*, American Crossroads 11 (Berkeley: University of California Press, 2002); Nancy Ordover, "Puerto Rico," The Eugenics Archives, accessed March 21, 2022, http://eugenics archive.ca/discover/connections/530ba18176f0db569b00001b.

11. Corey G. Johnson, "Female Inmates Sterilized in California Prisons without Approval," *Revealnews*, July 7, 2013, http://revealnews.org/article/female-inmates-sterilized-in-california -prisons-without-approval/; "Our Long, Troubling History of Sterilizing the Incarcerated," The Marshall Project, July 27, 2017, https://www.themarshallproject.org/2017/07/26/our-long -troubling-history-of-sterilizing-the-incarcerated; Rachel Treisman, "Whistleblower Alleges 'Medical Neglect,' Questionable Hysterectomies of ICE Detainees," *NPR*, September 16, 2020, sec. National, https://www.npr.org/2020/09/16/913398383/whistleblower-alleges-medical -neglect-questionable-hysterectomies-of-ice-detaine.

12. Anu Manchikanti Gomez, Liza Fuentes, and Amy Allina, "Women or LARC First? Reproductive Autonomy and the Promotion of Long-Acting Reversible Contraceptive Methods," *Perspectives on Sexual and Reproductive Health* 46, no. 3 (September 2014): 171–175, https://doi.org/10.1363/46e1614; "Policy Issues: Long-Acting Reversible Contraceptives (LARCs) | National Women's Health Network," accessed March 21, 2022, https:// nwhn.org/larcs/.

13. Melissa L. Gilliam, Amy Neustadt, and Rivka Gordon, "A Call to Incorporate a Reproductive Justice Agenda into Reproductive Health Clinical Practice and Policy," *Contraception* 79, no. 4 (April 1, 2009): 243–246, https://doi.org/10.1016/j.contraception.2008.12.004; Ushma D. Upadhyay, Alice F. Cartwright, and Daniel Grossman, "Barriers to Abortion Care and Incidence of Attempted Self-Managed Abortion among Individuals Searching Google for Abortion Care: A National Prospective Study," *Contraception* 106 (February 1, 2022): 49–56, https://doi.org/10.1016/j.contraception.2021.09.009; Gabriela Weigel et al., "Coverage and Use of Fertility Services in the U.S.," *KFF* (blog), September 15, 2020, https://www.kff .org/womens-health-policy/issue-brief/coverage-and-use-of-fertility-services-in-the-u-s/; Megan L. Kavanaugh, Rachel K. Jones, and Lawrence B. Finer, "Perceived and Insurance-Related Barriers to the Provision of Contraceptive Services in U.S. Abortion Care Settings," *Women's Health Issues* 21, no. 3 (May 2011): S26–S31, https://doi.org/10.1016/j.whi.2011.01.009; "Beyond the Numbers: Access to Reproductive Health Care for Low-Income Women in Five Communities—Executive Summary," *KFF* (blog), November 14, 2019, https://www.kff.org /report-section/beyond-the-numbers-access-to-reproductive-health-care-for-low-income -women-in-five-communities-executive-summary/.

14. Zakiya Luna and Kristin Luker, "Reproductive Justice," *Annual Review of Law and Social Science* 9, no. 1 (November 3, 2013): 327–352, https://doi.org/10.1146/annurev-lawsocsci -102612-134037; Loretta Ross and Rickie Solinger, "Reproductive Justice in the Twenty-First Century," in *Reproductive Justice: An Introduction* (Oakland, California: University of California Press, 2017), 58–116.

15. ACOG, "Ethical Decision Making in Obstetrics and Gynecology," 390 vols., ACOG Committee Opinion (American College of Obstetrics and Gynecology, 2007); ACOG, "The American College of Obstetricians and Gynecologists, Practice Bulletin 112: Emergency Contraception," *Obstetrics and Gynecology* 115, no. 5 (2010): 1100; Paul D. Blumenthal and Alison Edelman, "Hormonal Contraception," *Obstetrics & Gynecology* 112, no. 3

(2008): 670–684; Jenny A. Higgins, "Celebration Meets Caution: LARC's Boons, Potential Busts, and the Benefits of a Reproductive Justice Approach," *Contraception* 89, no. 4 (April 2014): 237–341, https://doi.org/10.1016/j.contraception.2014.01.027.

16. Christine Dehlendorf et al., "Recommendations for Intrauterine Contraception: A Randomized Trial of the Effects of Patients' Race/Ethnicity and Socioeconomic Status," *American Journal of Obstetrics and Gynecology* 203, no. 4 (October 2010): 319.e1-319.e8, https://doi.org/10.1016/j.ajog.2010.05.009.

17. Jacob Kohlhaas, "What Is Natural Law?" *U.S. Catholic* (blog), July 16, 2018, https://uscatholic.org/articles/201807/what-is-natural-law/.

18. Catholic Health Association, April 3, 2020, https://www.chausa.org/docs/default-source/advocacy/040420-cha-letter-to-senate-finance-committee-on-maternal-health.pdf?sfvrsn=2; Miranda R Waggoner, *The Zero Trimester: Pre-Pregnancy Care and the Politics of Reproductive Risk* (University of California Press, 2017).

19. R. E. Lawrence and F. A. Curlin, "Autonomy, Religion, and Clinical Decisions: Findings from a National Physician Survey," *Journal of Medical Ethics* 35, no. 4 (April 2009): 214–218, https://doi.org/10.1136/jme.2008.027565; Farr A. Curlin et al., "Religion, Conscience, and Controversial Clinical Practices," *New England Journal of Medicine* 356, no. 6 (February 8, 2007): 593–600, https://doi.org/10.1056/NEJMsa065316.

20. D. B. Stulberg et al., "Obstetrician-Gynecologists, Religious Institutions, and Conflicts Regarding Patient-Care Policies," *American Journal of Obstetrics and Gynecology* 207, no. 1 (2012): 73.e1-73.e5, https://doi.org/10.1016/j.ajog.2012.04.023; "Jewish Hospitals Keep Traditions Alive after Mergers," *Modern Healthcare*, October 6, 2017, https://www.modernhealthcare.com/article/20171007/NEWS/171009936/jewish-hospitals-keep-traditions-alive-after-mergers.

21. Ann Neumann, "The Limits of Autonomy: Force-Feedings in Catholic Hospitals and in Prisons," *New York Law School Law Review* 58 (2014 2013): 305; Tara Bannow, "Rural Oregonians Still Face Death with Dignity Barriers," *The Bulletin*, accessed March 21, 2022, https://www.bendbulletin.com/lifestyle/health/rural-oregonians-still-face-death-with-dignity-barriers/article_e41a5836-8bd6-5680-b37d-07517d3b9335.html.

22. John Rock, *The Time Has Come: A Catholic Doctor's Proposals to End the Battle over Birth Control* (New York: Avon Books, 1963).

23. "Humanae Vitae," July 25, 1968; "Paul VI," accessed March 21, 2022, https://www.vatican.va/content/paul-vi/en/encyclicals/documents/hf_p-vi_enc_25071968_humanae-vitae.html.

24. Leslie Woodcock Tentler, *Catholics and Contraception: An American History* (Cornell University Press, 2018).

25. Charles F. Westoff and Larry Bumpass, "The Revolution in Birth Control Practices of US Roman Catholics," *Science* 179, no. 4068 (1973): 41–44.

26. Pew Research Center, "Very Few Americans See Contraception as Morally Wrong," September 28, 2016, https://www.pewforum.org/2016/09/28/4-very-few-americans-see-contraception-as-morally-wrong/; Kimberly Daniels and Jo Jones, *Contraceptive Methods Women Have Ever Used: United States, 1982–2010*, 62 (US Department of Health and Human Services, Centers for Disease Control and . . . , 2013).

27. Catholic women use sterilization and contraception at nearly identical rates as the rest of the population. For example, in 2011, the Guttmacher Institute reported that 33 percent of all women were using sterilization, and 32 percent of Catholic women were using sterilization. Rachel K. Jones and Joerg Dreweke, "Countering Conventional Wisdom: New Evidence on Religion and Contraceptive Use," Report (Guttmacher Institute, 2011), https://www.guttmacher.org/sites/default/files/report_pdf/religion-and-contraceptive-use.pdf.

28. Brian A. Smoley and Christa M. Robinson, "Natural Family Planning," *American Family Physician* 86, no. 10 (November 15, 2012): 924–928; Grant M. Greenberg, "Is Natural Family Planning a Highly Effective Method of Birth Control? No: Natural Family Planning Methods Are Overrated," *American Family Physician* 86, no. 10 (November 15, 2012), https://www.aafp.org/afp/2012/1115/od2.html; "Understanding 'Abstinence': Implications for Individuals, Programs and Policies," (Guttmacher Institute), September 22, 2004, https://www.guttmacher.org/gpr/2003/12/understanding-abstinence-implications-individuals-programs-and-policies.

29. "Contraceptive Efficacy," *Contraceptive Technology* (blog), accessed March 23, 2022, http://www.contraceptivetechnology.org/the-book/take-a-peek/contraceptive-efficacy/.

30. "Fertility Awareness-Based Methods of Family Planning," accessed March 21, 2022, https://www.acog.org/en/womens-health/faqs/fertility-awareness-based-methods-of-family-planning.

31. American Board of Obstetrics and Gynecology, November 9, 2018, https://www.acgme.org/globalassets/PFAssets/ProposalReviewandComment/Complex_Family_Planning_LOIandProposal.pdf.

32. Ryan E. Lawrence et al., "Obstetrician-Gynecologists' Views on Contraception and Natural Family Planning: A National Survey," *American Journal of Obstetrics and Gynecology* 204, no. 2 (February 1, 2011): 124.e1–124.e7, https://doi.org/10.1016/j.ajog.2010.08.051.

33. Isabelle Côté, Philip Jacobs, and David C. Cumming, "Use of Health Services Associated with Increased Menstrual Loss in the United States," *American Journal of Obstetrics and Gynecology* 188, no. 2 (February 2003): 343–348, https://doi.org/10.1067/mob.2003.9; Wanda K. Nicholson et al., "Patterns of Ambulatory Care Use for Gynecologic Conditions: A National Study," *American Journal of Obstetrics and Gynecology* 184, no. 4 (March 2001): 523–530, https://doi.org/10.1067/mob.2001.111795.

34. For example, Dignity Health cited menorrhagia as an acceptable indication for contraception explicitly when reporting what reproductive services are available in one of their sole-provider hospitals when the California Attorney General assessed its proposal to merge with Catholic Health Initiatives; JD Healthcare Vizient, Inc., "Effect of the Ministry Alignment Agreement between Dignity Health and Catholic Health Initiatives on the Availability and Accessibility of Healthcare Services to the Communities Served by Dignity Health's Hospital Located in Santa Cruz County," September 10, 2018, accessed September 29, 2021, https://oag.ca.gov/sites/all/files/agweb/pdfs/charities/nonprofithosp/dignity-chi-santa-cruz-healthcare-impact-statement-report.pdf.

35. Barbara S. Apgar et al., "Treatment of Menorrhagia," *American Family Physician* 75, no. 12 (June 15, 2007): 1813–1919.

36. International Federation of Obstetrics and Gynecology International Consortium for Emergency Contraception, "Clinical Summary: Emergency Contraceptive Pills," December 2018, https://www.cecinfo.org/wp-content/uploads/2018/12/18-209_ICEC-Clinical-Summary_121918.pdf; Kristina Gemzell-Danielsson, Cecilia Berger, and P. G. Lalitkumar, "Emergency Contraception—Mechanisms of Action," *Contraception* 87, no. 3 (March 2013): 300–308, https://doi.org/10.1016/j.contraception.2012.08.021.

37. Kristina Gemzell-Danielsson, Cecilia Berger, and P. G. Lalitkumar, "Mechanisms of Action of Oral Emergency Contraception," *Gynecological Endocrinology: The Official Journal of the International Society of Gynecological Endocrinology* 30, no. 10 (October 2014): 685–687, https://doi.org/10.3109/09513590.2014.950648.

38. ACOG, "The American College of Obstetricians and Gynecologists, Practice Bulletin 112: Emergency Contraception," 112.

39. "The Emergency Contraception Question: When Is It Licit and When Is It Not?" *America Magazine*, March 5, 2013, https://www.americamagazine.org/issue/emergency-contraception-question.

40. "Access to Postpartum Sterilization," accessed March 21, 2022, https://www.acog.org/en/clinical/clinical-guidance/committee-opinion/articles/2021/06/access-to-postpartum-sterilization.

41. "Births Financed by Medicaid," *KFF* (blog), December 17, 2021, https://www.kff.org/medicaid/state-indicator/births-financed-by-medicaid/.

42. Clare Harney, Annie Dude, and Sadia Haider, "Factors Associated with Short Interpregnancy Interval in Women Who Plan Postpartum LARC: A Retrospective Study," *Contraception* 95, no. 3 (2017): 245–250, https://doi.org/10.1016/j.contraception.2016.08.012.

43. Edith Fox et al., "Client Preferences for Contraceptive Counseling: A Systematic Review," *American Journal of Preventive Medicine* 55, no. 5 (November 1, 2018): 691–702, https://doi.org/10.1016/j.amepre.2018.06.006; Lynn M. Yee and Melissa A. Simon, "Perceptions of Coercion, Discrimination, and Other Negative Experiences in Postpartum Contraceptive Counseling for Low-Income Minority Women," *Journal of Health Care for the Poor and Underserved* 22, no. 4 (2011): 1387–1400.

44. Maryam Guiahi et al., "Changing Depot Medroxyprogesterone Acetate Access at a Faith-Based Institution," *Contraception* 84, no. 3 (September 2011): 280–284, https://doi.org/10.1016/j.contraception.2010.12.003.

45. Poor birth outcomes (preterm birth, preeclampsia, neonatal intensive care unit admission) are more common in pregnancies with intervals less than eighteen months between births. However, there is debate about whether short interpregnancy intervals actually *cause* bad outcomes or are simply associated with them due to factors such as low income, health behavior, and access to contraception. Recent research shows that short intervals are associated with higher rates of gestational diabetes and obesity controlling for the other factors. See Gillian E. Hanley et al., "Interpregnancy Interval and Adverse Pregnancy Outcomes: An Analysis of Successive Pregnancies," *Obstetrics & Gynecology* 129, no. 3 (March 2017): 408–415, https://doi.org/10.1097/AOG.0000000000001891.

46. Kimberly Daniels and Joyce C. Abma, "Current Contraceptive Status among Women Aged 15–49: United States, 2017–2019," *NCHS Data Brief*, no. 388 National Center for Health Statistics (October 2020): 1–8.

47. S. Borrero, C. Nikolajski, K. L. Rodriguez, M. D. Creinin, R. M. Arnold, and S. A. Ibrahim, "Everything I Know I Learned from My Mother . . . or Not": Perspectives of African-American and White Women on Decisions about Tubal Sterilization, *Journal of General Internal Medicine* 24, no. 3 (2009): 312–319; J. E. Anderson, D. J. Jamieson, L. Warner, D. M. Kissin, A. K. Nangia, and M. Macaluso, "Contraceptive Sterilization among Married Adults: National Data on Who Chooses Vasectomy and Tubal Sterilization," *Contraception* 85, no. 6 (June 1, 2012): 552–557.

48. "What Is the Morally Acceptable Way of Ordering a Sperm Count as Part of the Evaluation of Infertility?" *Linacre Quarterly* 86, no. 1 (February 2019): 142, https://doi.org/10.1177/0024363919832764.

49. Gestating one or two babies maximum is considered safest for the pregnant woman. Of course, some choose to gestate more, assuming more risk. See "Multiple Pregnancy," accessed March 28, 2022, https://www.acog.org/en/womens-health/faqs/multiple-pregnancy.

50. United States Conference of Catholic Bishops, "Reproductive Technology (Evaluation & Treatment of Infertility) Guidelines for Catholic Couples," n.d., https://www.usccb.org/issues-and-action/human-life-and-dignity/reproductive-technology/upload/Reproductive-Technology-Evaluation-Treatment-of-Infertility-Guidelines.pdf.

51. "Family Building through Gestational Surrogacy," accessed March 21, 2022, https://www.acog.org/en/clinical/clinical-guidance/committee-opinion/articles/2016/03/family-building-through-gestational-surrogacy. Conflicts around care for surrogacy never arose in my physician interviews. This could be the case because people who pursue surrogacy generally learn from surrogacy resources that it would be problematic and have the means to avoid the Catholic hospital for delivery. One patient I interviewed was not so lucky; her story is shared in the next chapter.

52. Loyal | thisisloyal.com, "How Many Adults Identify as Transgender in the United States?" Williams Institute, accessed March 21, 2022, https://williamsinstitute.law.ucla.edu/publications/trans-adults-united-states/; American Medical Association, "Issue Brief: Health Insurance Coverage for Gender-Affirming Care of Transgender Patients," 2019, https://www.ama-assn.org/system/files/2019-03/transgender-coverage-issue-brief.pdf.

53. E. Coleman et al., "Standards of Care for the Health of Transsexual, Transgender, and Gender-Nonconforming People, Version 7," *International Journal of Transgenderism* 13, no. 4 (August 2012): 165–232, https://doi.org/10.1080/15532739.2011.700873; Wylie C. Hembree et al., "Endocrine Treatment of Gender-Dysphoric/Gender-Incongruent Persons: An Endocrine Society* Clinical Practice Guideline," *Journal of Clinical Endocrinology & Metabolism* 102, no. 11 (November 1, 2017): 3869–3903, https://doi.org/10.1210/jc.2017-01658; Kellan E. Baker, "The Future of Transgender Coverage," *New England Journal of Medicine* 376, no. 19 (May 11, 2017): 1801–1804, https://doi.org/10.1056/NEJMp1702427.

54. Juan Marco Vaggione, "The Conservative Uses of Law: The Catholic Mobilization against Gender Ideology," *Social Compass* 67, no. 2 (2020), https://doi.org/10.1177/0037768620907561.

55. In November 2021, the U.S. Supreme Court refused to hear Dignity Health's appeal of California's ruling in favor of Evan Minton's, allowing his victory at the California state level to stand. *Oliver Knight v. St. Joseph's* in Eureka, CA: Erin Allday, "Transgender Man Sues over Eureka Hospital's Refusal to Perform Hysterectomy," *San Francisco Chronicle*, March 25, 2019, https://www.sfchronicle.com/health/article/Transgender-man-sues-over-Eureka-hospital-s-13707502.php; *Evan Minton v Dignity* in Sacramento, CA: "Catholic Hospitals Dealt Blow in Transgender Discrimination Case," *Modern Healthcare*, September 18, 2019, https://www.modernhealthcare.com/legal/catholic-hospitals-dealt-blow-transgender-discrimination-case; *Jionni Conforti v St. Joseph's* in Paterson, NJ: "Catholic Hospital Approved His Hysterectomy, Then Refused because He Was Transgender, Suit Says," *Washington Post*, accessed March 21, 2022, https://www.washingtonpost.com/news/morning-mix/wp/2017/01/06/catholic-hospital-okd-his-hysterectomy-then-denied-him-because-he-was-transgender-suit-says/.

56. Elaine L. Hill, David J. G. Slusky, and Donna K. Ginther, "Reproductive Health Care in Catholic-Owned Hospitals," *Journal of Health Economics* 65 (2019): 48–62, https://doi.org/10.1016/j.jhealeco.2019.02.005.

57. Peter J. Cataldo, "Catholic Teaching on the Human Person and Gender Dysphoria" (Catholic Health Association of the United States), Summer 2019, https://www.chausa.org/docs/default-source/hceusa/catholic-teaching-on-the-human-person-and-gender-dysphoria.pdf?sfvrsn=cea2fbf2_2; Carol Bayley, "Transgender Persons and Catholic Healthcare," 2016, https://www.chausa.org/docs/default-source/hceusa/transgender-persons-and-catholic-healthcare.pdf.

58. Arlington Diocese, "A Catechesis on the Human Person and Gender Ideology," accessed March 21, 2022, https://www.arlingtondiocese.org/bishop/public-messages/2021/a-catechesis-on-the-human-person-and-gender-ideology/.

59. United States Conference of Catholic Bishops, "Questions and Answers about the Equality Act of 2019: Sexual Orientation, Gender Identity, and Religious Liberty Issues,"

n.d., https://www.usccb.org/issues-and-action/marriage-and-family/marriage/promotion
-and-defense-of-marriage/upload/Equality-Act-Backgrounder.pdf.

60. Elliott Louis Bedford, "The Reality of Institutional Conscience," *National Catholic Bioethics Quarterly* 16, no. 2 (2016): 255–272; Eric Plemons, "Not Here: Catholic Hospital Systems and the Restriction against Transgender Healthcare," *CrossCurrents* 68, no. 4 (December 2018), 533–549, https://doi.org/10.1111/cros.12341.

61. "FAQ: On Gender Identity Disorder and 'Sex-Change' Operations," National Catholic Bioethics Center, accessed March 21, 2022, https://www.ncbcenter.org/resources-and
-statements-cms/faq-on-gender-identity-disorder-and-sex-change-operations.

62. Vaggione, "The Conservative Uses of Law"; Plemons, "Not Here."

63. Movement Advancement Project, "Healthcare Laws and Policies: Medicaid Coverage for Transition-Related Care," accessed March 23, 2022, https://www.lgbtmap.org/img
/maps/citations-medicaid.pdf.

64. Nathaniel Blanton Hibner, "Discerning Scandal: Theological Scandal in Catholic Health Care Decision Making" (Saint Louis University, 2019).

65. Committee on Reproductive Health Services: Assessing the Safety and Quality of Abortion Care in the U.S. et al., *The Safety and Quality of Abortion Care in the United States* (Washington, DC: National Academies Press, 2018), https://doi.org/10
.17226/24950.

66. Father Tad Pacholczyk, "Making Sense of Bioethics: The Welcome Outreach of Perinatal Hospice" *Today's Catholic*, https://todayscatholic.org/the-welcome-outreach-of-peri
natal-hospice/; Mary Stachyra Lopez, "Perinatal Hosice Supports Parents When a Baby's Life is Short," July 12, 2017, https://www.catholicherald.com/article/local/perinatal-hospice
-supports-parents-when-a-babys-life-is-short/; Bryanna S. Moore et al., "Anticipation, Accompaniment, and a Good Death in Perinatal Care," *Yale Journal of Biology and Medicine* 92, no. 4 (December 20, 2019): 741–745.

67. A patient I interviewed found herself in this situation but had the means to find a private abortion provider and flew across the country to terminate a pregnancy in the third trimester. Many cannot or do not know how to find the resources to make it happen. See Katrina Kimport, *No Real Choice: How Culture and Politics Matter for Reproductive Autonomy*, Families in Focus (New Brunswick: Rutgers University Press, 2022).

68. Kathleen M. Joyce, "The Evil of Abortion and the Greater Good of the Faith: Negotiating Catholic Survival in the Twentieth-Century American Health Care System," *Religion and American Culture* 12, no. 1 (Winter 2002): 91–121.

69. ACOG, "Prelabor Rupture of Membranes: ACOG Practice Bulletin, Number 217," *Obstetrics & Gynecology* 135, no. 3 (2020): e80–e97, https://doi.org/10.1097/aog.0000000000003700.

70. American College of Obstetricians and Gynecologists' Committee on Practice Bulletins—Gynecology, "ACOG Practice Bulletin 193: Tubal Ectopic Pregnancy," *Obstetrics and Gynecology* 131, no. 3 (March 2018): e91–e103, https://doi.org/10.1097/AOG.000000
0000002560.

71. Catholic Medical Association, "Holy Alliance: Serving The Divine Physician," n.d., https://www.cathmed.org/assets/files/EntireBinder4-030617-SecuritySettingsOnForWeb.pdf.

72. Nicholas J. Kockler, "The Principle of Double Effect and Proportionate Reason," *AMA Journal of Ethics* 9, no. 5 (May 1, 2007): 369–374, https://doi.org/10.1001/virtualmentor
.2007.9.5.pfor2-0705.

73. D. B. Stulberg et al., "Obstetrician-Gynecologists, Religious Institutions, and Conflicts Regarding Patient-Care Policies," *American Journal of Obstetrics and Gynecology* 207, no. 1 (July 2012): 73 e1–e5, https://doi.org/10.1016/j.ajog.2012.04.023.

CHAPTER 3 — CONSUMER MEDICINE?

1. In her 2018 reporting on Catholic hospitals, *New York Times* reporter Katie Hafner wrote, "Most facilities provide little or no information up front about procedures they won't perform." Using a list from the CHA, she found that, on two-thirds of the 652 Catholic hospital websites, "it took more than three clicks from the home page to determine that the hospital was Catholic." Less than 3 percent had an easily locatable list of services not offered, but they were in Washington State where the lists were mandated. "In the rest of the country, such lists, if available, were posted only on the corporate parent's site, and they were often difficult to find." See Katie Hafner, "As Catholic Hospitals Expand, So Do Limits on Some Procedures," *New York Times*, August 10, 2018, sec. Health, https://www.nytimes.com/2018/08/10/health/catholic-hospitals-procedures.html.

2. Joelle Takahashi et al., "Disclosure of Religious Identity and Health Care Practices on Catholic Hospital Websites," *JAMA* 321, no. 11 (March 19, 2019): 1103, https://doi.org/10.1001/jama.2019.0133.

3. K. L. Edward et al., "Nursing Practices in Catholic Healthcare: A Case Study of Nurses in a Catholic Private Hospital," *Journal of Religious Health* 57, no. 5 (October 2018): 1664–1678, https://doi.org/10.1007/s10943-017-0520-z.

4. Melissa M. Garrido et al., "Hospital Religious Affiliation and Outcomes for High-Risk Infants," *Medical Care Research and Review* 69, no. 3 (June 2012): 316–338, https://doi.org/10.1177/1077558711432156l; Ann Kutney-Lee et al., "Distinct Enough? A National Examination of Catholic Hospital Affiliation and Patient Perceptions of Care," *Health Care Management Review* 39, no. 2 (2014): 134–144, https://doi.org/10.1097/HMR.0b013e31828dc491.

5. Luciana E. Hebert, Lori Freedman, and Debra B. Stulberg, "Choosing a Hospital for Obstetric, Gynecologic, or Reproductive Healthcare: What Matters Most to Patients?" *American Journal of Obstetrics & Gynecology MFM* 2, no. 1 (2020): 1–9, https://doi.org/10.1016/j.ajogmf.2019.100067.

6. The Pacific Northwest, which has heavy Catholic healthcare saturation but low religiosity, was intentionally underrepresented.

7. While hospital closure is increasing throughout the United States, an internet search suggests that this patient's non-Catholic option continues to exist. The more likely situation is that the doctor no longer held privileges there.

8. Grace Shih, David K Turok, and Willie J Parker, "Vasectomy: The Other (Better) Form of Sterilization," *Contraception* 83, no. 4 (2011): 310–315.

9. Sterilization is one of the most common contraceptive methods in the United States, although decreasing with greater use of long-acting reversible contraceptive methods. Among women at risk for pregnancy in 2014, 90 percent were using some form of contraception. Reliance on female sterilization decreased from 27 percent to 22 percent from 2008 to 2014. Male sterilization decreased from 10 percent to 7 percent in that time. Megan L. Kavanaugh and Jenna Jerman, "Contraceptive Method Use in the United States: Trends and Characteristics between 2008, 2012, and 2014," *Contraception*, October 2017, https://doi.org/10.1016/j.contraception.2017.10.003.

10. Katrina Kimport, "More than a Physical Burden: Women's Mental and Emotional Work in Preventing Pregnancy," *Journal of Sex Research* 55, no. 9 (2018): 1096–1105; Katrina Kimport, "Talking about Male Body-Based Contraceptives: The Counseling Visit and the Feminization of Contraception," *Social Science & Medicine* 201 (2018): 44–50.

11. Consumers are increasingly empowered to share negative healthcare experience through social media. See Sue Ziebland and Sally Wyke, "Health and Illness in a Connected

World: How Might Sharing Experiences on the Internet Affect People's Health?" *Milbank Quarterly* 90, no. 2 (2012): 219–249; Mark Schlesinger et al., "Taking Patients' Narratives about Clinicians from Anecdote to Science," *New England Journal of Medicine* 373, no. 7 (2015): 675–679.

12. For more about this pattern of self-blame in the data, see Jocelyn M. Wascher, Debra B. Stulberg, and Lori R. Freedman, "Restrictions on Reproductive Care at Catholic Hospitals: A Qualitative Study of Patient Experiences and Perspectives," *AJOB Empirical Bioethics* 11, no. 4 (October 1, 2020): 257–267, https://doi.org/10.1080/23294515.2020.1817173.

13. The following resource provides access to several summaries about religious traditions and their beliefs related to healthcare decision making: "Religious Beliefs & Health Care Decisions | Advocate Health Care," accessed March 23, 2022, https://www.advocatehealth.com/about-us/faith-at-advocate/office-for-mission-spiritual-care/spiritual-care/religious-beliefs-health-care-decisions.

14. "Long-Acting Reversible Contraception: Implants and Intrauterine Devices," November 2017, accessed March 23, 2022, https://www.acog.org/en/clinical/clinical-guidance/practice-bulletin/articles/2017/11/long-acting-reversible-contraception-implants-and-intrauterine-devices.

15. Kutney-Lee et al., "Distinct Enough?"

16. Regarding three separate cases: Maria Perez, "Transgender Man Sues California Hospital after Claiming He Was Denied Surgery Due to Catholic Ethics," *Newsweek*, March 22, 2019, https://www.newsweek.com/transgender-man-california-hospital-denied-surgery-catholic-ethics-1372233; Claudia Buck and Samantha Caiola, "Transgender Patient Sues Dignity Health for Discrimination over Hysterectomy Denial," *Sacramento Bee*, n.d., https://www.sacbee.com/news/local/health-and-medicine/article145477264.html; Sandhya Somashekhar, "Transgender Man Sues Catholic Hospital for Refusing Surgery," *Washington Post*, January 6, 2017, accessed March 23, 2022, https://www.washingtonpost.com/news/post-nation/wp/2017/01/06/transgender-man-sues-catholic-hospital-for-refusing-surgery/.

17. I intentionally omitted the country of origin for Kayden's privacy, but it is worth noting that the sterilization requirement for gender change in his country of origin, and in several other countries, is considered an abuse of human rights by advocacy groups. For more, see A. J. Lowik, "Reproducing Eugenics, Reproducing While Trans: The State Sterilization of Trans People," *Journal of GLBT Family Studies* 14, no. 5 (October 20, 2018): 425–445, https://doi.org/10.1080/1550428X.2017.1393361.

18. It is not entirely clear why Kayden says "hysterectomy" when Dr. Ward referenced the procedure as a removal of the ovaries, but I believe it was shorthand and familiar for Kayden, because that is the name his mother's procedure had. It is also possible Dr. Ward remembered incorrectly, but it does not change the point of the story either way.

19. Pew Research Center, "Views about Abortion," Religious Landscape Study, accessed March 23, 2022, https://www.pewforum.org/religious-landscape-study/views-about-abortion/.

20. In the 1980s and 1990s, news about "crack babies" created a racist moral panic. Later studies would show that crack and cocaine alone do not, in fact, result in terrible cognitive and physical deleterious effects in babies. However, some drug users combine multiple potentially hazardous substances that do cause birth defects, and many people struggling with addiction lack nutrition, which can increase the chance of premature birth.

21. M. Antonia Biggs et al., "The Fine Line between Informing and Coercing: Community Health Center Clinicians' Approaches to Counseling Young People about IUDs," *Perspectives on Sexual and Reproductive Health* 52, no. 4 (2020): 245–252; Kelly M. Hoffman et al., "Racial Bias in Pain Assessment and Treatment Recommendations, and False Beliefs

about Biological Differences between Blacks and Whites," *Proceedings of the National Academy of Sciences* 113, no. 16 (April 19, 2016): 4296–4301, https://doi.org/10.1073/pnas .1516047113.

22. From Desiree's description, this might have been a molar pregnancy, which is a nonviable pregnancy with tissue that can become cancerous. It often is treated with chemotherapy.

CHAPTER 4 — EMERGENCIES

1. Renee C. Fox, "Training for Uncertainty," in *The Student-Physician: Introductory Studies in the Sociology of Medical Education*, edited by Robert K. Merton, George G. Reader, and Patricia L. Kendall (Cambridge: Harvard University Press, 1957), 207–41; Robert Zussman, *Intensive Care: Medical Ethics and the Medical Profession* (Chicago: University of Chicago Press, 1992).

2. Renee C Fox, "Medical Uncertainty Revisited," *Handbook of Social Studies in Health and Medicine* 409 (2000): 425; Stefan Timmermans and Alison Angell, "Evidence-Based Medicine, Clinical Uncertainty, and Learning to Doctor," *Journal of Health and Social Behavior* (2001): 342–359.

3. Jocelyn M. Wascher et al., "Do Women Know Whether Their Hospital Is Catholic? Results from a National Survey," *Contraception* 98, no. 6 (2018): 498–503.

4. Debra B. Stulberg et al., "Women's Expectation of Receiving Reproductive Health Care at Catholic and Non-Catholic Hospitals," *Perspectives on Sexual and Reproductive Health* 51, no. 3 (2019): 135–142, https://doi.org/10.1363/psrh.12118.

5. Elaine L. Hill, David J. G. Slusky, and Donna K. Ginther, "Reproductive Health Care in Catholic-Owned Hospitals," *Journal of Health Economics* 65 (2019): 48–62, https://doi .org/10.1016/j.jhealeco.2019.02.005.

6. Coleman Drake et al., "Market Share of US Catholic Hospitals and Associated Geographic Network Access to Reproductive Health Services," *JAMA Network Open* 3, no. 1 (2020), https://doi.org/10.1001/jamanetworkopen.2019.20053.

7. Katherine Stewart, "Opinion | Why Was a Catholic Hospital Willing to Gamble with My Life?" *New York Times*, February 25, 2022, sec. Opinion, https://www.nytimes .com/2022/02/25/opinion/sunday/roe-dobbs-miscarriage-abortion.html; "Tamesha Means Lawsuit: Catholic Hospital 'Forced Miscarrying Woman to Deliver 18-Week Fetus," Daily Mail Online, accessed March 23, 2022, https://www.dailymail.co.uk/news/article-2517492 /Tamesha-Means-lawsuit-Catholic-hospital-forced-miscarrying-woman-deliver-18-week -fetus.html. Read more about Savita Halappanavar in the conclusion of this book, or see Kitty Holland Social Affairs Correspondent, "How the Death of Savita Halappanavar Revolutionised Ireland," *Irish Times*, accessed March 23, 2022, https://www.irishtimes.com /news/social-affairs/how-the-death-of-savita-halappanavar-revolutionised-ireland-1 .3510387.

8. Racial disparities in maternal health are increasingly documented in both the media and medical research. For example, see *New York Times* on COVID-related disparities: "She Was Pregnant with Twins during Covid. Why Did Only One Survive?" *New York Times*, August 6, 2020, accessed March 23, 2022, https://www.nytimes.com/2020/08/06 /nyregion/childbirth-Covid-Black-mothers.html. Also, an ob-gyn research synopsis on the topic warns: "Racial disparities in loss are also more pronounced between ten and twenty weeks, with self-reported black race conferring nearly double the adjusted hazard ratio as compared with white race." See Sarah Prager et al., "Pregnancy Loss (Miscarriage): Risk Factors, Etiology, Clinical Manifestations, and Diagnostic Evaluation," *UpToDate Internet*, 2018. See, also, Sudeshna Mukherjee et al., "Risk of Miscarriage among

Black Women and White Women in a US Prospective Cohort Study," *American Journal of Epidemiology* 177, no. 11 (2013): 1271–1278; Jonathan M. Metzl and Dorothy E. Roberts, "Structural Competency Meets Structural Racism: Race, Politics, and the Structure of Medical Knowledge," *AMA Journal of Ethics* 16, no. 9 (2014): 674–690; Dána-Ain Davis, "Obstetric .Racism: The Racial Politics of Pregnancy, Labor, and Birthing," *Medical, Anthropology* 38, no. 7 (2019): 560–573; Kelly M. Hoffman et al., "Racial Bias in Pain Assessment and Treatment Recommendations, and False Beliefs about Biological Differences between Blacks and Whites," *Proceedings of the National Academy of Sciences* 113, no. 16 (2016): 4296–4301; Juanita J. Chinn, Iman K. Martin, and Nicole Redmond, "Health Equity among Black Women in the United States," *Journal of Women's Health* 30, no. 2 (2020).

9. J. Trinder et al., "Management of Miscarriage: Expectant, Medical, or Surgical? Results of Randomised Controlled Trial (Miscarriage Treatment [MIST] Trial)," *BMJ* 332, no. 7552 (2006): 1235–1240.

10. Robin R. Wallace et al., "Counseling Women with Early Pregnancy Failure: Utilizing Evidence, Preserving Preference," *Patient Education and Counseling* 81, no. 3 (2010): 454–461, https://doi.org/10.1016/j.pec.2010.10.031; Margreet Wieringa-de Waard et al., "Expectant Management versus Surgical Evacuation in First Trimester Miscarriage: Health-Related Quality of Life in Randomized and Non-Randomized Patients," *Human Reproduction* 17, no. 6 (2002): 1638–1642; Lindsay F Smith et al., "Women's Experiences of Three Early Miscarriage Management Options a Qualitative Study," *British Journal of General Practice* 56, no. 524 (2006): 198–205.

11. United States Conference of Catholic Bishops, "Ethical and Religious Directives for Catholic Health Care Services (6th ed.)," 2018, https://www.usccb.org/about/doctrine /ethical-and-religious-directives/upload/ethical-religious-directives-catholic-health -service-sixth-edition-2016-06.pdf.

12. For a more detailed discussion of Catholic teachings on suffering in medical care, see Olivia Nyberg, "Women in Pain: How Narratives of Pain and Sacrifice Complicate the Debate over the Catholic Provision of Obstetrical Care," *Medical Humanities*, n.d., 2018–011606, https://doi.org/10.1136/medhum-2018-011606. She writes, "While secular medical practice devotes itself largely to the eradication of pain, labelling it solely as pathological, Catholic actors may adopt a more complicated, multifaceted notion of physical pain. Roman Catholic tradition is steeped with pain narratives which indicate that pain, rather than wholly negative, facilitates spiritual amelioration. That pain can mediate between the experience of the body and the growth of the soul is fundamental to understanding how pain can be interpreted as religiously valuable in a clinical situation, and can help elucidate how some religious patients, physicians and institutions translate potential pain and injury into spiritually formative experiences."

13. "Perinatal Mortality Rate (PMR)—DataForImpactProject," accessed March 23, 2022, https://www.data4impactproject.org/prh/womens-health/newborn-health/perinatal -mortality-rate-pmr/; Marcos Camacho-Ávila et al., "Experience of Parents Who Have Suffered a Perinatal Death in Two Spanish Hospitals: A Qualitative Study," *BMC Pregnancy and Childbirth* 19, no. 1 (December 19, 2019): 512, https://doi.org/10.1186/s12884-019 -2666-z.

14. Lori R Freedman et al., "Religious Hospital Policies on Reproductive Care: What Do Patients Want to Know?" *American Journal of Obstetrics & Gynecology* 218, no. 2 (2018): 251–e1.

15. Erin E Wingo et al., "Anticipatory Counseling about Miscarriage Management in Catholic Hospitals: A Qualitative Exploration of Women's Preferences," *Perspectives on*

Sexual and Reproductive Health 52, no. 3 (2020): 171–179. For more detail from this study, see Jocelyn M. Wascher, Debra B. Stulberg, and Lori R. Freedman, "Restrictions on Reproductive Care at Catholic Hospitals: A Qualitative Study of Patient Experiences and Perspectives," *AJOB Empirical Bioethics* 11, no. 4 (2020), https://doi.org/10.1080/23294515.2020 .1817173.

16. About 70 percent of women say where their doctor works is a key factor in choosing where to get reproductive care such as childbirth, and 20.1 percent say it is the most important factor, coming in third shortly after hospital reputation (33 percent) and insurance (20.4 percent). See Luciana E Hebert, Lori Freedman, and Debra B Stulberg, "Choosing a Hospital for Obstetric, Gynecologic, or Reproductive Healthcare: What Matters Most to Patients?" *American Journal of Obstetrics & Gynecology MFM* 2, no. 1 (2020).

17. Reluctance to discuss painful and/or stigmatized topics such as miscarriage (and even more so, abortion) can lead to a lack of familiarity with the issues and a perception of it being less common than it is. See Julia Frost et al., "The Loss of Possibility: Scientisation of Death and the Special Case of Early Miscarriage," *Sociology of Health & Illness* 29, no. 7 (2007): 1003–1022; Sarah K Cowan, "Secrets and Misperceptions: The Creation of Self-Fulfilling Illusions," *Sociological Science* 1 (2014): 466–492; Clare Bellhouse, Meredith J Temple-Smith, and Jade E Bilardi, "'It's Just One of Those Things People Don't Seem to Talk about . . .' Women's Experiences of Social Support Following Miscarriage: A Qualitative Study," *BMC Women's Health* 18, no. 1 (2018): 1–9.

18. Monica R. McLemore et al., "Health Care Experiences of Pregnant, Birthing and Postnatal Women of Color at Risk for Preterm Birth," *Social Science & Medicine (1982)* 201 (March 2018): 127–135, https://doi.org/10.1016/j.socscimed.2018.02.013; Molly R Altman et al., "Listening to Women: Recommendations from Women of Color to Improve Experiences in Pregnancy and Birth Care," *Journal of Midwifery & Women's Health* 65, no. 4 (2020): 466–473; Davis, "Obstetric Racism: The Racial Politics of Pregnancy, Labor, and Birthing."

19. Jessica Beaman et al., "Medication to Manage Abortion and Miscarriage," *Journal of General Internal Medicine* 35, no. 8 (August 1, 2020): 2398–2405, https://doi.org/10.1007 /s11606-020-05836-9; Sarah C. M. Roberts et al., "Miscarriage Treatment-Related Morbidities and Adverse Events in Hospitals, Ambulatory Surgery Centers, and Office-Based Settings," *Journal of Patient Safety* 16, no. 4 (December 2020): e317–e323, https://doi.org/10 .1097/PTS.0000000000000553; Ushma D. Upadhyay et al., "Abortion-Related Emergency Department Visits in the United States: An Analysis of a National Emergency Department Sample," *BMC Medicine* 16, no. 1 (June 14, 2018): 88, https://doi.org/10.1186/s12916-018-1072 -0; Ushma D Upadhyay et al., "Incidence of Emergency Department Visits and Complications after Abortion," *Obstetrics & Gynecology* 125, no. 1 (2015): 175–183.

20. See previous note. Angela Freeman, Elena Neiterman, and Shya Varathasundaram, "Women's Experiences of Health Care Utilization in Cases of Early Pregnancy Loss: A Scoping Review," *Women and Birth* 34, no. 4 (2020): 316–324; Adam James Janicki et al., "Obstetric Training in Emergency Medicine: A Needs Assessment," *Medical Education Online* 21, no. 1 (2016): 28930.

21. Pew Research Center, "Very Few Americans See Contraception as Morally Wrong," September 28, 2016, https://www.pewforum.org/2016/09/28/4-very-few-americans-see-contra ception-as-morally-wrong/.

22. See note about "The Principle of Double Effect" in chapter 2.

23. Christopher Kaczor, "Moral Absolutism and Ectopic Pregnancy" *Journal of Medicine & Philosophy* 26, no. 1 (2001): 61–74.

24. While Directive 48 prohibits "direct abortion" for ectopic pregnancies, the CHA has published a statement explicitly endorsing treatment with methotrexate. See "Catholic

Hospitals and Ectopic Pregnancies," accessed March 24, 2022, https://www.chausa.org /publications/health-care-ethics-usa/article/winter-2011/catholic-hospitals-and-ectopic -pregnancies. For further detail, see William E. May, "Ectopic Pregnancy: A. Arguments against Salpingostomy and Methotrexate," in *Catholic Health Care Ethics: A Manual for Practitioners* (The National Catholic Bioethics Center, 2009): 119–121; Edward J. Furton, "The Direct Killing of the Innocent," *Ethics and Medics* 35, no. 10 (October 2010): 1–2.

CHAPTER 5 — MOSTLY ABOVE-BOARD WORKAROUNDS

1. Steven Alter, "Theory of Workarounds," 2014. Communications of the Association for Information Systems: Vol. 34, Article 55, pp. 1041–1066.

2. Andrew Jameton, *Nursing Practice: The Ethical Issues* (Englewood Cliffs, NJ: Prentice-Hall, 1984), 331.

3. Alter, "Theory of Workarounds"; Alan Cribb, "Integrity at Work: Managing Routine Moral Stress in Professional Roles," *Nursing Philosophy* 12, no. 2 (2011): 119–127; Nancy Berlinger, *Are Workarounds Ethical?: Managing Moral Problems in Health Care Systems* (Oxford University Press, 2016).

4. I have been torn throughout the writing of this book about the ethics of bringing attention to workaround practices that are clearly done in the patient's best interest. If the bishops increase scrutiny and crack down on them in response, would I be responsible? I ultimately decided to include a discussion of practices that range from simply disadvantaging Catholic health systems (sending patients away to other doctors) to subterfuge (completely disregarding and breaking the rules) because, ultimately, all these practices have been written about before, both in the academic literature by me and my colleagues and in the Catholic blogosphere and Catholic journals by Catholics who feel their hospitals are not Catholic enough and want to strengthen surveillance and enforcement. They are referenced in many places on the web. This book, of course, lends credibility to those claims, but I include the data with the hope that shedding light on the problem will draw the attention of policymakers in a position to make change, and at minimum to help potential employees, potential patients, potential health system collaborators, and potential medical schools and residencies to make informed decisions about where to work.

5. Ob-gyns working in religious hospitals are as religiously diverse as the rest of the members of the specialty, and those who identify as Roman Catholic are no more likely to work in a Catholic hospital than those with no religious affiliation. D. B. Stulberg et al., "Obstetrician-Gynecologists, Religious Institutions, and Conflicts Regarding Patient-Care Policies," *American Journal of Obstetrics and Gynecology* 207, no. 1 (2012): 73.e1–73.e5, https://doi.org/10.1016/j.ajog.2012.04.023.

6. Sandra Hapenney, "Divergent Practices among Catholic Hospitals in Provision of Direct Sterilization," *Linacre Quarterly* 80, no. 1 (2013). 32–38. Dr. Hapenney researched sterilization practices of Catholic hospitals in seven states to determine if the hospitals were in compliance with the ERDs. Her webpage at Baylor University states: "Almost half were not. Her objective was to examine the threat posed to religious institutions based upon conscience clauses in U.S. law if hospitals do not comply with their stated religious beliefs . . . Her publications in the area have helped change the practices of a number of hospitals." Her data is stored on her website: catholichospitals.org managed by Dr. Hapenney and presents a summary of findings, https://www.baylorisr.org/scholars/h/sandra-hapenney/; "Researcher Defends Findings on Sterilizations at Catholic Hospitals | News Headlines," accessed March 25, 2022, https://www.catholicculture.org/news/headlines/index.cfm?storyid=13473.

7. "Catholic Hospitals Betray Mission–WikiLeaks," accessed March 25, 2022, https:// wikileaks.org/wiki/Catholic_hospitals_betray_mission; "Sterilization and Abortion Prac-

tices in Texas Catholic Hospitals–WikiLeaks," accessed March 25, 2022, https://wikileaks.org
/wiki/Sterilization_and_abortion_practices_in_Texas_Catholic_hospitals; "Texas Catholic
Hospitals Did Not Follow Catholic Ethics, Report Claims," July 2, 2008, Catholic News
Agency, https://www.catholicnewsagency.com/news/13120/texas-catholic-hospitals-did-not
-follow-catholic-ethics-report-claims.

8. David M. Cutler and Fiona Scott Morton, "Hospitals, Market Share, and Consolidation," *Jama* 310, no. 18 (2013): 1964–1970.

9. "Access to Postpartum Sterilization," accessed March 25, 2022, https://www.acog.org
/en/clinical/clinical-guidance/committee-opinion/articles/2021/06/access-to-postpartum
-sterilization; Sonya Borrero et al., "Medicaid Policy on Sterilization—Anachronistic or
Still Relevant?" *New England Journal of Medicine* 370, no. 2 (January 9, 2014): 102–104,
https://doi.org/10.1056/NEJMp1313325. Along with being constrained to religiously restrictive facilities, Medicaid requirements designed to protect women from sterilization abuse
can create insurmountable barriers. Some women struggle to obtain postpartum sterilization because they request sterilization too late in pregnancy or go into labor too early for
the required thirty-day waiting period to elapse, and some do not have the Medicaid form
present as required at the time of delivery. If these conditions are not met, payment for the
entire delivery becomes the responsibility of the patient (a prohibitive cost), so, instead,
women typically are denied the sterilization. While many still regard the policies as critical
protection against sterilization abuse, for an estimated 24 to 44 percent of women requesting sterilizations, practically speaking, they become unwanted barriers that women with
private insurance simply do not have.

10. Tess Solomon et al., "Bigger and Bigger: The Growth of Catholic Health Systems"
(Community Catalyst, 2020), https://www.communitycatalyst.org/resources/publications
/document/2020-Cath-Hosp-Report-2020-31.pdf.

11. Kira Shepherd, Elizabeth Reiner Platt, Katherine Franke, and Elizabeth Boylen, "Bearing Faith: The Limits of Catholic Health Care for Women of Color," Public Rights/Private
Conscience Project (Columbia Law School, January 19, 2018), https://lawrightsreligion.law
.columbia.edu/sites/default/files/content/BearingFaith.pdf.

12. Luciana E. Hebert et al., "Reproductive Healthcare Denials among a Privately
Insured Population," *Preventive Medicine Reports* 23 (2021): 101450; L. Hasselbacher et al.,
"P73 Employer vs. Employee Perspectives on Religious Healthcare Denials and Insurance
Networks: A Mixed Methods Study," *Contraception* 102, no. 4 (October 2020): 300–301,
https://doi.org/10.1016/j.contraception.2020.07.094.

13. Luciana E. Hebert, Lori Freedman, and Debra B Stulberg, "Choosing a Hospital for
Obstetric, Gynecologic, or Reproductive Healthcare: What Matters Most to Patients?"
American Journal of Obstetrics & Gynecology MFM 2, no. 1 (2020).

14. Office of the Commissioner, "Statement from FDA Commissioner Scott Gottlieb,
M.D., on Manufacturer Announcement to Halt Essure Sales in the U.S.; Agency's Continued Commitment to Postmarket Review of Essure and Keeping Women Informed," *FDA*,
March 24, 2020, https://www.fda.gov/news-events/press-announcements/statement-fda
-commissioner-scott-gottlieb-md-manufacturer-announcement-halt-essure-sales-us
-agencys; Center for Devices and Radiological Health, "Problems Reported with Essure,"
FDA, March 11, 2022, https://www.fda.gov/medical-devices/essure-permanent-birth-control
/problems-reported-essure; Center for Devices and Radiological Health, "Essure Permanent Birth Control," *FDA*, March 11, 2022, https://www.fda.gov/medical-devices/implants
-and-prosthetics/essure-permanent-birth-control.

15. T. Tam et al., "Post-Ablation Tubal Sterilization Syndrome (PATSS) Following Nova-
sure Endometrial Ablation: Two Case Reports and Review of Literature," *Journal of Minimally*

Invasive Gynecology 19, no. 6 (November 1, 2012): S112–S113, https://doi.org/10.1016/j.jmig
.2012.08.719.

16. Varvara B. Zeldovich et al., "Abortion Policies in US Teaching Hospitals: Formal and
Informal Parameters beyond the Law," *Obstetrics & Gynecology* 135, no. 6 (2020): 1296–
1305; L. Freedman et al., "Obstacles to the Integration of Abortion into Obstetrics and
Gynecology Practice," *Perspectives on Sexual and Reproductive Health* 42, no. 3 (September 2010): 146–151, https://doi.org/10.1363/4214610.

17. "New Catholic Directives Could Complicate Mergers and Partnerships," *Modern
Healthcare*, July 19, 2018, https://www.modernhealthcare.com/article/20180719/NEWS
/180719880/new-catholic-directives-could-complicate-mergers-and-partnerships.

18. The doctor was aware of it being used at least once for abortion. I was able to find
evidence of this particular entity online, but I do not give information about it here in
order not to draw attention to it, as it might not survive a challenge from the bishops.

19. U.S. health systems may have successfully managed to temper the impact on their
bottom line with creative IVF solutions. It is worth noting, however, that Catholic leadership in Belgium developed different religious policy than the U.S. bishops. The ERDs
regarding IVF possess a specific American rigidity due to their centralized medical
authority and decision making. Jessica Martucci, Ronit Y. Stahl, and Joris Vandendriessche, "One Religion, Two Paths: Making Sense of US and Belgian Catholic Hospitals'
Approaches to IVF," *Journal of Religious History* n/a, accessed August 31, 2022, https://doi
.org/10.1111/1467-9809.12878.

20. Directive 45, which addresses abortion, warns against material cooperation in abortion. Material cooperation refers to action taken with the same intent or toward the same
goal as the "wrongdoer." Thomas Kopfensteiner, "The Meaning and Role of Duress in the
Cooperation in Wrongdoing," *Linacre Quarterly* 70, no. 2 (May 2003): 150–158, https://doi
.org/10.1080/20508549.2003.11877672.

21. Charles Bouchard and Nathaniel Hibner, "US Bishops Revise Part Six of the 'Ethical
and Religious Directives'—An Initial Analysis by CHA Ethicists," *Health Care Ethics
USA*, 2018, 12–17.

22. F. A. Curlin, S. N. Dinner, and S. T. Lindau, "Of More than One Mind: Obstetrician-Gynecologists' Approaches to Morally Controversial Decisions in Sexual and Reproductive Healthcare," *Journal of Clinical Ethics* 19, no. 1 (Spring 2008): 11–21; S. K. Cowan, T. C.
Bruce, B. L. Perry, B. Ritz, S. Perrett, and E. M. Anderson, "Discordant Benevolence: How
and Why People Help Others in the Face of Conflicting Values," *Science Advances* 8, no. 7
(February 18, 2022): eabj5851, https://doi.org/10.1126/sciadv.abj5851; D. B. Stulberg, R. A.
Jackson, and L. R. Freedman, "Referrals for Services Prohibited in Catholic Health Care
Facilities," *Perspectives on Sexual and Reproductive Health* 48, no. 3 (September 2016):
111–117, https://doi.org/10.1363/48e10216; N. Homaifar, L. Freedman, and V. French, "'She's
on Her Own': A Thematic Analysis of Clinicians' Comments on Abortion Referral,"
Contraception 95, no. 5 (May 2017): 470–476, https://doi.org/10.1016/j.contraception.2017.01
.007.

23. E. Janiak and A. B. Goldberg, "Eliminating the Phrase 'Elective Abortion': Why Language Matters," *Contraception* 93, no. 2 (February 2016): 89–92, https://doi.org/10.1016/j
.contraception.2015.10.008; Katrina Kimport, Tracy A. Weitz, and Lori Freedman, "The
Stratified Legitimacy of Abortions," *Journal of Health and Social Behavior* 57, no. 4 (2016):
503–516, https://doi.org/10.1177/0022146516669970.

24. Secretariat of Pro-Life Activities, August 3, 2015, https://www.usccb.org/issues-and
-action/human-life-and-dignity/abortion/upload/s-1881-defund-planned-parenthood
-letter-august-3-2015.pdf; "We've Defunded Planned Parenthood 100 Times and Count-

ing," Catholic Investment Strategies, accessed March 25, 2022, https://www.catholicinvest
ments.com/catholic-investing/advocacy/defundplannedparenthood/.

25. F. A. Curlin et al., "Religion, Conscience, and Controversial Clinical Practices," *New England Journal of Medicine* 356, no. 6 (February 8, 2007): 593–600.

CHAPTER 6 — UNDER-THE-RADAR WORKAROUNDS

1. The principle of double effect holds that prohibited treatments are acceptable if done for a "moral" purpose, even though the "immoral" secondary effect will predictably follow. If a pregnant woman shows up to a Catholic hospital with an infected uterus or uterine lining (choreoamniotis), for example, it is allowable to evacuate the contents of the uterus, because doing so will achieve the "moral" purpose of saving the woman's life, even though treating the infection will kill the fetus in the process—an "immoral" secondary and indirect effect. Nicholas J. Kockler, "The Principle of Double Effect and Proportionate Reason," *AMA Journal of Ethics* 9, no. 5 (May 1, 2007): 369–374, https://doi.org/10.1001/virtualmentor.2007.9.5.pfor2-0705; John Seeds, "Direct Abortion or Legitimate Medical Procedure: Double Effect?" *Linacre Quarterly* 79, no. 1 (2012): 81–87.

2. Stephen M. Cherry, *Importing Care, Faithful Service: Filipino and Indian American Nurses at a Veterans Hospital* (Rutgers University Press, 2022); Ariana H. Bennett et al., "Interprofessional Abortion Opposition: A National Survey and Qualitative Interviews with Abortion Training Program Directors at US Teaching Hospitals," *Perspectives on Sexual and Reproductive Health* 52, no. 4 (2020): 235–244.

3. M. K. Wynia et al., "Physician Manipulation of Reimbursement Rules for Patients: Between a Rock and a Hard Place," *JAMA* 283, no. 14 (April 12, 2000): 1858–1865, https://doi.org/10.1001/jama.283.14.1858; Nicolas Tavaglione and Samia A. Hurst, "Why Physicians Ought to Lie for Their Patients," *American Journal of Bioethics* 12, no. 3 (March 2012): 4–12, https://doi.org/10.1080/15265161.2011.652797.

4. William J. Hall et al., "Implicit Racial/Ethnic Bias among Health Care Professionals and Its Influence on Health Care Outcomes: A Systematic Review," *American Journal of Public Health* 105, no. 12 (December 2015): e60–e76, https://doi.org/10.2105/AJPH.2015.302903.

5. Atul Gawande, *The Checklist Manifesto: How to Get Things Right*, 1st ed., A Metropolitan Book (New York: Picador, 2010).

CHAPTER 7 — SEPARATION OF CHURCH AND HOSPITAL

1. Barbara Bradley Hagerty, "Nun Excommunicated for Allowing Abortion," *NPR*, May 19, 2010, sec. Religion, https://www.npr.org/templates/story/story.php?storyId=126985072.

2. To be clear, both doctors reviewed this chapter and were comfortable with the content. Methodologically, it is questionable to potentially expose a study subject this way given that it might be possible for their colleagues to identify them through context. But they wanted this story told and reassured me it was worth it.

3. Kevin Deyoung, "What Constitutes a Pastoral Approach?" The Gospel Coalition, accessed March 30, 2022, https://www.thegospelcoalition.org/blogs/kevin-deyoung/what-constitutes-a-pastoral-approach/.

4. "The Practical Problems of the Pastoral Approach," Aleteia–Catholic Spirituality, Lifestyle, World News, and Culture, November 11, 2013, https://aleteia.org/2013/11/11/the-practical-problems-of-the-pastoral-approach/.

5. "What Is the Magisterium of the Catholic Church?" Aleteia–Catholic Spirituality, Lifestyle, World News, and Culture, July 2, 2020, https://aleteia.org/2020/07/02/what-is-the-magisterium-of-the-catholic-church/; "Teaching Authority of the Church (Magisterium) |

Encyclopedia.Com," accessed March 30, 2022, https://www.encyclopedia.com/religion /encyclopedias-almanacs-transcripts-and-maps/teaching-authority-church-magisterium; "Magisterium," Catholic Answers, accessed March 30, 2022, https://www.catholic.com /magazine/print-edition/magisterium.

6. Bishop O'Brien had been granted immunity for his role in covering up a child abuse scandal just before the hit-and-run incident. See Nick Madigan, "Phoenix Jury Finds Bishop Guilty in Fatal Hit-and-Run," *New York Times*, February 18, 2004, sec. U.S., https:// www.nytimes.com/2004/02/18/us/phoenix-jury-finds-bishop-guilty-in-fatal-hit-and-run .html.

7. As mentioned in chapter 5, Pope Benedict was known as Cardinal Ratzinger, Dean of the Cardinals in the United States, prior to his installment in 2005 as Cardinal Ratzinger. The cardinal was alarmed when a devout Catholic researcher, Sandra Hapenney, brought to his attention data showing that, between 2000 and 2003, sterilizations were happening in U.S. Catholic hospitals with regularity. The controversy is documented in Wikileaks and other publications noted below. New bishops were installed around that time in many locations. Practices seem to change shortly thereafter in many hospitals of the doctors I interviewed, similar to the way Dr. Murphy described. See Sandra Hapenney, "Divergent Practices among Catholic Hospitals in Provision of Direct Sterilization," *Linacre Quarterly* 80, no. 1 (2013): 32–38; Barbra Mann Wall, "Conflict and Compromise: Catholic and Public Hospital Partnerships," *Nursing History Review: Official Journal of the American Association for the History of Nursing* 18 (2010): 100–117; Catholic Medical Association, "Report of the Task Force on Ethical and Religious Directives," *Linacre Quarterly* 72, no. 2 (May 1, 2005), https://epublications.marquette.edu/lnq/vol72/iss2/4; "Catholic Hospitals Betray Mission— WikiLeaks," accessed March 25, 2022, https://wikileaks.org/wiki/Catholic_hospitals_betray _mission; "Sterilization and Abortion Practices in Texas Catholic Hospitals–WikiLeaks," accessed March 25, 2022, https://wikileaks.org/wiki/Sterilization_and_abortion_practices _in_Texas_Catholic_hospitals; Joseph Berger, "Vatican Tells Priest to Retract Views," *New York Times*, March 12, 1986, sec. U.S., https://www.nytimes.com/1986/03/12/us/vatican-tells -priest-to-retract-views.html; Samuel Koo, "Pope, Chastizing Dissident Theologian, Sends Message to U.S. Clergy," AP News, accessed March 30, 2022, https://apnews.com/article/3a9 6c0585b12dd24bb17542aec8c6d2e.

8. Bishop Thomas J. Olmsted, "Bishop Olmsted Statement in Response to Abortion Per- formed at St. Joseph's Hospital," *Arizona Republic*, May 18, 2010, https://www.catholicculture .org/culture/library/view.cfm?recnum=9323.

9. "Hospital Nun Rebuked for Allowing Abortion in Phoenix—USATODAY.Com," accessed March 30, 2022, https://usatoday30.usatoday.com/news/religion/2010-05-18-nun -abortion_N.htm.

10. The Daily Dish, "How Soon They Can Excommunicate," *The Atlantic*, May 18, 2010, https://www.theatlantic.com/daily-dish/archive/2010/05/how-soon-they-can-excommu nicate/186939/; Nicholas Kristof, "Opinion | Sister Margaret's Choice," *New York Times*, May 27, 2010, sec. Opinion, https://www.nytimes.com/2010/05/27/opinion/27kristof.html; Dan Harris and Claudia Morales, "Nun Excommunicated after Saving a Mother's Life with Abortion," *ABC News*, June 1, 2010, https://abcnews.go.com/WN/Media/church -excommunicates-nun-authorized-emergency-abortion-save-mothers/story?id=10799745.

11. The National Catholic Bioethics Center, "NCBC Commentary on the 'Phoenix Case,'" December 24, 2010, https://www.washingtonpost.com/wp-srv/health/documents/abortion /National-Catholic-Bioethics-Center-statement.pdf.

12. Hagerty, "Nun Excommunicated for Allowing Abortion."

13. A statement released to the press by CHW read, "At St. Joseph's Hospital and Medical Center, our highly-skilled clinical professionals face life and death decisions every day.

Those decisions are guided by our values of dignity, justice and respect, and the belief that all life is sacred . . . We have always adhered to the Ethical and Religious Directives for Catholic Health Care Services as we carry out our healing ministry and we continue to abide by them. As the preamble to the Directives notes, 'While providing standards and guidance, the Directives do not cover in detail all the complex issues that confront Catholic health care today.' In those instances where the Directives do not explicitly address a clinical situation—such as when a pregnancy threatens a woman's life—an Ethics Committee is convened to help our caregivers and their patients make the most life-affirming decision. "In this tragic case, the treatment necessary to save the mother's life required the termination of an 11-week pregnancy. This decision was made after consultation with the patient, her family, her physicians, and in consultation with the Ethics Committee, of which Sr. Margaret McBride is a member," https://www.reliasmedia.com/articles/20304 -nun-resigns-following-abortion-decision. Additionally, lengthy independent Catholic "moral analysis" of case by Dr. M. Therese Lysaught with more clinical detail, arguing why it was the right thing to do was posted on Dignity's website. M. Therese Lysaught, "A Moral Analysis of an Intervention Performed at St. Joseph's Hospital and Medical Center," Dignity Health, January 7, 2011, accessed April 1, 2022, https://www.dignityhealth.org /content/dam/dignity-health/pdfs/press-releases/2011/2011-01-07-independent-moral -analysis.pdf.

14. Bishop Thomas J. Olmsted, "Bishop Olmsted Statement in Response to Abortion Performed at St. Joseph's Hospital."

15. Harris and Morales, "Nun Excommunicated after Saving a Mother's Life With Abortion."

16. CNA, "Sister Violated More than Catholic Teaching in Sanctioning Abortion, Ethicist Says," Catholic News Agency, accessed March 30, 2022, https://www.catholicnewsagency .com/news/19716/sister-violated-more-than-catholic-teaching-in-sanctioning-abortion -ethicist-says; Diocese of Phoenix, "Abortion," Roman Catholic Diocese of Phoenix (blog), accessed March 30, 2022, https://dphx.org/respect-life/know-the-issues/abortion/.

17. Letter from Thomas Olmsted to Lloyd H. Dean, November 22, 2010, https://www .washingtonpost.com/wp-srv/health/documents/abortion/bishopletter.pdf.

18. Amanda Lee Myers, The Associated Press, "Phoenix Hospital Loses Catholic Status over Surgery," East Valley Tribune, accessed March 30, 2022, https://www.eastvalleytribune.com /local/the_valley/phoenix-hospital-loses-catholic-status-over-surgery/article_fb8a6996 -0d30-11e0-9f38-001cc4c03286.html.

19. "Phoenix Hospital Still Belongs to Catholic Health Association," National Catholic Reporter, 2:46 P.M., https://www.ncronline.org/news/phoenix-hospital-still-belongs-catholic -health-association.

20. "McBride Un-Excommunicated," America Magazine, December 14, 2011, https:// www.americamagazine.org/content/all-things/mcbride-un-excommunicated.

21. "Phoenix Bishop Removes Hospital's Catholic Status," National Catholic Reporter, December 21, 2010, https://www.ncronline.org/news/phoenix-bishop-removes-hospitals -catholic-status.

22. Blufish, "Linda Hunt, CEO, St. Joseph's Hospital And Medical Center," AZ Big Media, March 10, 2011, https://azbigmedia.com/business/health-care/linda-hunt-ceo-st -josephs-hospital/.

23. Sister McBride accepting The Call to Action Leadership Award in 2011: "I walked into the room and of course I burst into tears and she burst into tears, and she said, 'I'm so sorry for all these terrible things that happened to you. You saved my life, and all these terrible things happened to you,'" McBride said. "And if I were to say where I thought I was going to get my healing, it would have been from the church. But the healing really

came from the woman, who graciously told me that her life had been changed because of me, but that now she felt guilty that so many things had happened to me. And I told her 'you just don't see my support, you don't see the employees, you don't see the doctors, you don't see the board of directors and the Catholic Healthcare West who have supported me through this interesting time (coy smile, laughter) . . . not that I wish it on anybody else (bigger laughter) . . . as we move forward in this very disappointing time in our church, I think it's the time when we need to be the example of mercy and forgiveness and love. It is only by our example that the Church will change." See "Excommunicated Sister Finds Healing," *National Catholic Reporter*, 12:12 P.M., https://www.ncronline.org/news/people/excommunicated-sister-finds -healing; NCRonline, "Sister of Mercy McBride Receives Leadership Award at Call To Action 2011", 2011, https://www.youtube.com/watch?v=SVbIfjRRSf4.

24. "Excommunicated Sister Finds Healing," *National Catholic Reporter.*

25. In both number of hospitals and revenue, CommonSpirit ranks #2 in the United States, https://www.modernhealthcare.com/article/20190201/NEWS/190209994/catholic-health -initiatives-dignity-health-combine-to-form-commonspirit-health; "Catholic Health Initiatives, Dignity Health Combine to Form CommonSpirit Health," *Modern Healthcare*, February 1, 2019, https://www.modernhealthcare.com/article/20190201/NEWS/190209994/catholic -health-initiatives-dignity-health-combine-to-form-commonspirit-health; "Top 10 Largest Health Systems in the U.S.," *Definitive Healthcare*, accessed March 30, 2022, https://www .definitivehc.com/blog/top-10-largest-health-systems.

26. Bishop Olmsted resumed mass at St. Josephs: Diocese of Phoenix, "Bishop Olmsted Extends Permission for Eucharist, Mass at St. Joseph's Hospital and Medical Center," *Roman Catholic Diocese of Phoenix* (blog), March 24, 2020, https://dphx.org/bishop-olmsted -extends-permission-for-eucharist-mass-at-st-josephs-hospital-and-medical-center/; Samuel Leal, "COVID-19 Prompts Phoenix Diocese to Allow Mass at St. Joseph's Hospital after Revoking Privilege over Abortion Dispute," *Arizona Republic*, accessed November 4, 2021, https://www.azcentral.com/story/news/local/phoenix/2020/04/06/covid-19-prompts -phoenix-diocese-allow-mass-st-josephs-hospital/2945548001/.

27. "Dignity Health, Creighton University and the Diocese of Phoenix Form Collaborative Mission Committee to Better Serve the Community," accessed December 1, 2021, https://www.dignityhealth.org/arizona/locations/stjosephs/about-us/press-center/press -releases/dignity-health-forms-collaborative-mission-committee-to-better-serve-the -community.

28. Tony Gutiérrez, "Presence of Eucharist, Celebration of Mass Restored at St. Joseph Hospital," *Catholic Sun* (blog), March 26, 2020, https://www.catholicsun.org/2020/03/26 /presence-of-eucharist-celebration-of-mass-restored-at-st-joseph-hospital/.

29. "In 2017, Creighton University, Dignity Health St. Joseph's Hospital and Medical Center, Valleywise Health, and District Medical Group, entered into a strategic partnership to strengthen and expand the Graduate Medical Education programs offered by each institution. The move by the four core partners and affiliate member Dignity Health Medical Group brought together the administration of the residency and fellowship programs previously managed by each member under the Creighton University Arizona Health Education Alliance, with Creighton University serving as the sponsoring entity." See "Creighton University Arizona Health Education Alliance | Creighton University Arizona Health Education Alliance | Creighton University," accessed December 1, 2021, https:// alliance.creighton.edu/about/creighton-university-arizona-health-education-alliance.

30. "Linda Hunt, President and CEO of Dignity Health's Southwest Division, Retires after 51 Years of Health Care Service," accessed March 30, 2022, https://www.dignityhealth .org/arizona/about-us/press-center/linda-hunt--president-and-ceo-of-dignity-health-s -southwest-divi.

31. Katie Burke, "Preparing for a New Bishop with Gratitude and Trust," *Roman Catholic Diocese of Phoenix* (blog), accessed March 30, 2022, https://dphx.org/new-bishop/.

CONCLUSION

1. Kitty Holland and Paul Cullen, "Woman 'Denied a Termination' Dies in Hospital," *Irish Times*, accessed April 12, 2022, https://www.irishtimes.com/news/woman-denied-a-termination-dies-in-hospital-1.551412.

2. Holland and Cullen, "Woman 'Denied a Termination' Dies in Hospital."

3. Holland and Cullen.

4. Donna L. Hoyert, "Maternal Mortality and Related Concepts," *Vital & Health Statistics. Series 3, Analytical and Epidemiological Studies*, no. 33 (February 2007): 1–13.

5. "Maternal Mortality Rates in the United States, 2020," February 22, 2022, https://www.cdc.gov/nchs/data/hestat/maternal-mortality/2020/maternal-mortality-rates-2020.htm; "Maternal Mortality and Maternity Care in the United States Compared to 10 Other Developed Countries," November 18, 2020, https://doi.org/10.26099/411v-9255.

6. Melissa E. Bauer et al., "Maternal Sepsis Mortality and Morbidity during Hospitalization for Delivery: Temporal Trends and Independent Associations for Severe Sepsis," *Anesthesia & Analgesia* 117, no. 4 (October 2013): 944–950, https://doi.org/10.1213/ANE.0b013e3182a009c3.

7. "Irish Bishops Issue Statement on Death of Savita Halappanavar | Matthew Schmitz," First Things, accessed April 12, 2022, https://www.firstthings.com/blogs/firstthoughts/2012/11/irish-bishops-issue-statement-on-death-of-savita-halappanavar.

8. "U.S. Bishops Face a Lawsuit over Abortion Policies at Roman Catholic Hospitals," *Diane Rehm* (blog), December 4, 2013, accessed April 14, 2022, https://dianerehm.org/shows/2013-12-04/us-bishops-face-lawsuit-over-abortion-policies-roman-catholic-hospitals.

9. Molly Redden, "Abortion Ban Linked to Dangerous Miscarriages at Catholic Hospital, Report Claims," *The Guardian*, February 18, 2016, sec. US news, https://www.theguardian.com/us-news/2016/feb/18/michigan-catholic-hospital-women-miscarriage-abortion-mercy-health-partners.

10. It is possible that this case created bad law that will make it even harder to hold the bishops legally accountable. See "Federal Appeals Court Rejects ACLU-Backed Catholic Hospital Ethics Lawsuit," *Modern Healthcare*, September 9, 2016, https://www.modernhealthcare.com/article/20160909/NEWS/160909887/federal-appeals-court-rejects-aclu-backed-catholic-hospital-ethics-lawsuit.

11. "Health Care Denied," American Civil Liberties Union, accessed April 12, 2022, https://www.aclu.org/issues/reproductive-freedom/religion-and-reproductive-rights/health-care-denied.

12. Nina Martin, "At a Catholic Hospital, a Dispute over What a Doctor Can Do—and Say," ProPublica, accessed April 14, 2022, https://www.propublica.org/article/at-a-catholic-hospital-a-dispute-over-what-a-doctor-can-do-and-say?token=m1zeoMrj6m52j-J8AvluRGJmCGvDt8BG.

13. "Colorado Doctor Fired after Suing to Provide Aid-in-Dying Medication," *Time*, accessed April 13, 2022, https://time.com/5666225/colorado-doctor-fired-aid-in-dying-medication/.

14. Khiara Bridges, "The Deserving Poor, the Undeserving Poor, and Class-Based Affirmative Action," *Emory Law Journal* 66, no. 5 (January 1, 2017): 1049.

15. Kathleen M. Joyce, "The Evil of Abortion and the Greater Good of the Faith: Negotiating Catholic Survival in the Twentieth-Century American Health Care System," *Religion and American Culture* 12, no. 1 (Winter 2002): 91–121.

16. Lynn M. Morgan and Elizabeth F. S. Roberts, "Reproductive governance in Latin America." *Anthropology & Medicine* 19, no. 2 (2012): 241–254, https://doi.org/10.1080/1364 8470.2012.675046.

17. Ahmed Shaheed, "Freedom of Religion or Belief: Special Rapporteur on Freedom of Religion or Belief: Report on Restrictions Imposed on Expression on Account of Religion or Belief," 2019, https://tandis.odihr.pl/handle/20.500.12389/23006, https://www.guttmacher .org/gpr/2018/05/bad-faith-how-conservatives-are-weaponizing-religious-liberty-allow -institutions; K. Stewart, *The Power Worshippers: Inside the Dangerous Rise of Religious Nationalism* (Bloomsbury Publishing USA, 2020); Michelle Goldberg, *The Means of Reproduction: Sex, Power, and the Future of the World* (Penguin, 2009).

18. "Trump's 'Conscience' Rule for Healthcare Workers Struck Down by U.S. Judge," *Reuters*, November 6, 2019, sec. Healthcare & Pharma, https://www.reuters.com/article/us -usa-healthcare-religion-lawsuit-idUSKBN1XG2DD.

19. "A/HRC/43/48," accessed April 12, 2022, https://undocs.org/Home/Mobile?FinalSymbol =A%2FHRC%2F43%2F48&Language=E&DeviceType=Desktop&LangRequested=False; "OHCHR | Report on Freedom of Religion or Belief and Gender Equality," OHCHR, accessed April 12, 2022, https://www.ohchr.org/en/calls-for-input/reports/2020/report-freedom -religion-or-belief-and-gender-equality.

20. Davida Becker and Amy O. Tsui, "Reproductive Health Service Preferences and Perceptions of Quality among Low-Income Women: Racial, Ethnic and Language Group Differences," *Perspectives on Sexual and Reproductive Health* 40, no. 4 (2008): 202–211, https://doi .org/10.1363/4020208; Alison Norris et al., "Abortion Stigma: A Reconceptualization of Constituents, Causes, and Consequences," *Women's Health Issues, Abortion, Reproductive Rights and Health* 21, no. 3, Supplement (May 1, 2011): S49–S54, https://doi.org/10.1016/j.whi.2011.02.010.

21. "If Men Got Pregnant, Abortion Would Be Legal Everywhere," *New Statesman* (blog), December 4, 2015, https://www.newstatesman.com/politics/2015/12/if-men-got-pregnant-abor tion-would-be-legal-everywhere; Emma Brockes, "Gloria Steinem: 'If Men Could Get Pregnant, Abortion Would Be a Sacrament,'" *The Guardian*, October 17, 2015, sec. Books, https:// www.theguardian.com/books/2015/oct/17/gloria-steinem-activist-interview-memoir-my-life -on-the-road.

22. ACOG, "ACOG Committee Opinion 385 November 2007: The Limits of Conscientious Refusal in Reproductive Medicine," *Obstetric Gynecology* 110, no. 5 (November 2007): 1203–1208, https://doi.org/10.1097/01.AOG.0000291561.48203.27.

23. For one-stop shopping, Holly Fernandez Lynch, I. Glenn Cohen, and Elizabeth Sepper, *Law, Religion, and Health in the United States* (Cambridge University Press, 2017).

24. Lori R. Freedman et al., "Religious Hospital Policies on Reproductive Care: What Do Patients Want to Know?" *American Journal of Obstetrics & Gynecology* 218, no. 2 (2018): 251–e1, F. A. Chervenak and L. B. McCullough, "Professional Responsibility of Transparency of Obstetricians Practicing in Religious Hospitals," *American Journal of Obstetrics and Gynecology* 218, no. 2 (February 2018): 159–160, https://doi.org/10.1016/j.ajog.2017.12.216.

25. "Religious Liberties and the New Supreme Court: What's at Stake for Women and the LGBTQ+ Community," accessed April 12, 2022, https://www.americanbar.org/groups /diversity/women/publications/perspectives/2021/april/religious-liberties-and-new -supreme-court-whats-stake-women-and-lgbtq-community/.

26. Christina Maslach, Susan E. Jackson, and Michael P. Leiter, *Maslach Burnout Inventory Manual*, 3rd. ed. (Menlo Park, CA: Mind Garden, 2010); Committee on Systems Approaches to Improve Patient Care by Supporting Clinician Well-Being, National Academy of Medicine, and National Academies of Sciences, Engineering, and Medicine, *Taking Action against Clinician Burnout: A Systems Approach to Professional Well-Being* (Washington, DC: National Academies Press, 2019), https://doi.org/10.17226/25521.

27. To arrive at this percentage of 3 percent, I compared the Bureau of Labor Statistics on the number of doctors with the total membership of these two professional associations as documented on their websites or in news stories. See "Physicians and Surgeons: Occupational Outlook Handbook: U.S. Bureau of Labor Statistics," accessed October 28, 2021, https://www.bls.gov/ooh/healthcare/physicians-and-surgeons.htm; Ann Carey, "Catholic Medical Association Urges Sweeping Health Care Reforms," *Catholic News Service*, October 12, 2004, https://web.archive.org/web/20070608071755/http:/www.catholicnews.com/data/stories/cns/0405618.htm; "About CMDA–Christian Medical & Dental Associations® (CMDA)," accessed April 12, 2022, https://cmda.org/about-us/.

28. Eric Plemons, "Not Here: Catholic Hospital Systems and the Restriction against Transgender Healthcare," *CrossCurrents*, 2019, https://doi.org/10.1111/cros.12341; "Docket for 19–1135," accessed April 12, 2022, https://www.supremecourt.gov/docket/docketfiles/html/public/19-1135.html; "*Dignity Health v. Minton*—SCOTUSblog," accessed April 12, 2022, https://www.scotusblog.com/case-files/cases/dignity-health-v-minton/.

29. Early writing about institutional racism as a concept: Charles V. Hamilton and Kwame Ture, *Black Power: Politics of Liberation in America* (Vintage, 2011).

30. L. A. Penner et al., "Reducing Racial Health Care Disparities: A Social Psychological Analysis," *Policy Insights for the Behavioral and Brain Sciences* 1, no. 1 (October 2014): 204–212, https://doi.org/10.1177/2372732214548430.

31. Jonathan M. Metzl and Dorothy E. Roberts, "Structural Competency Meets Structural Racism: Race, Politics, and the Structure of Medical Knowledge," *AMA Journal of Ethics* 16, no. 9 (2014): 674–690; Juanita J. Chinn, Iman K. Martin, and Nicole Redmond, "Health Equity among Black Women in the United States," *Journal of Women's Health* 30, no. 2 (2020), https://doi.org/10.1089/jwh.2020.8868; Debra B. Stulberg et al., "Ectopic Pregnancy Rates in the Medicaid Population," *American Journal of Obstetrics and Gynecology* 208, no. 4 (April 1, 2013): 274.e1–274.e7, https://doi.org/10.1016/j.ajog.2012.12.038.

32. Jamila K. Taylor, "Structural Racism and Maternal Health among Black Women," *Journal of Law, Medicine & Ethics* 48, no. 3 (2020): 506–517.

33. Kira Shepherd, Elizabeth Reiner Platt, Katherine Franke, and Elizabeth Boylen, "Bearing Faith: The Limits of Catholic Health Care for Women of Color," Public Rights/Private Conscience Project (Columbia Law School, January 19, 2018), https://lawrightsreligion.law.columbia.edu/sites/default/files/content/BearingFaith.pdf.

34. Talcott Parsons, *The Social System* (Glencoe, IL: Free Press, 1951); Jody E. Steinauer et al., "Residents' Experiences of Negative Emotions toward Patients: Challenges to Their Identities," *Teaching and Learning in Medicine* 34, no. 5 (November 11, 2021): 1–9, https://doi.org/10.1080/10401334.2021.1988617.

35. Michelle Van Ryn and Steven S. Fu, "Paved with Good Intentions: Do Public Health and Human Service Providers Contribute to Racial/Ethnic Disparities in Health?" *American Journal of Public Health* 93, no. 2 (2003): 248–255; Sandra Bass, "Policing Space, Policing Race: Social Control Imperatives and Police Discretionary Decisions," *Social Justice* 28, no. 1 (2001): 156–176; Susan Nembhard and Lily Robin, "Racial and Ethnic Disparities throughout the Criminal Legal System," *Urban Institute*, August 2021.

36. K. R. White, J. W. Begun, and W. Tian, "Hospital Service Offerings: Does Catholic Ownership Matter?" *Health Care Management Review* 31, no. 2 (April 2006): 99–108.

37. Ann Kutney-Lee et al., "Distinct Enough? A National Examination of Catholic Hospital Affiliation and Patient Perceptions of Care," *Health Care Management Review* 39, no. 2 (2014): 134.

38. N. B. Thorne et al., "Reproductive Health Care in Catholic Facilities: A Scoping Review," *Obstetric Gynecology* 133, no. 1 (January 2019): 105–115, https://doi.org/10.1097/aog.0000000000003029.

39. Elaine L. Hill, David J. G. Slusky, and Donna K. Ginther, "Reproductive Health Care in Catholic-Owned Hospitals," *Journal of Health Economics* 65 (2019): 48–62.

40. Varvara B. Zeldovich et al., "Abortion Policies in US Teaching Hospitals: Formal and Informal Parameters beyond the Law," *Obstetrics & Gynecology* 135, no. 6 (2020): 1296–1305.

41. Lee A. Hasselbacher et al., "'My Hands Are Tied': Abortion Restrictions and Providers' Experiences in Religious and Nonreligious Health Care Systems," *Perspectives on Sexual and Reproductive Health* 52, no. 2 (July 2020): 107–115, https://doi.org/10.1363/psrh .12148; Yuan Liu et al., "'Am I Going to Be in Trouble for What I'm Doing?': Providing Contraceptive Care in Religious Health Care Systems," *Perspectives on Sexual and Reproductive Health* 51, no. 4 (December 2019): 193–199, https://doi.org/10.1363/psrh.12125; Elizabeth Sepper, "Zombie Religious Institutions," *Northwestern University Law Review*, 2018.

42. Elizabeth Reiner Platt, Katherine Franke, Candace Bond-Theriault, Lilia Hadjiivanova, and Amy Littlefield. "The Southern Hospitals Report: Faith, Culture, and Abortion Bans in the U.S. South" (The Law, Rights, and Religion Project: Columbia Law School, November 16, 2021), 77.

43. Office for Civil Rights (OCR), "Conscience Protections for Health Care Providers," Text, HHS.gov, October 14, 2010, https://www.hhs.gov/conscience/conscience-protections /index.html.

44. "Legal Fiction," LII / Legal Information Institute, accessed April 14, 2022, https:// www.law.cornell.edu/wex/legal_fiction.

45. "USCCB Poll: Americans Support Conscience Protection for Healthcare Professionals | USCCB," accessed April 14, 2022, https://www.usccb.org/news/2019/usccb-poll-americans -support-conscience-protection-healthcare-professionals.

46. "The Weldon Amendment: Interfering with Abortion Coverage and Care," July 2021, https://www.guttmacher.org/fact-sheet/weldon-amendment; Weldon Amendment, Consolidated Appropriations Act, 2009, Pub. L. No. 111–117, 123 Stat 3034, https://www.hhs.gov /sites/default/files/ocr/civilrights/understanding/ConscienceProtect/publaw111_117_123 _stat_3034.pdf.

47. "HHS Refuses to Enforce Weldon Amendment," United States Conference of Catholic Bishops, https://www.usccb.org/issues-and-action/religious-liberty/conscience-protection /upload/HHS-Refuses-to-Enforce-Weldon-Amendment-FACT-SHEET.pdf.

48. Hilary M. Schwandt, Bethany Sparkle, and Moriah Post-Kinney, "Ambiguities in Washington State Hospital Policies, Irrespective of Catholic Affiliation, Regarding Abortion and Contraception Service Provision," *Reproductive Health* 15, no. 1 (October 19, 2018): 178, https://doi.org/10.1186/s12978-018-0621-5; "Hospitals Now Required by Law to Disclose Which Reproductive Health Services They Offer," ACLU of Washington, September 24, 2019, https://www.aclu-wa.org/story/hospitals-now-required-law-disclose-which -reproductive-health-services-they-offer.

49. Amy Littlefield, "Oregon Will Protect Reproductive Health Care When Hospitals Merge," July 19, 2021, https://www.thenation.com/article/society/oregon-catholic-hospitals/; https://www.nysenate.gov/legislation/bills/2021/s1451; "Health Care Market Oversight," Oregon Health Authority, https://www.oregon.gov/oha/HPA/HP/Pages/health-care-market-over sight.aspx.

50. Elizabeth Sepper, "Taking Conscience Seriously," *Virginia Law Review* 98 (2012): 1501.

51. Watson, Katie. *Scarlet A: The Ethics, Law, and Politics of Ordinary Abortion* (Oxford University Press, 2018).

52. Diana Greene Foster, *The Turnaway Study: The Cost of Denying Women Access to Abortion* (Simon and Schuster, 2020); M. Antonia Biggs et al., "Women's Mental Health

and Well-Being 5 Years after Receiving or Being Denied an Abortion: A Prospective, Longitudinal Cohort Study," *JAMA Psychiatry* 74, no. 2 (February 1, 2017): 169–178, https://doi.org/10.1001/jamapsychiatry.2016.3478; Sarah C. M. Roberts et al., "Risk of Violence from the Man Involved in the Pregnancy after Receiving or Being Denied an Abortion," *BMC Medicine*, 2014, https://doi.org/10.1186/s12916-014-0144-z; Diana Greene Foster et al., "Comparison of Health, Development, Maternal Bonding, and Poverty among Children Born after Denial of Abortion vs. after Pregnancies Subsequent to an Abortion," *JAMA Pediatrics* 172, no. 11 (2018): 1053–1060.

53. Alexandra Desanctis, "The Disingenuous Debate over Ectopic Pregnancy and Miscarriage," National Review, July 27, 2022, https://www.nationalreview.com/corner/the-disingenuous-debate-over-ectopic-pregnancy-and-miscarriage/.

54. Eugene Declercq, Ruby Barnard-Mayers, Laurie Zephyrin, and Kay Johnson. "The Maternal Health Divide: The Limited Health Services and Worse Outcomes of States Proposing Abortion Restrictions" (The Commonwealth Fund, December 14, 2022), https://www.commonwealthfund.org/publications/issue-briefs/2022/dec/us-maternal-health-divide-limited-services-worse-outcomes. The study found: "Compared to states where abortion is accessible, states that have banned, are planning to ban, or have otherwise restricted abortion have fewer maternity care providers; more maternity care 'deserts'; higher rates of maternal mortality and infant death, especially among women of color; higher overall death rates for women of reproductive age; and greater racial inequities across their health care systems."

55. Kari White, Asha Dane'el, Elsa Vizcarra, Laura Dixon, et al., "Out-of-State Travel for Abortion Following Implementation of Texas Senate Bill 8," Texas Policy Evaluation Project, Research Brief, March 2022, https://sites.utexas.edu/txpep/files/2022/03/TxPEP-out-of-state-SB8.pdf; Lucy Kafanov, "Devastated Mom Forced to Travel Out of State for Abortion of Unviable Fetus," CNN, June 21, 2022, https://www.1011now.com/2022/06/21/devastated-mom-forced-travel-out-state-abortion-unviable-fetus/. See also: #WeCount, a study supported by the Society of Family Planning, conducted by public health researchers from multiple institutions, that is actively capturing the shifts in abortion volume, by state, following Dobbs: https://www.societyfp.org/wecount/.

56. Rania Soetirto and Sarah Kaufman, "Women Who've Tried 'Herbal Abortions' Urge Others Not to Follow their Lead," NBC News, July 22, 2022, https://www.nbcnews.com/health/health-news/women-ve-tried-herbal-abortions-urge-others-not-follow-lead-rcna39563; Erica Carbajal, "Experts Warn Against 'DIY Abortions' as Google Searches for Home Remedies Skyrocket," Becker's Hospital Review, July 8, 2022, https://www.beckershospitalreview.com/patient-safety-outcomes/experts-warn-against-diy-abortions-as-google-searches-for-home-remedies-skyrocket.html.

57. "Plan C" webpage, https://www.plancpills.org; Ushma D Upadhyay, Alice F. Cartwright, and Daniel Grossman, "Barriers to Abortion Care and Incidence of Attempted Self-Managed Abortion among Individuals Searching Google for Abortion Care: A National Prospective Study," *Contraception* 106 (February 1, 2022): 49–56, https://doi.org/10.1016/j.contraception.2021.09.009.

58. Abigail R. A. Aiken et al., "Self-Reported Outcomes and Adverse Events after Medical Abortion through Online Telemedicine: Population Based Study in the Republic of Ireland and Northern Ireland," *BMJ* 357 (May 16, 2017): j2011, https://doi.org/10.1136/bmj.j2011; Society of Family Planning Interim Recommendations, https://www.societyfp.org/wp-content/uploads/2022/06/SFP-Interim-Recommendation-Self-managed-abortion-07.14.22.pdf.

APPENDIX

1. Lori Freedman, *Willing and Unable: Doctors' Constraints in Abortion Care* (Nashville: Vanderbilt University Press, 2010).

2. I reported on these cases in my dissertation research, which became my first book, and in the *American Journal of Public Health* before collecting data used for this book: L. R. Freedman, U. Landy, and J. Steinauer, "When There's a Heartbeat: Miscarriage Management in Catholic-Owned Hospitals," *American Journal of Public Health*, 2008, https://doi.org/10.2105/AJPH.2007.126730.

3. Lori R. Freedman and Debra B. Stulberg, "Conflicts in Care for Obstetric Complications in Catholic Hospitals," *AJOB Primary Research* 4, no. 4 (2013): 1–10.

4. Katrina Kimport, Tracy A. Weitz, and Lori Freedman, "The Stratified Legitimacy of Abortions," *Journal of Health and Social Behavior* 57, no. 4 (2016): 503–516, https://doi.org/10.1177/0022146516669970; D. B. Stulberg, R. A. Jackson, and L. R. Freedman, "Referrals for Services Prohibited in Catholic Health Care Facilities," *Perspectives on Sexual and Reproductive Health* 48, no. 3 (September 2016): 111–117, https://doi.org/10.1363/48e10216; D. B. Stulberg et al., "Tubal Ligation in Catholic Hospitals: A Qualitative Study of Ob-Gyns' Experiences," *Contraception* 90, no. 4 (October 2014): 422–428, https://doi.org/10.1016/j.contraception.2014.04.015; Freedman and Stulberg, "Conflicts in Care for Obstetric Complications in Catholic Hospitals."

5. See acknowledgments.

6. M. Guiahi, J. Sheeder, and S. Teal, "Are Women Aware of Religious Restrictions on Reproductive Health at Catholic Hospitals? A Survey of Women's Expectations and Preferences for Family Planning Care," *Contraception* 90, no. 4 (October 2014): 429–434, https://doi.org/10.1016/j.contraception.2014.06.035.

7. Debra B. Stulberg et al., "Women's Expectation of Receiving Reproductive Health Care at Catholic and Non-Catholic Hospitals," *Perspectives on Sexual and Reproductive Health* 51, no. 3 (September 4, 2019): 135–142, https://doi.org/10.1363/psrh.12118.

8. Renee D. Kramer et al., "Prevalence and Experiences of Wisconsin Women Turned Away from Catholic Settings without Receiving Reproductive Care," *Contraception* 104, no. 4 (2021): 377–382, https://doi.org/10.1016/j.contraception.2021.05.007; Renee D. Kramer et al., "Expectations about Availability of Contraception and Abortion at a Hypothetical Catholic Hospital: Rural-Urban Disparities among Wisconsin Women," *Contraception* 104, no. 5 (2021): 506–511, https://doi.org/10.1016/j.contraception.2021.05.014.

9. Erin E. Wingo et al., "Anticipatory Counseling about Miscarriage Management in Catholic Hospitals: A Qualitative Exploration of Women's Preferences," *Perspectives on Sexual and Reproductive Health* 52, no. 3 (2020): 171–179; Jocelyn M. Wascher, Debra B. Stulberg, and Lori R. Freedman, "Restrictions on Reproductive Care at Catholic Hospitals: A Qualitative Study of Patient Experiences and Perspectives," *AJOB Empirical Bioethics* 11, no. 4 (2020), https://doi.org/10.1080/23294515.2020.1817173.

10. Lee A. Hasselbacher et al., "Beyond Hobby Lobby: Employer's Responsibilities and Opportunities to Improve Network Access to Reproductive Healthcare for Employees," *Contraception: X* 4 (2022): 100078.

11. Luciana E Hebert et al., "Reproductive Healthcare Denials among a Privately Insured Population," *Preventive Medicine Reports* 23 (2021).

12. Kellie E Schueler et al., "Denial of Tubal Ligation in Religious Hospitals: Consumer Attitudes When Insurance Limits Hospital Choice," *Contraception* (2021).

13. Zarina J. Wong et al., "What You Don't Know Can Hurt You: Patient and Provider Perspectives on Postpartum Contraceptive Care in Illinois Catholic Hospitals," *Contraception* 107 (March 2022): 62–67, https://doi.org/10.1016/j.contraception.2021.10.004.

14. In 2014, the lead ethicist of the Catholic Health Association wrote this piece in response to publications and talks by Dr. Stulberg and I. He accuses us of attacking Catholic health care and goes on to defend it. However, he also acknowledges that Catholic hospitals could do more to communicate how the doctrine can affect obstetric complications and to offer to transfer patients quickly. See R. Hamel, "Early Pregnancy Complications and the Ethical and Religious Directives," *Health Progress* 95, no. 3 (May 2014): 48–56.

15. Lori Freedman, "Open Forum: Affiliation with Dignity Health Is Too Risky for UCSF," *San Francisco Chronicle*, May 16, 2019, https://www.sfchronicle.com/opinion/openforum /article/Open-Forum-Affiliation-with-Dignity-Health-is-13849017.php; Jenny Gold, "Will Ties to a Catholic Hospital System Tie Doctors' Hands?" *California Healthline* (blog), April 29, 2019, https://californiahealthline.org/news/will-ties-to-a-catholic-hospital-system-tie-doctors -hands/.

Index

abortions and abortion care: ACA and, 9; access in Southside Chicago, 25; Church Amendment on, 19; Desiree's experiences with, 62–65; *Dobbs* on, xiii, 10–11, 157; for ectopic pregnancies, 89; in Ireland, 11, 144; in late 19th–early 20th c., 16–17, 171n8; legal access to, 4; Nadia on, 53, 55; outpatient referrals for, 95–97, 100–105; patients opinion on access to, 50, 54–55, 57–58, 63, 64–65, 67; by Planned Parenthood, 102–104; restrictions by non-Catholic hospitals, 154–155; *Roe v. Wade* on, 19, 148, 156; state restrictions on, 13, 154, 157, 197n54; training in, ix; workarounds for, 120–124, 157
above-board workarounds. *See* workarounds
abuse, 27, 61–62
Acker, Dr., 111, 120, 122–123
ACLU (American Civil Liberties Union), 145–146
ACOG. *See* American College of Obstetrics and Gynecology (ACOG)
activism. *See* anti-abortion activism; reproductive rights activism
advertising of health care services, 46–47
Affordable Care Act (ACA), 9, 40, 62, 65
Alaska, 2
Albu, Elena, 112–113, 119
Altera, Ana, 5–8, 168n18
America Magazine (publication), 36
American College of Obstetrics and Gynecology (ACOG), xv, 34, 36, 42, 43–44, 116, 150
American College of Surgeons (ACS), 17
American Medical Association, xv
American Public Health Association, xv
Amy, 5–8, 146
anesthesia, 17, 37, 96

anti-abortion activism, 11, 20–21, 63, 96–97, 157. *See also* reproductive rights activism
anticipatory guidance, 74–76
anti-Kell disorder, 12
antitrust laws, 21
Ascension Health, 25
author's positionality, 159–161
autonomy: as bioethics principle, xv; of patients, xv, 31–33, 42, 45, 52–55, 79, 149–150, 151; reproductive, xvi, 147. *See also* reproductive autonomy, as concept
Avera, 15

Baptist hospitals, 53, 66
Bari, Karen, 89, 90, 94, 96, 99, 100, 117, 123
Barrett, Amy Coney, 156
bathroom access for transgender people, 40
Battistelli, Molly, 160
Bayley, Carol, 22
beginning-of-life medical services, 9
Benedict XV (pope), 91, 129, 190n7
beneficence, xv
bioethics, xv, 150
biopower, 148
birth control. *See* contraception
Bishop of Arlington, 39–40
bishops, power and influence of, xvi, 9, 23, 150, 155. *See also* Catholic Health Association of the United States (CHA); Catholic healthcare system; ERDs (Ethical and Religious Directives for Catholic Health Care Services); Olmsted, Thomas J.; patriarchal religious governance
Black Lives Matter, 73
Black women and healthcare, 32, 63–64, 69–70, 76, 144, 153, 183n8. *See also* racial (in)justice; racist health care practices

blood transfusions, 11–12
Bob Wilson Memorial, 15
Bouchard, Charles, 46
Boyle, Philip, 98
breastfeeding, 2, 36
burnout, physician, 151

California, 156
California Women's Law Center, 21
Campos, Zina, 22–23
capitalism and healthcare business, 16, 18, 27, 50–52. *See also* consumer medicine; hospital mergers
Carrasco de Paula, Ignacio, 36
carve-out agreements, 21–24, 97–100, 150–151. *See also* workarounds
Catholic Health Association of the United States (CHA), 2, 9, 15, 17–19, 46, 89, 135. *See also* ERDs
Catholic healthcare system: advertising of, 46–47; carve-outs and controversies of, 19–24; charitable image of, 24–27, 148; effects of growth of, 12–14, 27; ERDs on, 9–10, 15, 18, 23; evolving role of, 147–149; institutional transformation of, 16–19; lawsuits against, 145–147; myths about, xiii–xv; overview of modern, 15–16, 147; specific clinical conflicts in, 10–12. *See also* ERDs; separation of church and hospital
Catholic Healthcare West (CHW), 18, 21–22, 126, 129, 134
Catholic Health Initiatives, 25, 137
Catholic Medical Association, 39, 152
Catholic Sun, The (publication), 138
cerclage, 72
Cesarean hysterectomy, 120
CHA. *See* Catholic Health Association of the United States (CHA)
Chamorro, Rebecca, 146
Chan, Sophia, 91, 92, 104–105, 112, 115
charitable image of Catholic hospitals, 24–27, 148
Chervenak, Frank, 150
CHI Health, 15
child abuse, 61–62
child custody, 56
Christian Medical and Dental Association, 152
Church, Frank, 19
Church Amendment (1973), 19
Church of Jesus Christ of Latter-Day Saints, 76, 77, 93, 101
citizenship, 59
client, as term, 4–5
collaborative agreements, 21–24, 97–100, 109
Colorado, 2
Columbia Law School, 154
CommonSpirit, xiv, 15, 137, 138, 142

Community Catalyst, 172n22
concealment strategy as workaround, 111, 115–119. *See also* workarounds
conscience rights, 24, 105, 148, 149, 167n8. *See also* ERDs
consolidations. *See* hospital mergers
consumer medicine, 46–48, 66–67. *See also* capitalism and healthcare business
contraception: access to, ix–x, xiii; Catholic doctrine conflicts with, 33–38; hospital mergers and, ix–x, 18, 19–23; rate comparison on, 165n5, 181n9; temporary types of, 1; workarounds for, 112, 116. *See also* emergency contraception (EC); *names of specific types;* sterilization
Creighton Alliance, 139–142, 192n29
Creighton University, 138–139, 141, 142
cross-sex hormone replacement, 39–40. *See also* transgender care

D&C (dilation and curettage), 11–12, 49, 78, 84
D&E (dilation and evacuation), 71
Dean, Lloyd, 134
Depo-Provera, 36
DeSanctis, Alexandra, 157
Desiree, 61–66
Dignity Health, 15, 18, 25–26, 46, 136, 137, 138, 177n34
Dignity Health v. Minton, 152–53
Directive 3, 24. *See also* ERDs
Directive 36, 35. *See also* ERDs
Directive 38, 38. *See also* ERDs
Directive 41, 38. *See also* ERDs
Directive 42, 56. *See also* ERDs
Directive 45, 41, 188n20. *See also* ERDs
Directive 47, 42, 43, 133, 134, 145. *See also* ERDs
Directive 48, 44, 81, 185n24. *See also* ERDs
Directive 50, 42. *See also* ERDs
Directive 52, 34, 128. *See also* ERDs
Directive 53, 37. *See also* ERDs
Directive 61, 71. *See also* ERDs
Directive 73, 100, 151. *See also* ERDs
Directive 74, 23. *See also* ERDs
Directive 75, 23. *See also* ERDs
discrimination, 152–154, 168n14. *See also* racist health care practices
diverting patients as workaround, 105–109. *See also* workarounds
divorce, 56, 127, 135
Dobbs v. Jackson Women's Health Organization, xiii, 10–11, 157
doctrinal iatrogenesis, xvi, 1, 5–9, 12, 13, 120, 150, 151
documentation practices, 17
domestic violence, xvi, 56
double effect principle, 44, 120, 133, 189n1
Drake, Theresa, 119

drug use, 62–63, 64, 182n20
dysfunctional bleeding, treatment of, 116–117

ectopic pregnancies, x, 40–44, 80–83, 85, 89, 98, 109, 124, 157
Ehrich, John, 132
elder care, 55. *See also* end-of-life medical services
elective, as term, 30
Elizabeth, 80–85
emergencies, ix–x, 16–17, 68–69, 85–86. *See also* miscarriages; pregnancy complications
emergency contraception (EC), ix–x, 35. *See also* contraception
Emergency Medical Treatment and Active Labor Act (1986), 80, 105
Emmanuel, Rahm, 25, 26
end-of-life medical services, xiv, 9, 16, 33, 167n8. *See also* elder care
ERDs (Ethical and Religious Directives for Catholic Health Care Services), 9–10, 15, 147; on abortions, 41; on contraception and sterilization, 34–38, 39; ethics committees and, 28–31; future of, 154–156; hospital mergers and, 19; on infertility, 38; revisions of, 23, 168n13. *See also* Catholic Health Association of the United States (CHA); workarounds; *specific directives*
Essure, 95–96, 97. *See also* sterilization
Ethical and Religious Directives for Catholic Health Care Services. *See* ERDs
ethics committees, 28–31, 105–106, 111, 132, 174n3. *See also* ERDs (Ethical and Religious Directives for Catholic Health Care Services)
eugenics, 32, 93
exclusive contracts of physicians, 107–108

fair share deficits, 24–25
Family Planning Advocates (FPA), 20
fertility care. *See* IVF (in vitro fertilization)
Fine, Noa, 106–108, 123
Fogel, Susan Berke, 21–22, 23
food restrictions, 33
forced sterilization, 32. *See also* sterilization
free will, 48–49

gay couples and reproductive rights, 10
gender-affirming surgery, 10, 39–40, 58–61, 146, 152–153, 182nn17–18. *See also* transgender care
gender binary and Catholic doctrines, 4, 133–134, 150, 151
gender discrimination, 152–153, 168n14
gender dysphoria, 39, 40. *See also* transgender care
"gender ideology," as term, 39, 168n14

gender nonbinary people, 4. *See also* transgender care
"gender theory," as term, 39
Gold, Pete, 112, 114, 118
Greenwall Foundation, 160
Groesbeck, Faith, 145
Guiahi, Maryam, 160

Hafner, Katie, 46, 181n1
Halappanavar, Savita, 11, 69, 144, 145, 146, 157
halo effect, 24–27, 148
Hass, John, 23–24, 98, 145
Hasselbacher, Lee, 154
healthcare business model, 16, 18, 27, 50–52. *See also* hospital mergers
health insurance, 1, 4, 8, 93–94, 149. *See also* Medicaid
Health Progress (publication), 27
hemolytic disease, 12
heterosexuality, 10
HHS. *See* U.S. Department of Health and Human Services (HHS)
Higgins, Jenny, 160
Hobby Lobby, 149
hormone replacement, 39–40, 59
Horn, Terry, 35, 93, 101–103
hospital mergers, ix–x, 18, 19–23, 93, 151, 156. *See also* healthcare business model; *names of specific groups*
"hospital within a hospital" method, 6. *See also* workarounds
Hudson Valley hospital merger, 20–21
Hunt, Linda, 134, 136, 137, 142
Hyde Amendment, 19, 156
hysterectomies, 32, 35, 39, 120. *See also* sterilization

iatrogenesis, as term, 5. *See also* doctrinal iatrogenesis
immigrant detention centers, 32
incest, 157
inequality of power, 4–5, 12
infertility, 10, 38
informed choice, 48, 53, 68–69
institutional conscience rights, 2, 16
insurance. *See* health insurance
interpregnancy intervals, 37, 178n45
in vitro fertilization, xiii, 10. *See also* contraception
Iowa, 2
Ireland, 11, 69, 144–145. *See also* Halappanavar, Savita
IUD (intrauterine device), 1, 35, 36, 53, 63. *See also* contraception
IVF (in vitro fertilization), 22, 38, 99, 188n19

Jaelyn, 69–74, 75, 146
Jay, Thomas, 90–91, 114, 118–119
Jennifer, 11–12
Jewish hospitals, 33
Johnson, Jana, 28–31
justice as bioethics principle, xv
justification strategy as workaround, 111,
    112–115. See also workarounds

Kaiser Health, 46
Katie, 113–114
Kayden, 58–61, 66, 146–147
Keehan, Carol, 9
Kim, Lisa, 43
Konrad, Julia, 41–42
kosher food policies, 33
Kramer, Renee, 160

Lange, Tracy, 91
lawsuits, 145–147, 169n25. See also names of
    specific cases
Lee, Adele, 126, 129–130, 139, 141
Leonard Hospital, 20, 172n28
levonorgestrel EC, 36
Little Sisters of the Poor, xiv
long-acting contraception, x
Los Angeles Times (publication), 22
Lown Institute Hospitals Index, 24

Magnusson, Sara, 160
marriage, Catholic doctrine on, 10
material cooperation, 188n20
maternal morbidity and mortality: case of
    Halappanavar, 11, 69, 144, 145, 146, 157;
    racial disparities in, 12–13, 32, 63–64, 69–70,
    76, 144, 153, 183n8
McBride, Margaret, 101, 126, 132, 135, 137,
    140, 191n23
McCullough, Laurence, 150
McManus, Robert, 23
Means, Tamesha, 69, 145–146
Medicaid: Catholic hospital care for those
    on, xiv, 24–27; Desiree's experience of, 62,
    64–65; patient population on, 13; steriliza-
    tion and, 187n9. See also health insurance
medical aid-in-dying, xiv
medical insurance. See health insurance
menorrhagia, 35, 177n34
menstrual irregularities, 112
Mercy Health Partners, 145–146
Mercy Hospital, 15, 58, 59
MergerWatch, ix–x, 19–21
methotrexate, 44, 81, 83, 185n24
Meyer, Harris, 98
military medical insurance, 1
Minton, Evan, 146, 152–153
Mirena (intrauterine device) IUD, 53, 63

miscarriages, x; access to care after, 10–11;
    of Elizabeth, 80–85; of Jaelyn, 69–74; of
    Jennifer, 11–12; of Rosemary, 48–52; of
    Samantha, 77–80; workarounds for
    management of, 114–115; of Zia's friend,
    75–76. See also emergencies; pregnancy
    complications; suffering
misoprostol, 78
Missouri, 2
molar pregnancy, 183n22
moral distress, 150–152
morning after pill. See emergency contra-
    ception (EC)
Murphy, William, 89, 126–143
Muskegon, Michigan, 145–146
myths, xiii–xv

Nadia, 52–55, 66
Natchitoches Regional Medical Center, 15
National Catholic Bioethics Center (NCBC),
    23, 39, 40, 98, 132
National Review (publication), 157
natural family planning (NFP), 34
Nebraska, 2
New York, 156
New York Times (publication), 15, 46
nonmaleficence as bioethics principle, xv
Norris, Jennafer, 146
"Nun Excommunicated after Saving a Mother's
    Life with Abortion" (ABC News), 133
Nygren, David, 27

O'Brien, Bishop, 128–129, 190n6
obstetric emergencies. See emergencies
Olmsted, Thomas J., 126, 129, 132–133, 134,
    138–140, 142. See also bishops, power and
    influence of
Oregon, 2, 156
OSF Healthcare, 15
outpatient care as workaround, 94–97. See also
    workarounds

pain: Black women and tolerance of, 63–64,
    69–70; Catholic doctrines on, 184n12
Patel, Akshun, 43, 99, 108
paternalism, 32, 36, 53–54, 63–64
patient, as term, 4–5
patient autonomy, xv, 31–33, 42, 45, 52–55, 79,
    149–150, 151. See also autonomy; reproduc-
    tive autonomy, as concept
Patient Awareness of Religious Restrictions
    in Catholic Healthcare (PARRCH), 160
patient dumping, 106–108
patriarchal religious governance, 4, 89–90,
    133–134, 150, 151. See also bishops, power
    and influence of
Paul IV (pope), 34

physician burnout, 151
Pitocin, 29
Plan B. *See* emergency contraception (EC)
Planned Parenthood, 63, 102–104
Platt, Elizabeth Reiner, 154
Plemons, Eric, 40
Pontifical Academy for Life, 36
post-partum trauma, 72–73
poverty: Catholic hospitals and charitable
    image on, 24–27, 148; Murphy on health-
    care and, 89–90; reproductive autonomy
    and risks with, xvi
power dynamics, 4–5. *See also* paternalism;
    patriarchal religious governance
pregnancy, defined, 35
pregnancy complications: ectopic, 40–44,
    80–83, 85, 89, 98, 109, 124, 157; ERD
    conflicts with, 28–31; miscarriages, 48–52.
    See also emergencies
Presence Health, 25
Preserve Medical Secularity (P.M.S.), 20
prison health care, 32
pro-choice activism, 20–21, 23, 32, 144
Protestant hospital, 154
Providence Health, 25, 46
provider bias, 88, 118. *See also* racist health
    care practices
PTSD (post traumatic stress disorder), 61, 64
Puerto Rico, 32

Quarles, Franklin, 103–104

racial (in)justice, 12–13, 73; 93, 144
racist health care practices, 32, 63–64, 69–70,
    76, 93–94, 152–154. *See also* provider bias
rape, ix–x, 35–36, 64, 157
Ratzinger (cardinal), 91, 190n7. *See also*
    Benedict XV (pope)
rebellion strategy as workaround, 111, 122–125.
    See also workarounds
referrals as workaround, 100–105. *See also*
    workarounds
Rehm, Diane, 145
Reich, Adam, 47
religious faith: of Elizabeth, 80; of Jaelyn,
    69; of Nadia, 52, 66; of Rosemary, 48; of
    Samantha, 76, 77; of Zia, 55–56
religious freedom, 65–66, 148–149
renaming strategy as workaround, 111,
    119–122. *See also* workarounds
reproductive autonomy, as concept, xvi, 147.
    See also autonomy; patient autonomy
reproductive injustice, 147, 152–154
reproductive rights activism, 12–13, 20–21, 23,
    24, 32, 144. *See also* anti-abortion activism
research methods, 4, 10, 159–161
resource-poor health settings, xvi

Roe v. Wade, 19, 148, 156
Rosemary, 48–52, 66
Roy, Hakeem, 108

Samantha, 76–80
Save Sur Services (S.O.S.), 20
scandal, defined, 41
scholarly journey, 159–61
separation of church and hospital, 126–127,
    142–143; disaffiliation, 134–137; reaffiliation,
    138–142; rupture, 131–134; as troubled
    relationship, 127–131. *See also* Catholic
    healthcare system
sex, Catholic doctrine on, 10
sexual abuse, ix–x, 27, 35–36, 61–62, 64, 157
Sheila, 116–117
Sherman, Sara, 6, 8
Sisters of Mercy, 135
Smith, JoAnn, 20
Society for Family Planning, 160
South Dakota, 2, 167n7
South Hampton Memorial, 15
"standard of care," as term, xv, 31, 174n7
state abortion restrictions, 13, 154, 157, 197n54.
    See also abortions and abortion care
Statement of Common Values (SCVs), 22
sterilization, x, xiii; Catholic hospital
    restrictions on, 1, 5–8, 22–23, 49, 52–55, 66;
    ERDs on, 33–38, 39; by Essure, 95–96;
    factors of women choice for, 4; hysterec-
    tomies, 32, 35, 39, 120; in prisons, 32; rate
    comparison of, 165n5, 168n11, 168n12;
    WikiLeaks scandal on, 91–92; workarounds
    for, 90–96, 118–120. *See also* contraception;
    tubal ligation
St. Joseph's Hospital (Phoenix, Arizona),
    126–143, 190n13
Stulberg, Debra, ix–xi, 159, 160, 161
suffering, 69–74. *See also* miscarriages
surrogacy, 10, 56–57, 66
Sutter Health, 46
Swank, Mindy, 146

Teel, Miriam, 103
temporary contraception, 1. *See also*
    contraception
therapy, 59, 64
"tired uterus" condition, 120
transgender care, 4, 26, 39–40, 58–61, 146–147,
    152–153. *See also* gender-affirming surgery
Tricare, 1
Trinity Health, 98
Trump administration, 149
tubal ligation, x, 1–2, 22–23, 49–50, 92, 118–119;
    postpartum surgery of, 167n5; workarounds
    for, 90–91, 95, 129, 168n18. *See also*
    contraception

UCSF medical centers, 25–26
uncertainty *vs.* informed choice, 68–69
under-the-radar workarounds. *See*
 workarounds
United States Conference of Catholic
 Bishops (USCCB), 39–41; about, xiii,
 4; ERDs (ethical and religious directives)
 by, 18; lawsuit against, 145–146; on
 Planned Parenthood funding, 103;
 power and influence of, 13, 32, 33, 155;
 Subcommittee on Health Care Issues,
 168n14; on transgender care, 39. *See also*
 ERDs
United States Supreme Court, 10
University of California medical centers,
 25–27
University of Chicago, 154
Unni, Nancy, 108–109, 124
U.S. Department of Health and Human
 Services (HHS), 19, 156
'uterine isolation committee,' 119–120
'uterine separation' procedure, 119
Uttley, Lois, 19–21

vasectomy, 1, 19, 50, 66, 95, 98
Vijay, Neysa, 97

Ward, Tim, 38, 58–61, 94, 96, 117
Washington, 2, 156, 181n1
Weber, Katie, 44
Weldon Amendment, 19, 156
"When There's a Heartbeat: Miscarriage
 Management in Catholic Hospitals"
 (Freedman), x
WikiLeaks scandal, 91–92
Willa, 1–2, 5, 8
Wisconsin, 2
women, as term, 4–5
workarounds, xiii, 87–88, 109–110, 125, 152;
 carve-out and collaborative agreements
 as, 21–24, 97–100, 150–151; concealment
 strategy as, 111, 115–119; diverting patients
 as, 105–109; justification strategy as, 111,
 112–115; outpatient care as, 94–97; rebellion
 strategy as, 111, 122–125; referrals, 100–105;
 renaming strategy as, 111, 119–122; scholarship and publicity on, 186n4; taking
 patients elsewhere, 90–94, 129. *See also*
 ERDs (Ethical and Religious Directives
 for Catholic Health Care Services)

Zander, Deborah, 115, 120–122
Zia, 55–58, 66, 75–76

About the Author

Lori Freedman is a sociologist, bioethicist, and professor of obstetrics, gynecology, and reproductive sciences with the Advancing New Standards in Reproductive Health (ANSIRH) program of the Bixby Center for Global Reproductive Health at the University of California, San Francisco. Her work investigates how our social structure and medical culture shape the delivery of reproductive care. Her first book, *Willing and Unable: Doctors' Constraints in Abortion Care*, is a qualitative investigation of the challenges of integrating abortion into physician practice.

Available titles in the Critical Issues in Health and Medicine series

Janet Greenlees, *When the Air became Important: A Social History of the New England and Lancashire Textile Industries*

Gerald N. Grob and Howard H. Goldman, *The Dilemma of Federal Mental Health Policy: Radical Reform or Incremental Change?*

Gerald N. Grob and Allan V. Horwitz, *Diagnosis, Therapy, and Evidence: Conundrums in Modern American Medicine*

Rachel Grob, *Testing Baby: The Transformation of Newborn Screening, Parenting, and Policymaking*

Mark A. Hall and Sara Rosenbaum, eds., *The Health Care "Safety Net" in a Post-Reform World*

Laura L. Heinemann, *Transplanting Care: Shifting Commitments in Health and Care in the United States*

Rebecca J. Hester, *Embodied Politics: Indigenous Migrant Activism, Cultural Competency, and Health Promotion in California*

Laura D. Hirshbein, *American Melancholy: Constructions of Depression in the Twentieth Century*

Laura D. Hirshbein, *Smoking Privileges: Psychiatry, the Mentally Ill, and the Tobacco Industry in America*

Timothy Hoff, *Practice under Pressure: Primary Care Physicians and Their Medicine in the Twenty-First Century*

Beatrix Hoffman, Nancy Tomes, Rachel N. Grob, and Mark Schlesinger, eds., *Patients as Policy Actors*

Ruth Horowitz, *Deciding the Public Interest: Medical Licensing and Discipline*

Powel Kazanjian, *Frederick Novy and the Development of Bacteriology in American Medicine*

Claas Kirchhelle, *Pyrrhic Progress: The History of Antibiotics in Anglo-American Food Production*

Rebecca M. Kluchin, *Fit to Be Tied: Sterilization and Reproductive Rights in America, 1950–1980*

Jennifer Lisa Koslow, *Cultivating Health: Los Angeles Women and Public Health Reform*

Jennifer Lisa Koslow, *Exhibiting Health: Public Health Displays in the Progressive Era*

Susan C. Lawrence, *Privacy and the Past: Research, Law, Archives, Ethics*

Bonnie Lefkowitz, *Community Health Centers: A Movement and the People Who Made It Happen*

Ellen Leopold, *Under the Radar: Cancer and the Cold War*

Barbara L. Ley, *From Pink to Green: Disease Prevention and the Environmental Breast Cancer Movement*

Sonja Mackenzie, *Structural Intimacies: Sexual Stories in the Black AIDS Epidemic*

Stephen E. Mawdsley, *Selling Science: Polio and the Promise of Gamma Globulin*

Frank M. McClellan, *Healthcare and Human Dignity: Law Matters*

Michelle McClellan, *Lady Lushes: Gender, Alcohol, and Medicine in Modern America*

David Mechanic, *The Truth about Health Care: Why Reform Is Not Working in America*

Richard A. Meckel, *Classrooms and Clinics: Urban Schools and the Protection and Promotion of Child Health, 1870–1930*

Terry Mizrahi, *From Residency to Retirement: Physicians' Careers over a Professional Lifetime*

Manon Parry, *Broadcasting Birth Control: Mass Media and Family Planning*

Alyssa Picard, *Making the American Mouth: Dentists and Public Health in the Twentieth Century*

Heather Munro Prescott, *The Morning After: A History of Emergency Contraception in the United States*

Sarah B. Rodriguez, *The Love Surgeon: A Story of Trust, Harm, and the Limits of Medical Regulation*

David J. Rothman and David Blumenthal, eds., *Medical Professionalism in the New Information Age*

Andrew R. Ruis, *Eating to Learn, Learning to Eat: School Lunches and Nutrition Policy in the United States*

James A. Schafer Jr., *The Business of Private Medical Practice: Doctors, Specialization, and Urban Change in Philadelphia, 1900–1940*

Johanna Schoen, ed., *Abortion Care as Moral Work: Ethical Considerations of Maternal and Fetal Bodies*

David G. Schuster, *Neurasthenic Nation: America's Search for Health, Happiness, and Comfort, 1869–1920*

Karen Seccombe and Kim A. Hoffman, *Just Don't Get Sick: Access to Health Care in the Aftermath of Welfare Reform*

Leo B. Slater, *War and Disease: Biomedical Research on Malaria in the Twentieth Century*

Piper Sledge, *Bodies Unbound: Gender-Specific Cancer and Biolegitimacy*

Dena T. Smith, *Medicine over Mind: Mental Health Practice in the Biomedical Era*

Kylie M. Smith, *Talking Therapy: Knowledge and Power in American Psychiatric Nursing*

Matthew Smith, *An Alternative History of Hyperactivity: Food Additives and the Feingold Diet*

Paige Hall Smith, Bernice L. Hausman, and Miriam Labbok, *Beyond Health, Beyond Choice: Breastfeeding Constraints and Realities*

Susan L. Smith, *Toxic Exposures: Mustard Gas and the Health Consequences of World War II in the United States*

Rosemary A. Stevens, Charles E. Rosenberg, and Lawton R. Burns, eds., *History and Health Policy in the United States: Putting the Past Back In*

Marianne Sullivan, *Tainted Earth: Smelters, Public Health, and the Environment*

Courtney E. Thompson, *An Organ of Murder: Crime, Violence, and Phrenology in Nineteenth-Century America*

Barbra Mann Wall, *American Catholic Hospitals: A Century of Changing Markets and Missions*

Frances Ward, *The Door of Last Resort: Memoirs of a Nurse Practitioner*

Jean C. Whelan, *Nursing the Nation: Building the Nurse Labor Force*

Shannon Withycombe, *Lost: Miscarriage in Nineteenth-Century America*